Introduction to Human and Social Biology

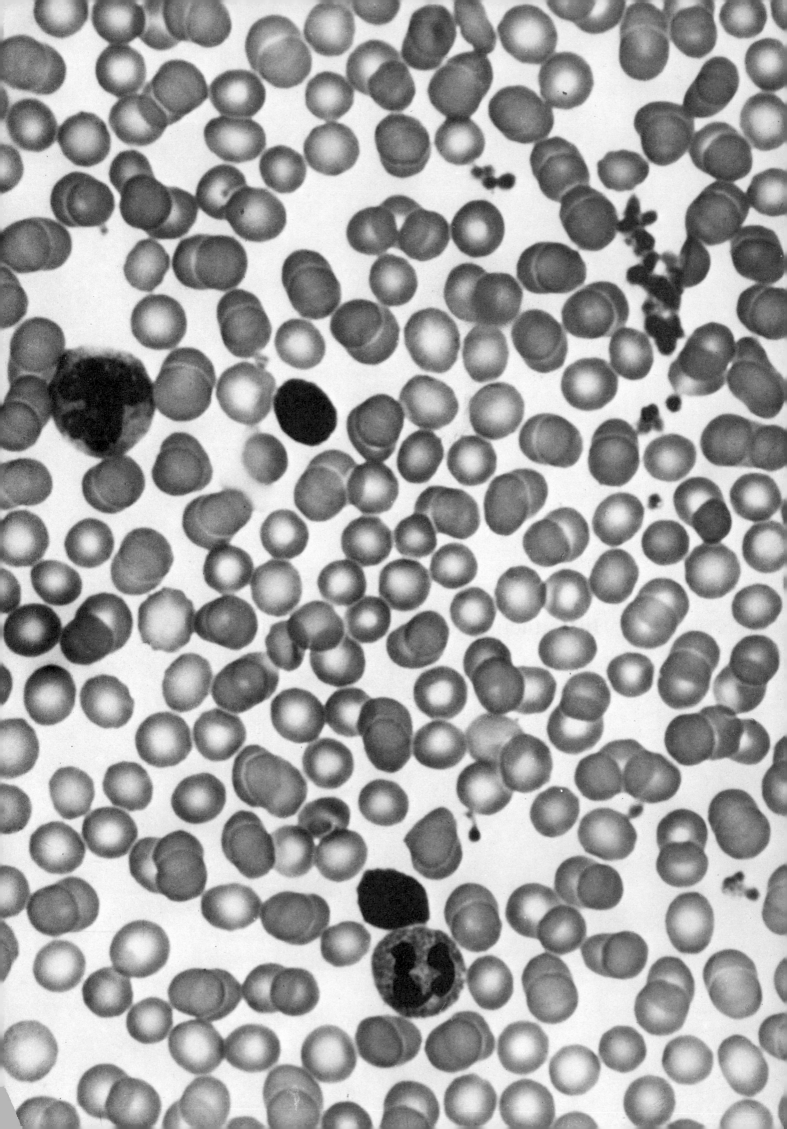

Introduction to Human and Social Biology

Don Mackean BA, FIBiol
Sir Frederic Osborn School, Welwyn Garden City

Brian Jones BSc, FIBiol
Dulwich College

John Murray   Albemarle Street   London

Other books by Don Mackean

Introduction to Biology, 5th edition
Introduction to Biology: New Tropical edition
Introduction to Biology: West African edition
Introduction to Biology: Colour edition
   One of the most widely used biology books
   in the English-speaking world

Introduction to Genetics, 3rd edition
Enquiries in Biology (with Stephen W. Hurry)

Experimental Work in Biology
   1 *Food Tests*
   2 *Enzymes*
   3 *Soil*
   4 *Photosynthesis*
   5 *Germination and Tropisms*
   6 *Diffusion and Osmosis*
   7 *Respiration and Gaseous Exchange*
   8 *Human Senses*

© Don Mackean & Brian Jones 1975
Reprinted with corrections 1976, 1977, 1979

Printed in Great Britain by Jarrold and Sons Ltd, Norwich

ISBN 0 7195 3209 4

Contents

Acknowledgements

The authors would like to thank the following who read various sections of the manuscript and made many constructive criticisms. We greatly value the contribution they have made to the accuracy and clarity of the text;

Mr S. W. Hurry (physiology)
Dr C. O. Carter (genetics)
Dr P. R. Travers (posture and exercise)
Mr G. T. Creber

We are also extremely grateful to all those who have supplied photographs. They have taken a great deal of trouble to supply us with prints, some of which were specially prepared for this book. They are acknowledged individually on the pages where the illustrations appear.

Thanks are also due to the following who supplied photographs for the cover:

Heather Angel; Brian Bracegirdle; Philip Harris Biological; Professor Hamilton; Henry Brandt; MacMillan & Co. Ltd; Rank Organization; Shell; Rentokil; Radio Times Hulton Picture Library; St. Bartholomew's Hospital; World Health Organization; Barnaby's Picture Library; J. Allan Cash.

Preface

Introduction to Human and Social Biology is primarily a textbook for students following courses leading to 'O' and 'AO' examinations in the General Certificate of Education. The contents cover the Human and Social Biology syllabuses of the Cambridge and the London Overseas examinations, and also the Human Biology syllabuses at 'O' and 'AO' level in Great Britain. It is expected that the book will also be useful for pre-nursing courses and as a general reference book for a variety of other social and biological studies.

Human Biology is of universal significance and though it is often necessary to quote examples peculiar to certain regions, the facts presented in this book are relevant to human society in all parts of the world. It is as valid for a student in Britain to learn about the problems of disease and food production in tropical countries as it is for a student in Malaysia to study the dangers of pollution and faulty nutrition in the Western Hemisphere.

Our objective has been to present the facts as clearly as possible, without advocating any particular order or method of study (although a knowledge of the facts and principles described in the early chapters is taken for granted in the later sections). The extensive use of cross-references and the presence of a glossary should make it relatively easy to use the book for reference at any point.

The questions at the ends of chapters are designed to make the reader use, reorganize or appraise the information in the text rather than simply replicate it. Some of the essay questions set by the main examining boards in recent years have been reproduced at the end of the book.

The suggestions for practical work have been kept as simple as possible so that the students can attempt the experiments with a minimum of apparatus.

Don Mackean
Brian Jones

1
Living Organisms

Characteristics of living organisms

Biology is the study of life (Greek *bios* = life, *logos* = knowledge) which, in practice, means the study of living things.

In most animals, the characteristics by which we know they are alive are self-evident: they move about, they feed, they have young, and they respond to changes in their surroundings.

These features are less obvious in plants and certain small animals; and when dealing with organisms like bacteria and viruses the distinctions between living and non-living can often be drawn only by a trained scientist with the appropriate apparatus and techniques at his disposal. The main differences between living organisms and non-living objects can be summarized as follows:

1 **Respiration.** This is the process by which energy is made available as a result of chemical changes within the organism, the commonest of which is the chemical decomposition of food as a result of its combination with oxygen. This is not a particularly obvious occurrence in plants and animals; but it is fairly easy to demonstrate that living creatures take in air, remove some of the oxygen from it and increase the volume of carbon dioxide in it. More simply expressed it can be said that living organisms take in oxygen and give out carbon dioxide. Sometimes this takes place with obvious breathing movements. Respiration also results in a rise of temperature, which is more easily detectable in animals than in plants.
2 **Feeding.** This is an essential preliminary to respiration, since energy comes ultimately from food. The feeding of a tree by its leaves is less obvious than that of an animal, which moves actively in search of food. Feeding may also result in growth.
3 **Excretion.** Living involves a vast number of chemical processes, including respiration, many of which produce substances that are poisonous when moderately concentrated. The elimination of these from the organism is called excretion.
4 **Growth.** Strictly, growth is simply an increase in size, but it usually implies also that the organism is becoming more complicated and more efficient. An illustration of this is an animal which changes its form from larva to adult, for example, a frog or a butterfly.
5 **Movement.** An animal can generally move its whole body, whereas the movements of the higher plants are usually restricted to certain parts such as the opening and closing of petals, or to movements of parts as a result of growth.
6 **Reproduction.** No organism has a limitless life, but although individuals must die sooner or later their life is handed on to new individuals by reproduction, resulting in the continued existence of the species.

7 **Irritability** (Sensitivity). Irritability is the ability to respond to a stimulus. Obvious signs of sensitivity are the movements made by animals as a result of noises, on being touched or on seeing an enemy. Fully grown plants do not show such responses under casual observation, but during growth they respond to the direction of light, gravity and moisture.

Differences between animals and plants

Both plants and animals have in common, to a greater or lesser extent, all the features listed above, but there are some fundamental differences between them, of which one of the most important is the method of feeding.

1 **Method of feeding.** Animals take in food that is chemically very complicated (i.e. composed of large molecules); it consists either of plant products or of other animals. This food is reduced to simpler material by the process of digestion, and in this form it can be taken up by the body.

Plants, in general, take in very simple substances that are composed of small molecules, namely carbon dioxide from the air, and water and dissolved salts from the soil. In their leaves they combine this carbon dioxide and water into sugar, using sunlight as a source of energy. From the sugar so produced, and the salts taken in from the soil, green plants can make all of the substances needed for their existence. The feeding of animals thus involves a breaking-down process, while that of plants is a building-up, or synthesis.

2 **Chlorophyll.** The green colour found in most plants is important for the absorption of sunlight and is due to chlorophyll, which is not present in any animal. This difference is one indication of the fundamental difference in feeding. (However, many plants such as fungi do not possess chlorophyll.)

3 **Cellulose.** In their structures, notably their cell walls, plants have a large quantity of a substance called cellulose, which is never present in animal structures.

4 **Movement.** Unlike animals, most of the familiar plants do not move about as complete organisms, but certain microscopic plants move as actively as microscopic animals.

5 **Sensitivity.** Although both plants and animals respond to stimuli, the response of an animal usually follows almost immediately after the application of even a very brief stimulus. In plants, on the other hand, a response may take place over a matter of hours or days, and then only if the stimulus persists for a relatively long time.

The varieties of living organisms

The earth is populated by enormous numbers of different kinds of plants and animals. When these organisms are studied and described it becomes apparent that they can be divided into groups. In each group of plants or animals the members show strong likenesses to each other. These similarities are not always immediately obvious but become clearer when the characteristics of the group are known. Bees and butterflies, for example, though differing considerably in appearance, size, colour and habits, belong to the same group, insects, because they both have hard outer skeletons and three distinct regions in their bodies, the middle region carrying six legs and two pairs of wings.

The largest division of organisms is into the plant and animal kingdoms. The next distinct groups are phyla (singular *phylum*); for example, the first ten groups of animals listed in the table. The smallest natural group of animals or plants is the *species*. For example, birds are not a species but house sparrows are. Generally speaking, all members of a species look and behave alike in all important respects and can breed among themselves. Breeding between members of different species does not happen very frequently in nature.

Placing an organism in a particular category is not always easy. For example, certain single-celled creatures are not definitely animals or plants but possess characteristics of both. Fungi and bacteria are placed in the plant kingdom, although they do not contain chlorophyll and differ considerably from the green plants in their methods of obtaining food.

The table of living organisms given below does not conform to any strict biological classification but offers a simplified and convenient scheme. For example, the vertebrate groups—fish, amphibia, reptiles, birds and mammals—are not phyla but only subdivisions of a phylum called *Chordata*. Also, although ten invertebrate phyla are listed there are at least seven others which have not been mentioned because the animals concerned are unlikely to be familiar to anyone other than an experienced zoologist.

ANIMALS

A—Animals without vertebral columns: invertebrates (Fig. 1.1 *a–h*)

1 **Single-celled animals.** Very abundant, microscopic animals living in water and body fluids.

2 **Coelenterates.** Examples are the sea anemones, jelly-fish, coral-building 'anemones' and hydra. Most coelenterates live in the sea.

3 **Flatworms.** Mostly small freshwater and marine animals called planarians, often found under stones and floating leaves in streams. The group includes parasitic tapeworms and flukes.

4 **Nematodes** or 'round worms'. Very widely distributed worms, often parasitic, e.g. elephantiasis and hookworm disease are caused by nematodes.

5 **(True) Worms.** This phylum includes the earthworm, many little worms that live in ponds, lugworms, ragworms and bristle-worms of the sandy coasts.

6 **Molluscs.** In this phylum are snails, slugs, whelks, oysters, and other 'shellfish'; squid and octopus.

7 **Crustacea.** Familiar crustaceans are crabs, lobsters, crayfish, prawns, shrimps, many small freshwater creatures such as the freshwater shrimp, water-flea and water-louse.

8 **Insects** possess six legs and usually wings. Examples are: ants, bees, grasshoppers, flies, mosquitoes and beetles.

9 **Arachnids** have four pairs of walking legs and no wings. The group includes spiders, scorpions, ticks and mites.

10 **Echinoderms.** Included among these marine animals are the starfish and sea-urchin.

B—Animals with vertebral columns: vertebrates (Fig. 1.2 *a–e*)

I *Poikilothermic* (variable body temperature)

1 **Fish** breathe by means of gills and have bodies covered with scales. Examples: shark, guppy, sardine, mudfish.

2 **Amphibia** (e.g. frogs and toads) have no scales on their bodies; they spend much of their lives on land but usually breed in water.

3 **Reptiles** are land-dwelling animals with scaly bodies. Examples: lizards, snakes, turtles, crocodiles.

II *Homoiothermic* (constant body temperature)

4 **Birds** have bodies that are covered with feathers. Examples: crow, duck, egret.

5 **Mammals** have bodies that are covered with fur; their young are born alive and suckled with milk. Examples: cows, dogs, cats, whales, seals, apes, man.

PLANTS

A—Plants which do not have flowers

1 **Single-celled plants** are similar to single-celled animals, but they are green and obtain their food differently. When in great numbers they often make pond-water look green. They also occur as a green powdery dust on tree trunks.

2 The **algae** include the green slimy filaments on ponds. Seaweeds are also algae.

3 **Fungi** include moulds, toadstools, mushrooms, bracket fungi and yeasts.

4 **Liverworts** are small, flat, green, leaf-like plants found in clusters in damp places, stream banks, and in cellars and caves to which light has access.

5 **Mosses.** Small green plants growing in dense colonies, e.g. eyelid moss which grows on oil palms.

6 **Ferns.** These range from floating, water-ferns to large tree ferns which resemble palms. Many grow on the trunks and branches of forest trees.

7 **Cone-bearing plants,** Pine, Cypress, cycads, Ginkgo.

B—Flowering plants

1 **Monocotyledons.** Narrow leaves with parallel veins and only one cotyledon in their seeds. Examples: grasses, cereals, reeds, lilies and palms.

2 **Dicotyledons.** Broad-leaved plants, net-veined and with two cotyledons in their seeds.

  (i) *Herbaceous plants*. Examples: Salvia, Sunflower, Tribulus.

  (ii) *Shrubs*. Woody, bushy plants. Examples: Hibiscus, Bauhinia, Caesalpinia, privet.

  (iii) *Deciduous trees*. Examples: Delonix (flamboyante), Ceiba (silk cotton), oak, ash, beech.

  (iv) *Evergreen trees*. Examples: Mango, Cassia, holly.

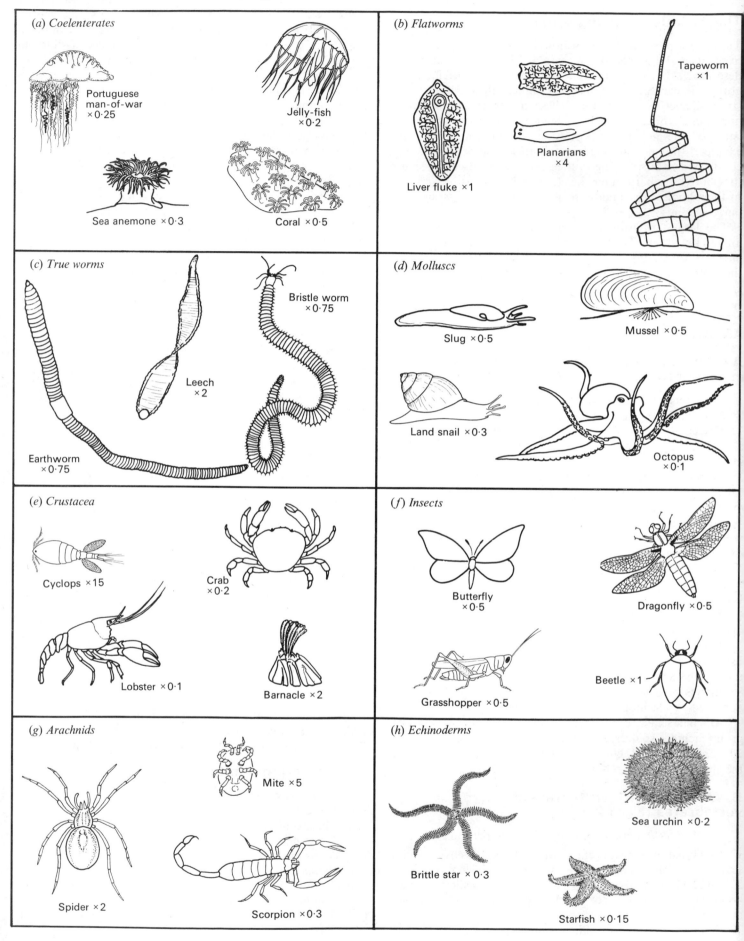

Fig. 1.1 Invertebrates

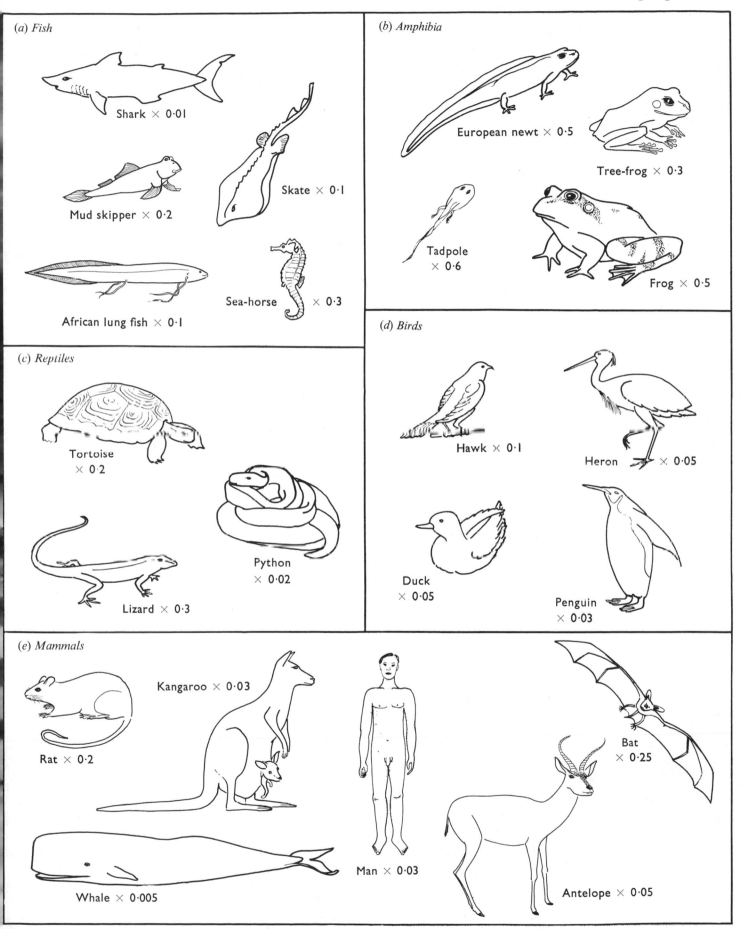

(a) Fish

Shark × 0·01

Mud skipper × 0·2

Skate × 0·1

African lung fish × 0·1

Sea-horse × 0·3

(b) Amphibia

European newt × 0·5

Tree-frog × 0·3

Tadpole × 0·6

Frog × 0·5

(c) Reptiles

Tortoise × 0·2

Python × 0·02

Lizard × 0·3

(d) Birds

Hawk × 0·1

Heron × 0·05

Duck × 0·05

Penguin × 0·03

(e) Mammals

Rat × 0·2

Kangaroo × 0·03

Bat × 0·25

Whale × 0·005

Man × 0·03

Antelope × 0·05

Fig. 1.2   Vertebrates

2
Cells

If almost any structure from a plant or an animal is examined microscopically it will be seen to consist of more or less distinct units—cells—which, although too small to be seen individually, in large numbers make up the structure or organ (Fig. 2.1a and b).

Methods of studying cells

Cells are too small to be seen with the naked eye so they must be magnified, at least × 100 and usually much more, in order to get any idea about their structure. To make a microscopic examination it is necessary to direct light through the tissue being studied and so the layer of tissue must be very thin. This may be achieved by squashing or smearing the tissue thinly on a glass slide, as in the case of cells from the lining of the mouth, or cells in the blood. In most cases, however, the tissue is cut into very thin slices, 10 μm* thick or less. The slices or *sections* are passed through one or more dyes (*stains*) which show up their outlines and their contents more clearly, then mounted on a glass slide and sealed under a thin glass cover slip (Fig. 2.2).

The kind of microscopes available in schools and colleges are

* A micrometre, symbol μm, (often called a micron) is one-thousandth of a millimetre.

light microscopes. Tissues are studied by passing light through them or reflecting light off them. The light microscope will magnify up to × 1 500. Magnifications up to × 200 000 can be achieved by using the electron microscope, which passes a

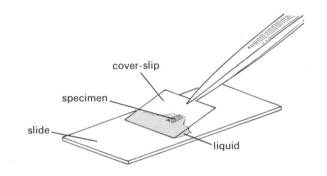

Fig. 2.2 Mounting a specimen for examination under the microscope

beam of electrons rather than rays of light through the object and takes a photograph of the image. Modern knowledge of cell structure is largely due to studies with the electron microscope.

Fig. 2.1 Plant and animal cells

(a) Cells in plant stem. The photograph shows part of a very thin slice taken across the stem. The cell contents are not visible at this magnification.
(G.B.I. Laboratories Ltd)

(b) Cells from the human adrenal gland (magnification much greater than in (a)).
(Brian Bracegirdle)

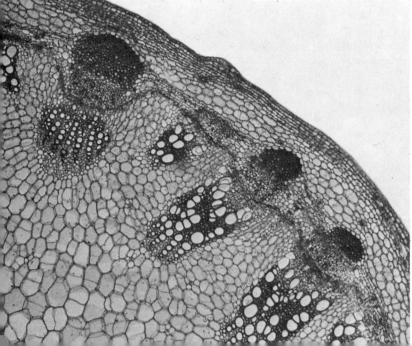

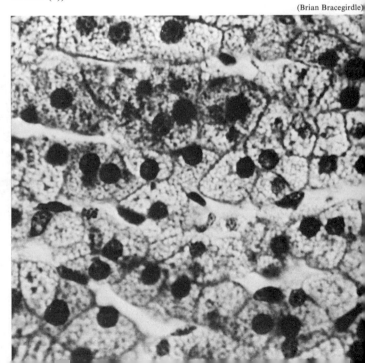

Cell structure

The size of human cells varies according to the type of cell being considered. One of the smallest is the red blood cell (p. 70) which is 7.5 μm in diameter and 2.2 μm thick. The largest human cell is probably the female egg, or ovum, (p. 102) which is 100 μm across. The average diameter of human cells is therefore probably 10–30 μm.

The shape also depends on the type of cell. A cell of a gland such as the salivary gland may be more or less spherical, but a nerve cell in the leg having a diameter of only 10 μm can be over one metre long, because it runs from the foot to the spinal cord. Since the cells of any organ are usually specially developed in their size, shape and chemistry to carry out one particular function there is, strictly speaking, no such thing as a typical cell. Nevertheless, all animal cells have certain important features in common. They all consist of an outer membrane enclosing a mass of cytoplasm in which is contained a nucleus. It is these common features which are illustrated in Fig. 2.3a.

Cell membrane. This forms the outer boundary of the cell and keeps the cell contents intact, preventing them from mixing with the medium outside the cell or with the contents of neighbouring cells. Under the light microscope the cell membrane appears as little more than a line, but the electron microscope shows it to be a structure about 1/100 000 mm (10 nanometres) thick. One of its principal functions is to exercise control over which substances enter and leave the cell. The wrong type or quantity of a substance entering the cell could upset its delicately balanced chemistry.

Cytoplasm. Under the light microscope, this appears to be a uniform, semifluid, structureless substance containing a variety of particles and occupying most of the space inside the cell. The electron microscope, however, shows that it is by no means a structureless jelly but consists of a variety of folded membranes forming tubes and passages, called the *endoplasmic reticulum*, which communicate with the external medium and the nucleus (Figs. 2.3*b* and 2.4). In addition to the internal system of membranes, there are other structures or *organelles* in the cytoplasm. Two examples of organelles are the *mitochondria* and the *ribosomes*, both involved in essential chemical processes for the maintenance of life.

The ribosomes play a part in building up proteins, complex chemicals from which all cells and tissues are constructed. In the mitochondria, food substances such as sugar are broken down chemically to release the energy that is needed to drive the reactions in the cell.

In addition to these and other organelles in the cytoplasm there may be *inclusions* of non-living material. Depending on the cell there might be food reserves such as oil droplets or glycogen granules (p. 16). Sometimes droplets of fluids collect in the cytoplasm and form vacuoles.

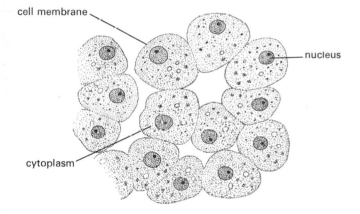

(a) Generalized animal cells as seen with the light microscope.

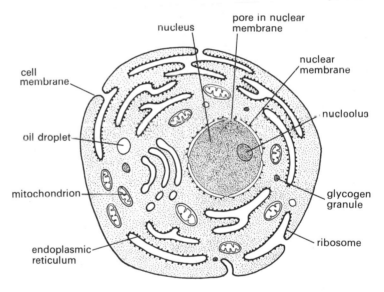

(b) Generalized animal cell as seen with the electron microscope (the mitochondria and endoplasmic reticulum change their shape and appearance continuously in many living cells).

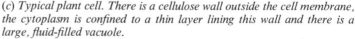

(c) Typical plant cell. There is a cellulose wall outside the cell membrane, the cytoplasm is confined to a thin layer lining this wall and there is a large, fluid-filled vacuole.

Fig. 2.3   Generalized cells

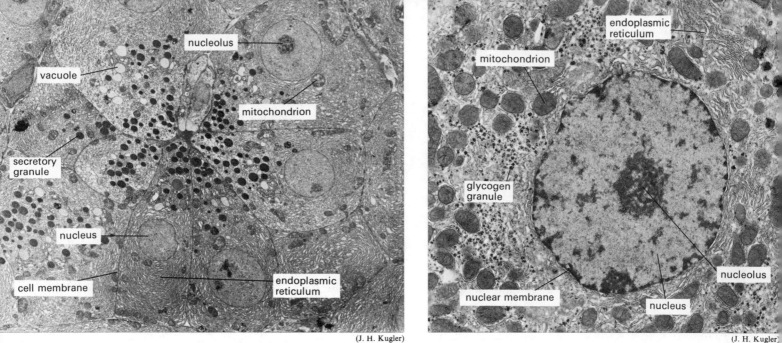

(a) Cells from the pancreas. (J. H. Kugler)

(b) Part of a liver cell. (J. H. Kugler)

Fig. 2.4   Human cells as seen under the electron microscope

The nucleus is a large spherical or ovoid body enclosed in the cytoplasm but separated from it by a membrane similar to the cell membrane, Fig. 2.4(b). The contents are more acid than the cytoplasm and so react differently to the stains used in making microscopical preparations. The stains are selected because they are taken up more strongly by the nucleus. Consequently in most microscopical preparations (and hence in most drawings and photographs of cells) the nucleus is seen as a dark object in the cytoplasm.

In the nucleus there are a number of fine thread-like bodies called *chromosomes* (p. 162). These cannot normally be seen with either the light microscope or the electron microscope unless the nucleus is dividing, but there is plenty of evidence that they are there all the time and produce substances that pass into the cytoplasm and control the chemical reactions going on there.

It is the nucleus that ultimately determines the shape and function of the cell. A cell may live for a time without its nucleus but it cannot divide and produce new cells.

Protoplasm. The cytoplasm and nucleus are often collectively described as protoplasm.

Cell division

Animals and plants grow as a result of cell division and cell enlargement. Most animals begin their existence as a single cell, i.e. a fertilized egg. This cell divides into 2, 4, 8, 16, 32 and so on to produce a body consisting of millions of cells, specialized for particular functions. These become grouped into tissues, organs and systems. Cell division begins by the nucleus dividing into two, followed by the cytoplasm dividing, so

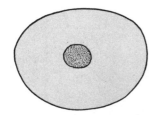

(a) Animal cell about to divide.

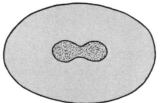

(b) The nucleus divides first.

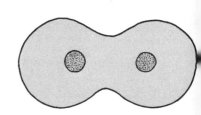

(c) The daughter nuclei separate.

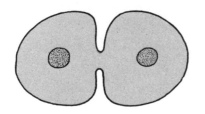

(d) The cytoplasm constricts between the nuclei.

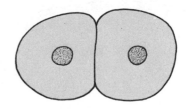

(e) Two cells are formed; one may retain the ability to divide and the other may become specialized.

Fig. 2.5   Cell division (animal cell)

forming two smaller cells which will then grow to the size of the parent (Fig. 2.5). In the early stages of development all the cells are able to reproduce, but as they become specialized to form bone, muscle, blood and so on, they lose the ability to divide. This power is retained by certain cells only; for example, there are cells in the bone marrow that constantly produce new blood cells, cells in the skin that continuously replace the outer layers as they wear away, and cells in the reproductive organs that produce sperms or eggs.

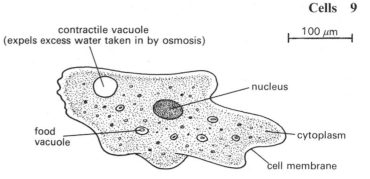

(a) An amoeba is a single-celled animal. Different species of amoeba live in fresh water, sea water or soil. Some related species are parasitic, e.g. the dysentery amoeba.

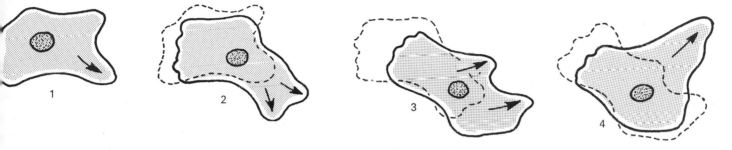

(b) The amoeba moves as a result of its cytoplasm flowing into a protuberance from its surface.

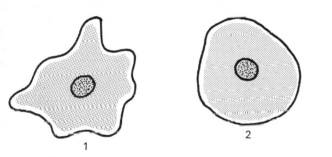

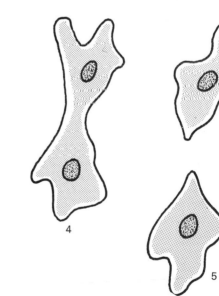

(c) Amoebae reproduce by cell division. First the nucleus divides and then the cytoplasm.

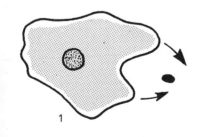

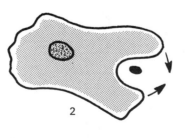

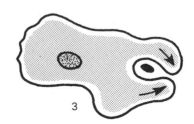

(d) In feeding, an amoeba 'flows' towards and around microscopic plants, engulfing them in a food vacuole where they are digested and absorbed.

Fig. 2.6   Amoeba

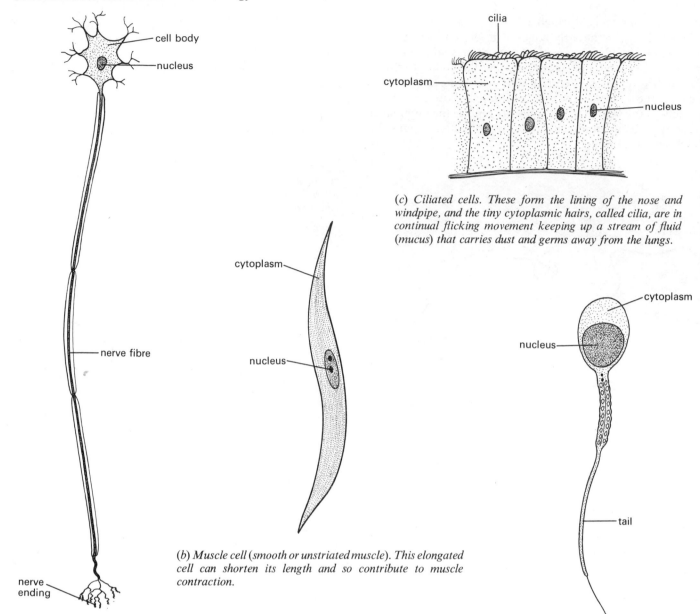

(c) Ciliated cells. These form the lining of the nose and windpipe, and the tiny cytoplasmic hairs, called cilia, are in continual flicking movement keeping up a stream of fluid (mucus) that carries dust and germs away from the lungs.

(b) Muscle cell (smooth or unstriated muscle). This elongated cell can shorten its length and so contribute to muscle contraction.

(a) Nerve cell. Specialized for conducting impulses of an electrical nature along the axon. A nerve consists of hundreds of axons bound together. The fibres may be very long, e.g. from the foot to the spinal column.

(e) Sperm cell. The movements of the tail help the sperm to reach the female's egg and fertilize it.

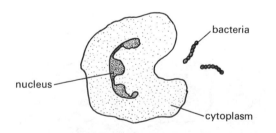

(d) White blood cell. Occurs in the blood stream and is specialized for engulfing harmful bacteria. It is able to change its shape and move about, even through the walls of blood vessels into the surrounding tissues.

Fig. 2.7   Specialized cells

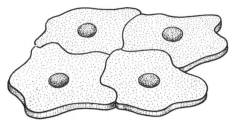

(*a*) *Cells forming an epithelium, a thin layer of tissue, e.g. that lining the mouth cavity.*

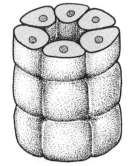

(*b*) *Cells forming a fine tube, e.g. a kidney tubule (p. 93).*

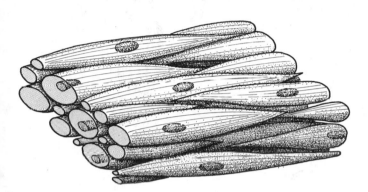

(*c*) *Unstriated muscle cells forming a sheet of muscle tissue. Blood vessels, nerve fibres and connective tissues will also be present.*

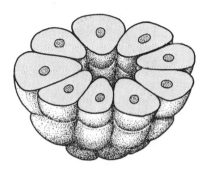

(*d*) *Cells forming part of a gland. The cells make chemicals which are released into the central space and are carried away by a tubule such as shown in (b).*

Fig. 2.8   How cells form tissues

Specialized cells

As already implied, cells have different functions and consequently different shapes and internal chemistry. A single-celled animal such as *Amoeba* (Fig. 2.6) can carry out all the processes necessary for its existence; it can move about, capture and digest its food, and reproduce. A specialized cell, on the other hand, has usually developed one particular function: e.g. a muscle cell can contract, a nerve cell can conduct impulses and a gland cell can produce chemical substances. Once a cell has become specialized it does not usually reproduce although specialized cells can still carry out all other normal cell functions. Some examples of specialized cells are shown in Fig. 2.7.

Relation of cells to the organism as a whole

Although each cell can carry on the vital chemistry of living, it is not capable of existence on its own. A muscle cell cannot obtain its own food or oxygen. These materials are supplied by the blood and transported or made available by the activities of other specialized cells. Unless individual cells are grouped together in large numbers and made to work together by the co-ordinating mechanisms of the body, they cannot exist for long.

Tissue. A tissue such as bone, nerve or muscle is made up of many hundreds of cells of one or a few types (Fig. 2.8), each type being more or less identical in structure and activity so that the tissue can also be said to have a specific function, e.g. nerves conduct impulses, muscles contract, glands secrete chemicals. The structures of tissues such as blood, bone, cartilage, muscle and nerve are described more fully in the chapters dealing with human physiology.

Organs consist of several tissues grouped together making a functional unit; for example, a muscle is an organ containing long muscle cells held together with connective tissue and permeated with blood vessels and nerve fibres. The arrival of a nerve impulse causes the muscle to contract, using the food and oxygen brought by the blood vessels to provide the necessary energy.

System. A system is usually a series of organs whose functions are co-ordinated to produce effective action in the organism; for example, the heart and blood vessels constitute the circulatory system; the brain, spinal cord and nerves make up the nervous system (Fig. 2.9).

Organism. A multicellular organism is formed from a number of organs and systems whose working is efficiently co-ordinated. It is able to reproduce its own kind.

Plant cells

Although a plant cell has a nucleus, cytoplasm, organelles and cell membranes, it differs from an animal cell in having a cellulose wall outside its cell membrane and usually a large central vacuole in its cytoplasm (Fig. 2.3*c*).

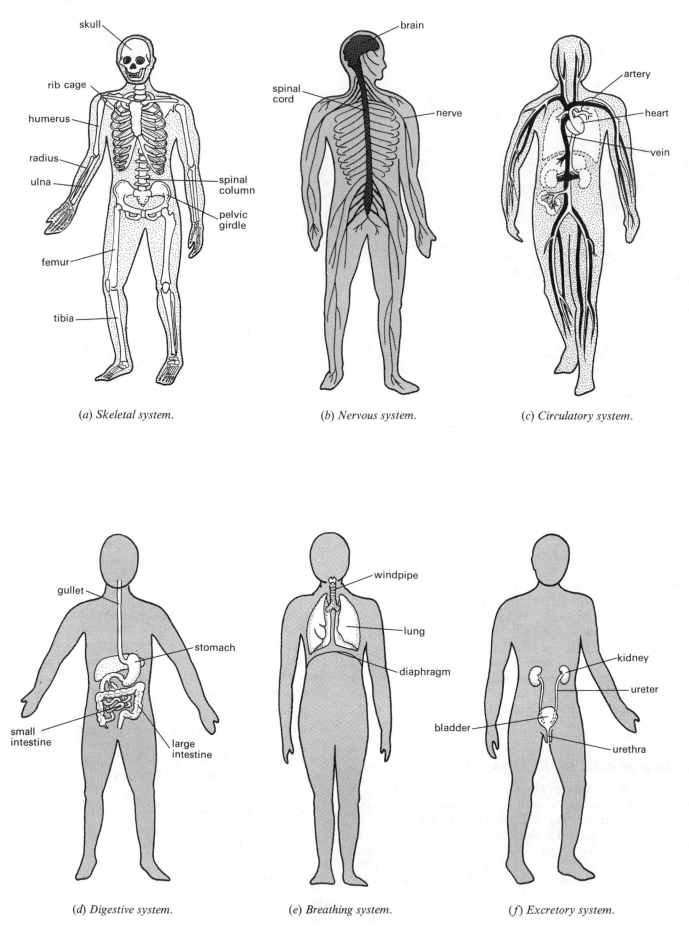

(a) *Skeletal system.*

(b) *Nervous system.*

(c) *Circulatory system.*

(d) *Digestive system.*

(e) *Breathing system.*

(f) *Excretory system.*

Fig. 2.9   Some of the systems of the body

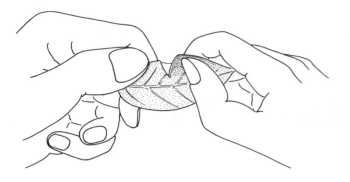

(a) Tear the leaf to expose the lower epidermis.

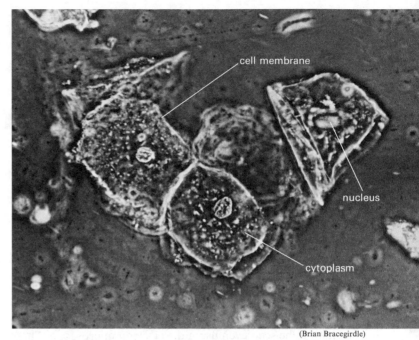

(Brian Bracegirdle)

Fig. 2.11   Cells from the cheek lining

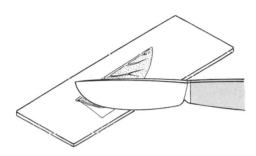

(b) Trim away the thick portion.

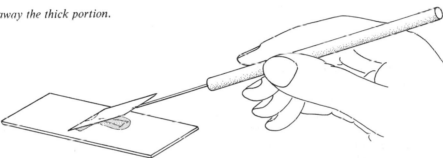

(c) Lower the cover-slip carefully to exclude air bubbles.

Fig. 2.10   Preparing plant cells for microscopic study

Practical Work

Experiment 1   Plant cells

The epidermis can be stripped fairly easily from a bulb scale, for example an onion, or from the lower surface of many leaves (Fig. 2.10). Since the epidermis is only one cell thick, the cells can be seen in transparency if a small piece of the tissue is placed flat on a microscope slide, covered with a drop of water and examined under the low power of the microscope. A little iodine solution may stain the nuclei light brown and any starch grains present will turn dark blue. Cells and chloroplasts may be seen in a moss leaf if it is mounted flat on a slide with a drop of water.

Experiment 2   Animal cells

If a finger is run round the inside of the cheek, and the fluid so collected is smeared on to a slide, examination under the low power of the microscope will show numbers of epithelial cells scraped from the mouth lining (Fig. 2.11). The nuclei can be seen without staining but will show up more clearly if a drop of methylene blue solution is placed on the slide for about one minute, and the slide is then tilted to let the stain run off. The cytoplasm and the nuclei will both take up the stain but the nuclei will be darker.

Questions

1   What features are (a) possessed by both plant and animal cells, (b) possessed by plant cells only?
2   With what materials must cells be supplied if they are to live and grow?
3   In what ways would you say that the white blood cell (Fig. 2.7d) is less specialized than the nerve cell (Fig. 2.7a)?
4   In many microscopical preparations of animal tissues, it is difficult to make out the cell boundaries and yet the disposition and numbers of cells can usually be determined. Which cell structure makes this possible?
5   At one time it was thought that cytoplasm was a kind of structureless jelly. At the same time it was difficult to understand how a complicated series of ordered chemical reactions could take place in such an amorphous fluid. How do you think that electron microscope studies of the cell have helped to resolve this problem?
6   Most mature cells are incapable of dividing to produce new cells. In which parts of the human body in (a) a baby, (b) an adult, would you expect cells to retain their power of division?
7   The systems illustrated in Fig. 2.9 seem to be independent of each other but, in fact, they are closely interconnected. Say how the functions of any one system might influence or be influenced by any of the other systems.

3

The Chemicals of Living Cells

The preceding chapter described cells as the units which, in their thousands, go to make up the bodies of plants and animals. By suitably magnifying the cells they can be seen to consist of nucleus and cytoplasm, containing smaller units such as ribosomes and mitochondria. These subcellular structures are themselves built up from particles, which for the most part are too small to be seen even using the electron microscope. These particles are the molecules of the various chemical substances that contribute to the structures listed above. Chemical substances can conveniently be considered under the headings of *elements* and *compounds*.

Elements

An element is a substance that cannot be split up into two other substances. Copper, iron, sulphur and carbon are examples of solid elements; oxygen and nitrogen are gaseous elements.

The smallest particle of an element is an *atom*, and so elements can be visualized as consisting of countless millions of atoms, all of the same kind, and with a good deal of space between them. When describing and explaining chemical reactions, the atom of an element is represented by a letter, often the initial letter of the element, e.g. C represents an atom of carbon, O represents an atom of oxygen, S sulphur, H hydrogen and N nitrogen.

Compounds

When two or more elements combine chemically they make a compound. If the elements carbon and oxygen combine they make the compound carbon dioxide. Since each element consists of atoms, it is assumed that the combination takes place between the atoms of the different elements (Fig. 3.1).

In many cases, one atom of an element will combine with more than one atom of another element. The atoms may be linked in small, discrete groups called *molecules* or con-

tinuously throughout the material in a three-dimensional array described as a *giant structure*. A molecule of carbon dioxide thus consists of one carbon atom joined to two oxygen atoms, and for simplicity can be visualized as in Fig. 3.2. In silicon dioxide, there are two oxygen atoms to each silicon atom but they are linked in a giant structure (Fig. 3.4).

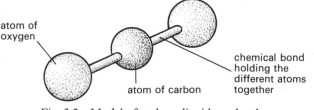

Fig. 3.2   Model of carbon dioxide molecule

In describing compounds and their reactions, the molecules are represented by the letters of their constituent atoms. Carbon dioxide is depicted as CO_2, the figure 2 after the C signifying that there are two atoms of oxygen in the molecule; CO_2 is called the *formula* of carbon dioxide. The formula for silicon dioxide, SiO_2, represents the simplest ratio of atoms present in the giant structure. It so happens that the smallest particle of many gases, including oxygen and nitrogen, consists of two atoms joined together, i.e. it is a molecule, so that the formula of oxygen is O_2 and for nitrogen is N_2 (i.e. N—N).

Gases, liquids and solids

Gases. The molecules of a gas are spaced very far apart and move about rapidly in all directions. If the gas is heated the molecules move faster and further apart, and so the gas expands (Fig. 3.3, Experiment 1). If the gas is cooled the molecules slow down and the gas contracts. Because the molecules are so far apart, it is not difficult to push them closer

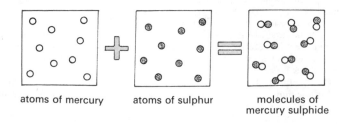

Fig. 3.1   Combination of atoms to make molecules

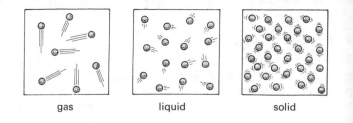

Fig. 3.3   Movement and spacing of molecules in solid, liquid and gas

together by applying pressure to the gas. Thus a gas is easily compressed (Experiment 2). Also, being so far apart, free to move and not greatly attracted to each other, the molecules of a small quantity of gas released into a large space will spread out until they are uniformly distributed through that space (*see* diffusion, p. 22).

Liquids. In liquids the molecules are closer together than they are in a gas but they are still free to move at random. Hence a liquid can flow, though it cannot be compressed.

Solids. The molecules of a solid are much closer together (although there is still a great deal of space between them) and are not free to move, apart from vibrating. Usually they are held in a three-dimensional pattern which gives the substance a crystalline structure (Fig. 3.4, Experiment 3).

Organic and inorganic chemicals

The distinction between these two classes of chemicals was made originally because it was thought that the organic chemicals were produced only by living organisms and could not be made artificially in a laboratory. Although this is not true, there are still significant differences between the two types of chemicals. Inorganic chemicals are substances such as the compounds of metals, for example copper sulphate or sodium chloride. Their molecules are usually small, consisting of up to ten atoms; or, in giant structures, the ratio of the different atoms is small.

Organic chemicals

Organic molecules are usually large, sometimes consisting of hundreds or thousands of atoms. Examples are sugar, starch, oil, fat and protein. The principal chemical feature that identifies organic compounds is that they consist for the most part of carbon atoms joined to each other in chains or rings.

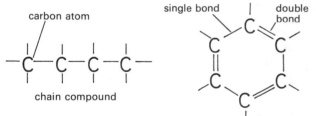

The lines in the formulae represent the chemical bonds holding the atoms together. The 'spare' bonds sticking out from the two formulae above would normally be holding hydrogen, oxygen, nitrogen, phosphorus or other carbon atoms.

Note that each carbon atom has four chemical bonds for holding other atoms, including carbon atoms, in place. Each bond must be used in some way for combining with other

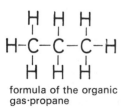

formula of the organic gas-propane

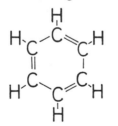

formula of the organic liquid benzene

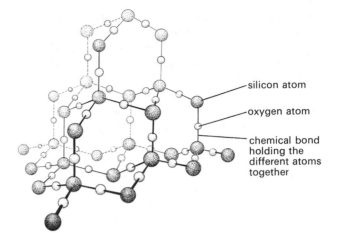

This shows the arrangement of atoms in a tiny part of a crystal of silica (silicon oxide). The atoms are geometrically spaced as shown and thus, in their millions, produce regular crystals.

Fig. 3.4 Atoms in a crystal lattice

atoms. One, two or three bonds, depending on the compound, may be used for holding other carbon atoms. The chain compound, propane, has only single bonds between carbon atoms in its molecule. In the benzene molecule, however, there are three *double bonds*.

The organic molecules which constitute the greater part of living cells are classified as carbohydrates, fats and proteins.

Carbohydrates

Carbohydrate molecules consist of chains of usually six or more carbon atoms combined with hydrogen and oxygen atoms only. The principal groups of carbohydrates are sugar, starch, glycogen and cellulose. Apart from cellulose in plant cell walls, the carbohydrates do not form permanent structures in cells but are used in chemical reactions to provide energy for driving other reactions.

Sugar. One of the simplest and most important sugars is *glucose*. Its formula is $C_6H_{12}O_6$; i.e. a molecule of glucose contains six carbon atoms, twelve hydrogen atoms and six oxygen atoms. It is sometimes represented structurally as

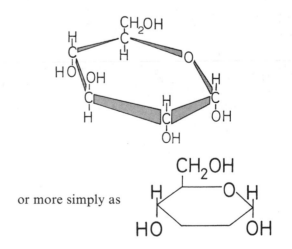

or more simply as

showing only the reactive parts of the molecule.

There are other C_6 sugars (monosaccharides) with the same $C_6H_{12}O_6$ formula but with different arrangements of these atoms in their molecules, which makes them react differently from glucose. Two examples are *fructose* and *galactose*.

Maltose has the formula $C_{12}H_{22}O_{11}$ and is made up from two glucose molecules. Some cells can build up a maltose molecule by combining two glucose molecules. The reaction

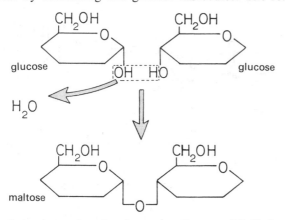

proceeds by removing the elements of water (H_2O) from the two glucose molecules (an —OH from one and an —H from the other). The reaction will not take place spontaneously; that is, when two glucose molecules meet they will not combine to form maltose of their own accord. Another type of chemical in the cell, called an *enzyme* (p. 27), is responsible for making this reaction occur.

There are other C_{12} sugars (disaccharides) of which the most important is *sucrose* (cane sugar), consisting of a glucose and a fructose molecule combined.

Starch. The starch molecule is very large, being made up of a long chain of 300 or more glucose molecules linked together as in maltose, (Experiment 6). Starch is a common storage material in plant cells.

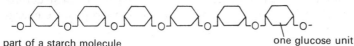

part of a starch molecule   one glucose unit

Glycogen. Animal cells cannot make or store starch. Their storage carbohydrate is usually glycogen which, like starch, has a large molecule built up from thousands of glucose molecules joined together in a branching chain. Glycogen granules occur as inclusions in animal cells.

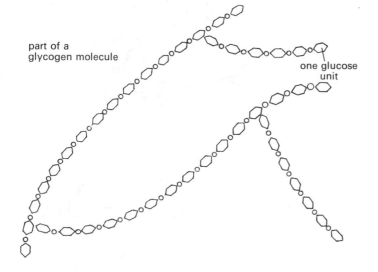

part of a glycogen molecule

one glucose unit

Cellulose is chemically similar to starch in that it consists of one thousand or more glucose units, but the units are joined together in a slightly different way so that the chemical and physical properties of cellulose are different from starch. Only plants can make cellulose and they incorporate it in their cell walls (p. 7), the long molecules being packed together in bundles to make tough micro-fibrils which give the cell wall its strength. Textile fibres such as cotton and flax, made from plant materials, consist largely of cellulose.

Starch, glycogen and cellulose are sometimes called *poly-saccharides*.

Hydrolysis of carbohydrates. Just as the disaccharides and polysaccharides can be built up from glucose and fructose molecules joined together by eliminating the elements of water (—OH and —H), they can be broken down again by reacting them with water (Experiment 5). This process, called hydrolysis

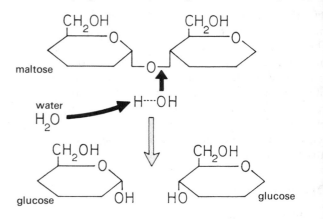

(Greek *hydro* = water, *lysis* = breakdown), does not take place spontaneously in cells but requires the intervention of a particular enzyme. In human saliva there is an enzyme which brings about the hydrolysis of starch to maltose.

part of a starch molecule

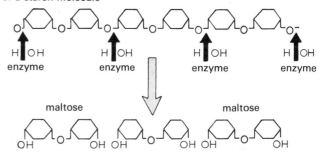

Fats

Like carbohydrates, fats contain atoms of only carbon, hydrogen and oxygen, but there are four distinct parts to a fat molecule. One of these is *glycerol* and the other three are organic acids called *fatty acids*.

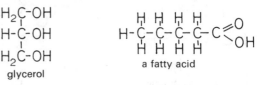

glycerol

a fatty acid

C_4H_9COOH

shorter formula of same acid

The short formula is written in this way and not as $C_5H_{10}O_2$ because there could be other compounds with this formula but with quite different properties, e.g.

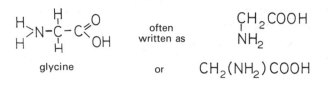

It is the —COOH group at the end of a fatty acid molecule that gives it its characteristic properties.

The reactive parts of the glycerol and the fatty acid are the —OH groups at the ends of the molecules. By removing the elements of water, an —H from the glycerol and an —OH from the fatty acid, the glycerol molecule can be made to combine with three molecules of a fatty acid such as stearic acid to make a *triglyceride*, one form of fat. In the formula below, the —COOH group of the fatty acid is written in reverse to show the reaction with glycerol more clearly.

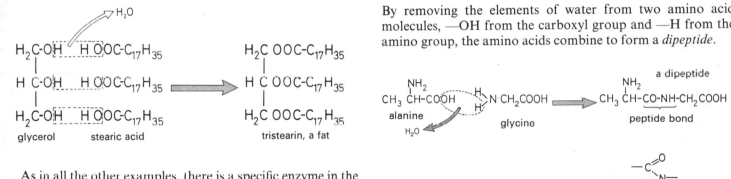

glycerol   stearic acid   tristearin, a fat

As in all the other examples, there is a specific enzyme in the cell that brings about this reaction. Most natural fats have more than one kind of fatty acid combined in the molecule, and whether they are hard fats or liquid oils will depend on which particular fatty acids are involved.

Fats can be hydrolysed by the appropriate enzymes to split them up into fatty acids and glycerol once again.

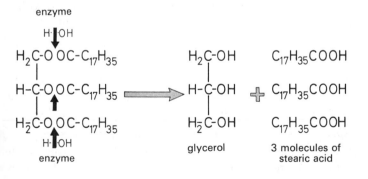

glycerol   3 molecules of stearic acid

Fats form part of the permanent structures of the cell, particularly the cell membrane and the internal membranes. Oil droplets may be present as inclusions in cells, and both plant and animal cells break down fats in chemical reactions to obtain energy from them.

Proteins

In addition to atoms of carbon, hydrogen and oxygen, protein molecules contain atoms of nitrogen and, sometimes, sulphur. The units from which protein molecules are built are called *amino acids* and the simplest of these is *glycine*.

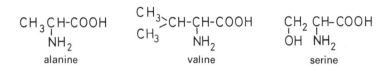

As with fatty acids, the reactive —H of the —OH group confers acidic properties but the —H of the —NH$_2$ is also reactive. The —COOH group is called the *carboxyl* group and the —NH$_2$ is the *amino* group. The amino group is always attached to the carbon atom next to the carboxyl group, as shown in the formulae of alanine, valine and serine.

$$CH_3\,CH\text{-}COOH \qquad {}^{CH_3}_{CH_3}\!\!>CH\text{-}CH\text{-}COOH \qquad CH_2\ CH\text{-}COOH$$

alanine   valine   serine

By removing the elements of water from two amino acid molecules, —OH from the carboxyl group and —H from the amino group, the amino acids combine to form a *dipeptide*.

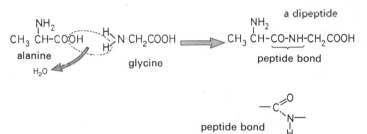

Three amino acids joined in this way will form a *tripeptide* and numerous amino acids will form a *polypeptide*. A protein molecule is a long polypeptide chain containing fifty or more amino acids, but instead of being a straight chain, the molecule is often branched and folded or coiled up because of cross-linkages which form between amino acids at different parts of the chain. Some amino acids such as *cysteine* contain sulphur atoms which are important in forming these cross links. There are twenty different commonly occurring amino acids, and the relative numbers of each amino acid, the order in which they are joined up and the folding and cross-linkages which subsequently form, determine the type of protein and its properties (Fig. 3.5).

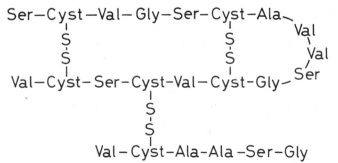

Fig. 3.5 A small imaginary protein made from only five different amino acids

In cells, proteins are built up by the ribosomes. Amino acids in the cytoplasm surrounding the ribosomes are assembled in the 'correct' order to make a particular protein. The correct order is dictated by chemical messengers (RNA) produced in the nucleus and taken up by the ribosomes.

Cells can also break down proteins into their constituent amino acids by hydrolysis in the presence of the appropriate enzymes.

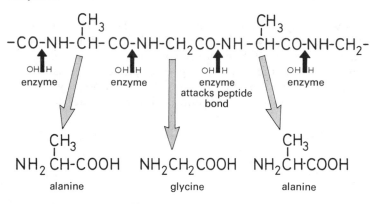

Although proteins and amino acids can be broken down to provide energy, their principal value in cells is as the material from which the cell is constructed. They contribute very largely to the cytoplasm and its membranes, the mitochondria, ribosomes, the nucleus and its chromosomes, and the enzymes themselves which control the direction and rate of all of the chemical reactions in the cell.

Unlike fats and carbohydrates, proteins are adversely affected by rising temperature. Sugar, starch and fat can be subjected to temperatures of 100 °C without their decomposing, other than by a slow hydrolysis, but proteins exposed to temperatures even above 50 °C for any length of time are irreversibly altered. The folds and cross-linkages of the molecule are disarranged and the protein is said to be *denatured*. In this case, the structural proteins of the cell membranes are damaged and the protein of enzymes rendered ineffective. As a result, the cell can no longer function properly and will die. This is the prime reason why continued exposure to temperatures above 50 °C ultimately proves lethal to most living organisms.

Practical Work

Experiment 1   Expansion of air and water

Fit a small bottle or 250 cm³ flask with a bung and glass delivery tube, as shown in Fig. 3.6a. Remove the bung and delivery tube, dip the bung in a jar of water so that water rises in the tube, place your finger over the top of the tube, and replace the bung and tube in the mouth of the bottle (Fig. 3.6b). In this way, a short column of liquid will be trapped in the tube. Make sure that the liquid column is neither rising nor falling and then clasp the bottle in your hands. The warmth of your hands will reach the air in the bottle and make it expand as shown by the upward movement of the liquid column.

Remove the bung and tube and fill the bottle with cold water. When the bung is replaced, the water will rise some way up the tube. Make a mark on the tube at the water level and again

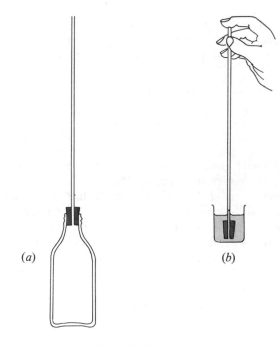

(a)   (b)

Fig. 3.6   Expansion of air

warm the bottle with your hands. As the heat expands the water in the bottle, the water will rise up the tube but not nearly so far as when the bottle contained air. The expansion can be increased by placing the bottle in water at 40–50 °C, or the expansion can be magnified by substituting a capillary tube for the delivery tube.

Experiment 2   Compressibility of gases and liquids

Select a large plastic syringe, 5 or 10 cm³, without a needle and in which the plunger moves freely in the barrel. Withdraw the plunger, place a finger firmly over the short tube at the end and push the plunger in. The gas can fairly easily be compressed in this way to half its original volume and will return to its first volume when the plunger is released.

Now draw up water with the syringe to fill it. Expel air bubbles by pointing the syringe upwards and depressing the plunger slightly. If the syringe opening is now blocked with a finger or thumb, it will be found impossible to compress the water.

Experiment 3   Crystals

Examine a few grains of salt and sugar with a × 10 hand lens or, better still, with a microscope. Many of the particles will be seen to have the regular shape characteristic of crystals.

Experiment 4   The presence of carbon in organic substances

Heat very small samples of food on a tin lid from below with a bunsen flame. Steam and smoke will be produced, but in each case there will be a black residue of carbon. This experiment produces strong smells and is best conducted in a fume cupboard, outside the laboratory or at the end of a school session when the laboratories can be cleared.

Experiment 5   The hydrolysis of starch by acid

Place 5 cm³ of 3 per cent starch solution in each of three test-tubes labelled 1 to 3. Add 1 cm³ dilute (2M) hydrochloric acid to each and place all three in a water bath of boiling water (Fig. 3.7). Remove tube 1 after 5 minutes in the water bath, tube 2 after 10 minutes and tube 3 after 15 minutes. Cool the

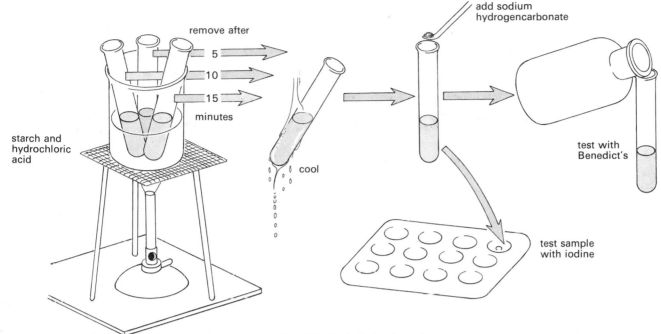

remove after

5

10

15

minutes

starch and hydrochloric acid

cool

add sodium hydrogencarbonate

test with Benedict's

test sample with iodine

Fig. 3.7   Hydrolysis of starch

tubes under the cold tap or by dipping in a jar of cold water, and then add solid sodium hydrogencarbonate, a little at a time, until all fizzing stops and the acid is neutralized. With a dropping pipette take a sample of the liquid from each tube and add it to a little iodine solution in a test-tube or on a tile. Look for the presence or absence of a blue colour. Now add 3 cm³ Benedict's solution to each tube and return them to the boiling water bath for 5 minutes. After this time examine the tubes for evidence of a sugar.

Result. A red precipitate after heating with Benedict's solution indicates that sugar is present (*see* p. 38). A blue colour with iodine shows that starch is present. There should be evidence of an increasing quantity of sugar in tubes 1 to 3 and a decrease in the amount of starch.

Interpretation. Heating with dilute hydrochloric acid converts starch to sugar by hydrolysis (*see* p. 16). The longer the heating is maintained the further the reaction proceeds.

(*Note.* Experiments involving hydrolysis by enzymes can be found on p. 30 and p. 69.)

Experiment 6   **Building up starch from glucose**

The glucose used in this experiment is glucose-l-phosphate, a reactive compound of glucose. The reaction is brought about by an enzyme (*see* p. 27) extracted from potatoes.

A cube of potato of side about 2 cm is crushed in a mortar with 10 cm³ distilled water and a little clean sand. The liquid is filtered into a clean test-tube through a filter paper and will contain, amongst other substances, the enzyme *starch phosphorylase*. Half the solution is poured into another test-tube and boiled over a low bunsen flame. A dropping pipette is used to place two rows of four single drops of a 5 per cent solution of glucose-l-phosphate on a cavity tile. One drop of unboiled potato extract is added to each drop of glucose-l-phosphate in the top row and one drop of boiled extract to each drop of glucose-l-phosphate in the bottom row. After 5 minutes one drop of iodine solution is placed on the first drop in each row. Five minutes later the second drop in each row is similarly tested, and so on at 5-minute intervals

until all the drops have been tested. A sample of the potato extract and the glucose-l-phosphate solution is tested separately to show that no starch is present to begin with.

Result. In the top row, the iodine test should produce first a mauve and then a blue colour which becomes more intense with successive samples. The bottom row should give no blue colour.

Interpretation. Since no starch was present to start with in either solution, it is reasonable to infer that starch molecules have been built up from glucose-l-phosphate units (*see* p. 16). This inference is strengthened by the fact that when the liquid thought to contain the enzyme is boiled, it fails to produce starch with glucose-l-phosphate. This supports the idea that it is an enzyme that causes the glucose units to combine.

The formulae for the chemicals and reagents mentioned in the practical work will be found on p. 268. For other experiments involving enzymes, giving fuller practical details, see Experimental Work in Biology No. 2, *Enzymes* (p. 269).

Questions

1   Which of the following are elements and which are compounds: sugar, carbon dioxide, silver, water, iodine, calcium, benzene?

2   What are the differences between a molecule and an atom?

3   The molecule of sodium carbonate contains two sodium atoms, one carbon atom and three oxygen atoms. Write a formula for this compound (sodium = Na, carbon = C, oxygen = O).

4   Give three general differences between organic and inorganic compounds. Why is there no such thing as an organic element?

5   In what way do maltose, starch, glycogen and cellulose resemble each other?

6   The formula on p. 17 represents a molecule of one kind of fat. Write the formula for a different fat using palmitic acid, $C_{15}H_{31}COOH$, instead of stearic acid.

7   What is the final product of hydrolysis of glycogen, starch and cellulose?

8   A molecule of starch consists of hundreds of glucose units joined together. A molecule of protein consists of perhaps hundreds of amino acids joined together. In what way is the joining-up process similar, and in what way do the final products differ?

9   Write the formula for a dipeptide made from joining valine and serine.

4

Solutions, Diffusion and Osmosis

Before a substance can enter a cell it must dissolve. Moreover, all the chemical reactions in a cell take place in solution. For these and many other reasons it is desirable for a biologist to understand some of the chemical and physical properties of solutions.

When sugar is thoroughly mixed with water the solid crystals of sugar disappear and samples from all parts of the liquid will taste equally sweet. The sugar molecules are evenly dispersed throughout the liquid, and the sugar–water mixture is called a *solution*. The sugar is said to have *dissolved* in the water (Fig. 4.1).

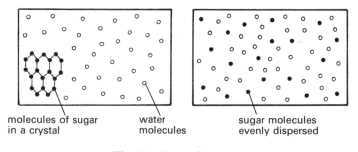

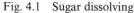

molecules of sugar in a crystal   water molecules   sugar molecules evenly dispersed

Fig. 4.1   Sugar dissolving

The liquid part of the mixture, in this case water, is called the *solvent* and the solid which dissolves is called the *solute*. Because the sugar will dissolve in water it is said to be *soluble*, while a substance like sand which does not dissolve is described as *insoluble* in water (Experiment 1*a*).

Although the terms 'soluble' and 'solubility' nearly always refer to water, it is important to realize that other liquids can act as solvents. Sugar is insoluble in petrol; fats and oils, however, dissolve readily in this solvent though they are insoluble in water (Experiment 1*b*).

Since living organisms consist of about 70 per cent water, it is the solubility of substances in water that is of prime importance. The cell membrane, however, contains fats, and consequently substances that can dissolve in fats and oils will sometimes penetrate the membrane more readily than water-soluble substances. Also there are a number of vitamins which are fat-soluble and therefore present only in natural fats and oils such as butter and fish-liver oils.

The process of digestion in animals is generally concerned with turning a variety of insoluble compounds into other compounds that are soluble in water and can therefore be carried in solution in the blood stream.

Solubility. There is a limit to the weight of solute that will dissolve in a given volume of water. If too much solute is added, it will remain undissolved. A solution that can dissolve no more solute is called *saturated*. Some substances are more soluble than others; sodium nitrate, for example, is much more soluble than lead chloride. In 100 g water at 20 °C it is possible to dissolve 87 g sodium nitrate, but in the same conditions only 2 g lead chloride will dissolve before the solution is saturated. In general, the higher the temperature of the solution, the larger the amount of solute that can be dissolved i.e. solubility increases with temperature (Experiment 1*c*).

The quantity of solute dissolved in a solution is referred to as its *concentration*. A solution of 80 g sodium nitrate in 100 g water is more concentrated than one containing only 8 g sodium nitrate.

Gases in solution. It is not only solids that can dissolve in water; so can liquids and gases (Experiments 2*b* and 2*c*). The gases which concern the biologist are those present in the atmosphere—oxygen, carbon dioxide and nitrogen—and their solubilities are given in the table below.

	cm^3 gas in 1 cm^3 water	
	at 0 °C	*at 15 °C*
carbon dioxide	1.8	1.0
oxygen	0.05	0.035
nitrogen	0.023	0.017

The table shows that carbon dioxide is the most soluble and nitrogen the least soluble of the atmospheric gases, and also that the solubility of these gases *decreases* with rise in temperature (Experiment 2*a*). It is the carbon dioxide dissolved in water which enables aquatic plants to make their food by photosynthesis (p. 40) and the oxygen dissolved in water which is used by all aquatic organisms for their respiration (p. 27). In fact, the oxygen and carbon dioxide entering and leaving all cells in the body must be in solution, irrespective of whether the animal lives in water or on land.

If a gas is in contact with a liquid and the pressure of the gas is increased, more gas will dissolve. The carbon dioxide in fizzy drinks has been dissolved under high pressure so that when the stopper is removed the gas escapes from solution as bubbles. The air supplied to a diver has to be delivered at high pressure in order to force it down to him against water pressure. At high pressure, more of all the atmospheric gases will dissolve in the blood. The oxygen and carbon dioxide are taken out of solution by chemical reactions but not the nitrogen. Consequently, if the diver surfaces too rapidly, the nitrogen that has dissolved in his blood comes out of solution and the bubbles get trapped in small blood vessels in the limbs giving intense pain known as the 'bends' or decompression sickness. The symptoms can be avoided by bringing the diver to the surface slowly, or counteracted by placing him in a pressure tank when he surfaces and reducing the pressure slowly so that the surplus nitrogen can escape from his blood as it passes through the lungs rather than coming out of solution in the body tissues and blood vessels.

Ions in solution. In most cases where a compound has a giant structure the linking arises because the atoms develop electrical charges when they combine. In the salt sodium chloride, the sodium atoms become positively charged and the chlorine atoms negatively charged. Such charged atoms are called *ions*. Because positive and negative charges strongly attract one another, the ions are held by the attractive forces in a continuous regular array. When such compounds are dissolved in water the giant structure breaks down and the ions become free to move independently in solution. The compound is said to have *dissociated*. The properties of ions are very different from atoms (Experiment 3). For example, sodium atoms react violently with water but sodium ions are quite stable in water. Chlorine atoms are combined in pairs and constitute a gas; chloride ions, on the other hand, exist singly and remain in solution.

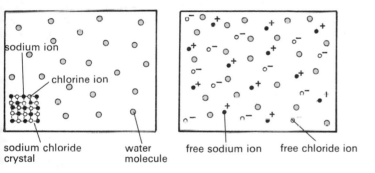

Fig. 4.2 Sodium chloride dissolving

Ions are not necessarily single atoms but may themselves be discrete groups of atoms that carry electrical charges. Potassium nitrate, for example, has the formula KNO_3 and is composed of potassium and nitrate ions.

$$KNO_3 \longrightarrow K^+ + NO_3^-$$
potassium nitrate   potassium ion   nitrate ion

Nitrate, NO_3, cannot exist as a compound on its own but it is perfectly stable as an ion in solution.

Most inorganic salts dissociate into free ions when dissolved in water. If both sodium chloride and potassium nitrate are dissolved in water, the solution will contain ions of sodium, potassium, chloride and nitrate (Fig. 4.3). In such a case, it would be impossible to say whether the salts originally dissolved had been sodium chloride and potassium nitrate or sodium nitrate and potassium chloride. Since the ions formed from a substance behave more or less independently in solution, the biologist is more concerned with, say, the reactions involving chloride ions and sodium ions in the blood than with the reactions of sodium chloride as a compound.

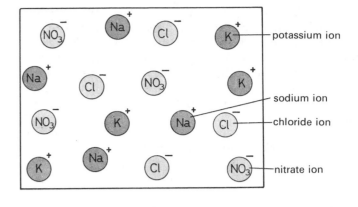

Fig. 4.3 Two salts ionized in solution (water molecules not represented)

When some compounds composed of molecules dissolve in water, the process of dissolving may split at least some of the molecules into ions, even though the atoms in the molecules were originally uncharged and not present as ions. The dissociation of the molecules in a compound may be complete or only partial so that not all the molecules dissolved form ions.

Acids and alkalis

When acids are dissolved in water, they dissociate to form hydrogen ions, e.g.

$$HCl \longrightarrow H^+ + Cl^-$$
hydrochloric acid   hydrogen ion   chloride ion

$$H_2SO_4 \longrightarrow H^+ H^+ + SO_4^-$$
sulphuric acid   two hydrogen ions   sulphate ion

With an acid such as hydrochloric acid, 90 per cent of the HCl molecules in solution will be dissociated into ions, but in sulphuric acid of the same concentration only 50 per cent of the molecules will form ions. Because, at a given concentration, hydrochloric acid produces more ions than does sulphuric acid, the former is said to be the stronger acid.

Organic acids such as fatty acids and amino acids are very weak acids. Acetic (ethanoic) acid, one of the simplest fatty acids, will have only 6 out of every 1 000 molecules dissociated in a solution of the same concentration as the hydrochloric and sulphuric acids mentioned above.

Water is very slightly dissociated to H^+ and OH^- ions which enables it to take part in reactions such as the hydrolysis described on p. 16.

Alkalis such as sodium hydroxide, NaOH, dissociate into a positive ion and a negative OH^- (hydroxyl) ion.

$$NaOH \longrightarrow Na^+ + OH^-$$
sodium hydroxide   sodium ion   hydroxyl ion

pH

The acidity of a compound is determined by how many hydrogen ions it produces. The strong acids such as hydrochloric acid, which dissociate almost completely, produce a high concentration of H^+ ions. Similarly, the alkalinity of a compound depends on the concentration of OH^- ions that it can produce. The degree of acidity or alkalinity of a compound is expressed as a *pH value* (Experiment 9).

When there are equal numbers of OH^- and H^+ ions, the solution is said to be *neutral* and its pH value is 7; e.g. pure water ($H_2O \rightarrow H^+ + OH^-$) has this pH value. As the proportion of OH^- ions increases, the pH value rises (up to 14). With a rise in the proportion of H^+ ions, the pH value falls (to 1). The scale is logarithmic, i.e. there are ten times more H^+ ions in a solution of pH 3 than there are in a solution of pH 4, and one hundred times more than in a solution of pH 5. A solution of pH 2 is strongly acid and one of pH 6 is weakly acid. The pH of a solution can be measured approximately by use of dyes called *indicators*. A familiar pH indicator is litmus, which is red in solutions of pH 5 or less (acid) and blue at pH 8 or more.

The reactions which take place in cells, particularly those involving enzymes, are very sensitive to changes in pH (*see* p. 27). A marked change of pH in a cell can have very harmful effects, and one function of many organ systems in the body is to keep the pH of the blood, tissue fluid and cells within very narrow limits (*see* homeostasis, p. 92).

Diffusion

If a lump of sugar is placed in a bowl of water and left without stirring or disturbing in any way, the sugar will dissolve. At first, the sugar solution in the immediate neighbourhood of the lump will be very concentrated and the concentration will lessen as the distance from the lump increases. Eventually, however, the sugar molecules will distribute themselves evenly through the water so that all samples of the liquid will have the same concentration (Fig. 4.4).

The difference in concentration which brings about diffusion is called a *diffusion gradient*; the greater the difference in the two concentrations the 'steeper' is the gradient and the more rapidly will diffusion occur (Fig. 4.5).

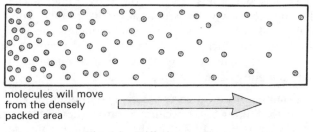

molecules will move from the densely packed area

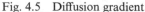

Fig. 4.5   Diffusion gradient

Diffusion can account for the movement of oxygen and carbon dioxide within the alveoli of a lung (p. 86) and, to some extent, for the exchange of dissolved gases between the blood and tissue fluid (*see* p. 83) and the movement of substances within cells.

Osmosis

Osmosis can be regarded as a special case of diffusion: the diffusion of water from a weaker to a stronger solution. A weak solution of salt, for example, will contain relatively less salt and more water than a strong solution of salt. Thus, the diffusion gradient for salt is from the strong to the weak solution, but for water the diffusion gradient is from the weak to the

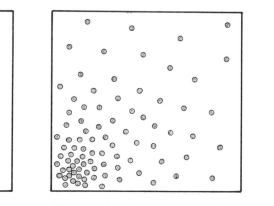

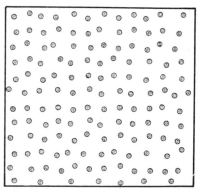

(a)   (b) *Sugar dissolves; molecules diffuse.*   (c) *Sugar molecules evenly spaced.*

Fig. 4.4   Diffusion (water molecules not represented)

This kind of directional movement of molecules is called *diffusion* and occurs because the molecules of solute are in constant motion (Experiment 5). Although molecules move in random directions, each molecule will continue in a straight line until it is deflected from its path by colliding with other molecules or the wall of the container. This will go on until the solute molecules are evenly distributed.

The same phenomenon occurs with gases (Experiment 4a and b). If a small quantity of oxygen is introduced into a container full of nitrogen, the oxygen molecules will diffuse until they are uniformly spaced throughout the container.

strong solution. If two such solutions were in contact, the water molecules would move one way and the salt molecules the other until both were evenly distributed. If, however, the two solutions are separated by a membrane that allows water molecules to pass through more easily than salt, water will diffuse out of the weak solution more rapidly than salt will diffuse into it. Such a membrane is said to be *differentially permeable* or *selectively permeable*, and the water movement is called osmosis (*see* Fig. 4.6). Osmosis, then, is the passage of water across a selectively permeable membrane from a weak to a strong solution (Experiment 8).

Selectively permeable membranes. It is not very clear what the properties are that make a membrane selectively permeable. One theory supposes that the membrane acts as a molecular sieve, having tiny pores in it which are too small to allow large molecules like sugar, $C_{12}H_{22}O_{11}$, to pass through easily but large enough to let small water molecules, H_2O, go through quite rapidly (Fig. 4.6). Another theory suggests that the solvent actually dissolves in the membrane and seeps through it by diffusion while the solute molecules dissolve less readily in the membrane.

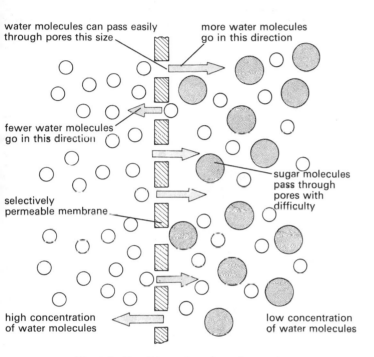

water molecules can pass easily through pores this size

more water molecules go in this direction

fewer water molecules go in this direction

selectively permeable membrane

sugar molecules pass through pores with difficulty

high concentration of water molecules

low concentration of water molecules

Fig. 4.6   Possible explanation of osmosis

Osmotic pressure. If a strong solution of sugar is enclosed in a bag made from selectively permeable material such as cellophane and immersed in water, molecules of water will pass through the membrane into the sugar solution faster than they will pass out (Fig. 4.7). Consequently the volume of water

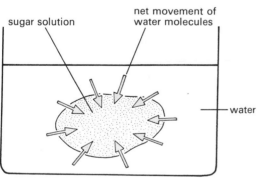

sugar solution

net movement of water molecules

water

Fig. 4.7   Osmotic pressure

inside the membrane will increase, and this increase in volume will be accompanied by an increase in pressure which may swell the bag or burst it. The pressure that does this is called the

osmotic pressure of the sugar solution. The more concentrated the solution, the higher is its osmotic pressure (Experiment 7).

If the bag of sugar solution is removed from the water, osmosis cannot take place and pressure will not build up. Even when separated, however, the water and the sugar solution are said to have an *osmotic potential* because they can cause osmosis in the appropriate situation. The water has a higher osmotic potential than the sugar solution because the diffusion gradient for water molecules is from the pure water to the solution.

Osmosis in cells. The cell membrane has selectively permeable properties, and the cytoplasm inside it contains many substances in solution. The cell thus has a low osmotic potential and if it is surrounded by a solution weaker than that in the cytoplasm, water will pass into it by osmosis. If surrounded by a solution stronger than that in the cytoplasm, the cell will lose water by osmosis through its membrane and shrink. Loss or gain of water in this way will distort the cell and may damage its internal structure, affecting the important chemical reactions taking place. It is vital, therefore, that the tissue fluid which surrounds the cells does not become appreciably weaker or stronger than the cytoplasm. The composition of the tissue fluid depends on the composition of the blood, and the latter is kept within narrow limits by the combined action of the brain, kidneys and liver (*see* pp. 72 and 92). The osmotic potential of the blood is also thought to play a part in the exchange of water between the capillaries and the tissue fluid (p. 83).

Practical Work

Experiment 1   **Solubility of solids**

(a) *Salt and sand.* Make marks on three test-tubes, 1 cm and 7 cm from the base. Pour salt (sodium chloride) into two of the tubes up to the 1-cm mark and the same depth of sand into the third tube. In the tube with sand and one of the tubes with salt pour water up to the 7-cm mark. In the remaining tube of salt pour ethanol (industrial methylated spirit will do) up to the 7-cm mark. Cork each tube or cover the mouth with your thumb, shake them vigorously for about 30 seconds and then let them settle down. Examine the contents of each tube and record your conclusions on the solubility of salt and sand in water and the solubility of salt in ethanol.

(b) *Fats.* Select two clean, dry test-tubes. Into one pour about 5 cm water and into the other a similar quantity of iso-propyl alcohol (propan-2-ol). Use a dropping pipette to add 10 drops of vegetable oil to each tube. Observe the effects in each tube both before and after shaking them to mix the contents. What conclusions do you reach about the solubility of oil in (i) water, and (ii) isopropyl alcohol?

(c) *Temperature and saturation.* Select two clean, dry test-tubes. In one tube place some potassium nitrate to a depth of 1 cm. In the other, place potassium nitrate to a depth of 2 cm. Add water to both to a depth of 5 cm. Shake the tubes for a few seconds to mix the contents and notice that the smaller quantity of nitrate dissolves entirely in the water, while in the other tube some salt is left undissolved, i.e. the solution is saturated at room temperature. Heat the second tube with a bunsen flame or place it in a water bath at 100 °C and observe that all the solid dissolves when the temperature of the solution is increased.

Experiment 2   **Solubility of atmospheric gases in water**

(a) *Extracting dissolved air from water*. The apparatus is set up as in Fig. 4.8 and filled completely with tap water. The water

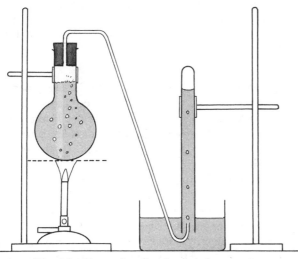

Fig. 4.8   Extracting dissolved air from water

in the flask is heated to boiling point and heating is continued for another ten minutes. A mixture of steam and air enters the trough but the steam condenses in the cold water while the air collects in the inverted tube. When the heating is stopped, the steam left in the flask condenses and water is sucked back to fill the apparatus once again. The gas collected in the tube is a mixture similar in composition to air but containing a different proportion of each gas. It will contain little nitrogen as this is the least soluble of the three important atmospheric gases.

(b) *Dissolving air in water*. For this experiment, a supply of boiled and cooled water is needed. Water is boiled for five minutes to expel most of the dissolved gases. The boiled water is allowed to cool to about 40 °C and stored in stoppered bottles. The bottles are filled to the top, the tops securely replaced and left to stand for 24 hours to acquire room temperature.

A small, screw-top bottle is two-thirds filled with the boiled water, the stopper replaced and the bottle shaken for about thirty seconds. The bottle is then held upside down and the screw cap slowly loosened. Bubbles of air are seen to enter, replacing the air that has dissolved in the water during shaking. If the experiment is repeated using tap water instead of boiled water, no bubbles will enter because the tap water is already saturated with oxygen (see Experiment 2c) and no more will dissolve.

(c) *Solubility of carbon dioxide*. A small screw-top bottle is two-thirds filled with tap water. Carbon dioxide from a cylinder or a carbon dioxide generator (Fig. 4.9) is run into the air space at the top of the bottle for about fifteen seconds. The stopper is replaced and the bottle shaken for a few seconds. When the bottle is held upside down and the screw cap loosened, there will be an inward rush of air to replace the carbon dioxide that has dissolved in the water. This shows that the tap water was by no means saturated with carbon dioxide. Thus, in Experiment 2b the principal gas dissolving must have been oxygen; the 0.04 per cent carbon dioxide in the atmosphere would produce so little change in volume when it dissolved that no air would enter the bottle to replace it.

Experiment 3   **Ionization**

A piece of iron or steel, e.g. a large nail, is cleaned with sandpaper until it is bright. It is then dipped for five seconds in a strong solution of copper sulphate. When it is withdrawn it is seen to be coated with copper. This shows that copper is present in the blue solution but in a very different form from the familiar metal. It is the ions of copper which are present in the solution (p. 21) and which are deposited on the iron as copper atoms.

Experiment 4   **Diffusion of gases**

(a) *Carbon dioxide*. Two gas jars or jam jars are washed and dried. One of the jars is filled with carbon dioxide by placing the tube from a cylinder or carbon dioxide generator (Fig. 4.9) in it for about fifteen seconds. The other jar is now placed

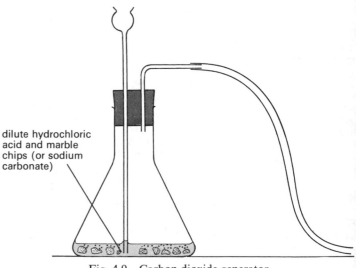

dilute hydrochloric acid and marble chips (or sodium carbonate)

Fig. 4.9   Carbon dioxide generator

upside down over the one filled with carbon dioxide and left for five minutes (Fig. 4.10). After this time, the jars are separated, a little lime water is poured into each and swilled around. Although, originally, only the bottom jar contained carbon dioxide which is heavier than air, the lime water in both jars will go milky showing that the gas has diffused into the top jar.

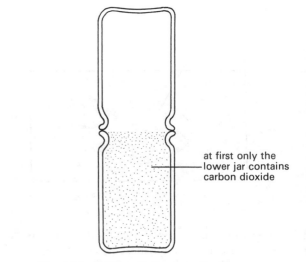

at first only the lower jar contains carbon dioxide

Fig. 4.10   Diffusion of carbon dioxide

(b) *Ammonia.* Squares of wetted red litmus paper are pushed with a glass rod or wire into a wide glass tube, corked at one end, so that they stick to the side and are evenly spaced out (Fig. 4.11). The open end of the tube is closed with a cork carrying a plug of cotton wool saturated with a strong solution of ammonia. The alkaline ammonia vapour diffuses along inside the tube at a rate which can be determined by observing the time when each square of litmus paper turns completely blue. If the experiment is repeated using a more dilute solution of ammonia the rate of diffusion is seen to be slower.

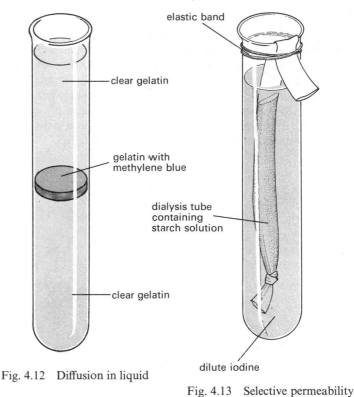

Fig. 4.12　Diffusion in liquid

Fig. 4.13　Selective permeability

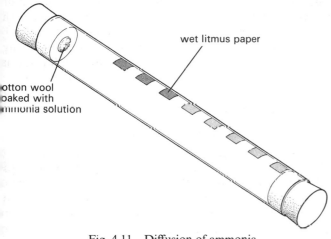

Fig. 4.11　Diffusion of ammonia

Experiment 5　Diffusion in a liquid

Diffusion in a liquid is slow and liable to be affected by convection currents or other physical disturbances in the liquid. In this experiment the water is 'kept still' so to speak, by dissolving gelatin in it. 10 g gelatin is dissolved in 100 g hot water and the solution is poured into test-tubes to half fill them. Some of the liquid gelatin remaining is coloured with methylene blue and when the first layer of gelatin in the test-tube has set firmly, a narrow layer of blue gelatin is poured into it. When the blue layer of gelatin is cold and firm, the test-tube is filled with cool but liquid gelatin and cooled quickly so that the blue gelatin is sandwiched between two layers of clear gelatin (Fig. 4.12). After a week, the blue dye is seen to have diffused into the clear gelatin, upwards and downwards to equal extents.

Experiment 6　Selective permeability

A 15-cm length of 6 mm dialysis tubing (Cellophane or Visking tubing) is cut, soaked in water for a few minutes, and a knot tied tightly near one end. Using a dropping pipette, the tubing is partly filled with 1 per cent starch solution, placed in a test-tube and held in place by an elastic band as shown in Fig. 4.13. The test-tube and dialysis tube are now washed with water from a running tap to remove any starch solution that may have escaped from the dialysis tubing. Fill the test-tube with water, add one or two drops of iodine solution, sufficient to colour the water yellow, and leave the tube in a rack for 10–15 minutes. After this time it will be seen that the starch inside the dialysis tube has turned blue but the iodine outside remains yellow.

When iodine mixes with starch or starch mixes with iodine, a blue colour results. In this experiment, the simplest interpretation of the result is that the dialysis tubing allows iodine

through to reach the starch but does not allow starch out to reach the iodine. Since the starch molecules are hundreds of times larger than the iodine molecules this might be the reason for their failure to pass through the membrane of the dialysis tubing.

Experiment 7　Osmotic pressure

A 20-cm length of 6 mm dialysis tubing is cut, soaked in water, and securely knotted near one end. The tube is then partly filled with a strong solution of syrup or sugar and the open end tightly knotted. The tube should be flabby and easily bendable (Fig. 4.14). Immerse the dialysis tube in a test-tube full of

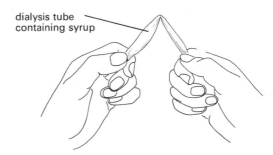

Fig. 4.14　The partly filled tube is flexible enough to bend

water and leave it for 30–45 minutes. When it is removed from the water the dialysis tubing will be taut and full. Water has been taken in by osmosis and has thus increased the pressure inside the tubing.

Experiment 8   **Osmosis**

A length of dialysis tubing (6 mm Cellophane or Visking tubing) is soaked in water, securely knotted at one end, filled with a strong solution of syrup or sugar, and fitted over the end of a capillary tube with the aid of an elastic band (Fig. 4.15). The dialysis tube is lowered into a beaker or jar of water and clamped vertically. In a few minutes, the level of liquid is seen to rise up the capillary tube and may continue to do so for a metre or more according to the length of the tube.

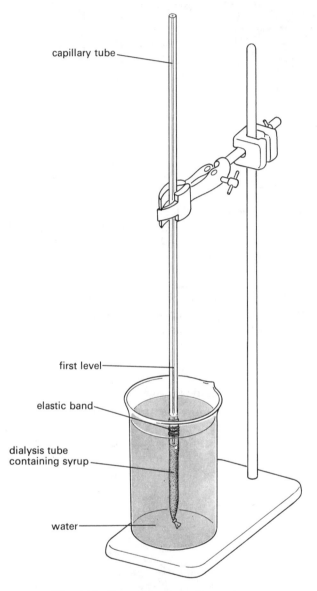

capillary tube

first level

elastic band

dialysis tube
containing syrup

water

Fig. 4.15   Demonstration of osmosis

Interpretation. The most plausible interpretation is that water molecules have passed through the cellophane tubing into the sugar solution, increasing its volume and forcing it up the capillary tube. This movement should theoretically continue until the pressure of the column of syrup in the capillary is equal to the diffusion pressure of the water entering the dialysis tube. In practice, the dialysis tubing does allow sugar molecules to pass through into the water but more slowly

than it allows water molecules in. Eventually, the concentrations of sugar in the beaker and the dialysis tubing would become the same.

Experiment 9   **pH and universal indicator**

Fill three test-tubes to a depth of about 5 cm with tap water. To each add 10 drops of universal indicator. Using a dropping pipette add dilute (M/10) hydrochloric acid, two drops at a time, to one of the tubes. Shake the tube after each addition and note any change in colour by comparing it with the other tubes. Continue adding the acid until there is no further colour change. Wash the pipette and use it to add dilute (M/20) sodium carbonate solution (an alkali), two drops at a time to one of the remaining tubes. Again, compare the colours with the third tube and go on adding the alkali until no further colour change occurs. If the colours produced are compared with a special colour chart for this indicator, the pH represented by each colour can be seen. Approximately, pink is pH 4, yellow is 6 orange 5, green 7, blue 8–9 and purple 10.

Experiment 10   **Carbon dioxide and pH**

Two test-tubes are half filled with tap water, and carbon dioxide from a cylinder or carbon dioxide generator (Fig. 4.9) is bubbled through one of them for a minute. Ten drops of universal indicator are added to each tube and the colour compared with the results of Experiment 9. The experiment may also be tried by bubbling carbon dioxide through hydrogencarbonate indicator (*see* p. 268). It will be seen that carbon dioxide makes an acid solution when it dissolves in water.

Further experiments on diffusion and osmosis, with more detailed instructions, can be found in Experimental Work in Biology No. 6, *Diffusion and osmosis* (*see* p. 269).

Questions

1   Rubber dissolves in benzene, chloroform dissolves Perspex, salt and water make a solution. In each case, say which substance is the solvent and which the solute.
2   Which of the following solutions is the more concentrated: 10 g potassium chloride in 50 g water, or 25 g potassium chloride in 130 g water?
3   The dissolved air in the water of a pond and the air in the atmosphere above it are in equilibrium, i.e. the gases are escaping from the water at the same rate as they are dissolving in it. Nevertheless, the proportions of oxygen, carbon dioxide and nitrogen in the air and pond water are quite different. Suggest a reason for this.
4   What ions will form when the following salts dissolve in water: potassium chloride, KCl; copper nitrate, $CuNO_3$; zinc sulphate, $ZnSO_4$; nitric acid, HNO_3; potassium hydroxide, KOH?
5   Which is the more acid, a solution of pH 6 or a solution of pH 4?
6   As a general rule diffusion takes place in gases and liquids but not in solids. Why is this so?
7   Which system offers the steeper diffusion gradient: (a) a solution containing 200 g salt per litre in contact with one containing 20 g per litre, or (b) a solution containing 20 g per litre in contact with one containing 2 g per litre?
8   A solution of salt (sodium chloride) is separated by a differentially permeable membrane from a solution of sugar of equal concentration (equimolecular, i.e. the same number of molecules in a given volume). Discuss whether osmosis is likely to take place, assuming that the sodium chloride molecule is far smaller than the sugar molecule. Justify your conclusions.
9   A strong solution of sodium chloride is sometimes used as an antiseptic, i.e. it destroys certain bacteria. Suggest, in terms of osmosis, how it might achieve its effect.
10   What activities in man are likely to (a) increase and (b) decrease the osmotic potential of his blood and body fluids?

5
Reactions in the Cell

Chapters 3 and 4 dealt with the structures of the cell and the chemicals of which it is composed or which take part in reactions inside it. These reactions are necessary (a) to enable the cell to grow and reproduce, (b) to produce energy for driving other reactions and (c) to carry out special functions of the cell such as contraction or conduction. Some of these reactions will be considered in more detail but first it is necessary to describe the chemicals which control and direct all the reactions in a cell, the *enzymes*.

Enzymes

Enzymes are proteins made in the cell and they have the function of accelerating chemical reactions. Chemicals that affect the speed of reactions but are not themselves used up in the reaction are called *catalysts*, and enzymes are organic catalysts in cells.

Catalytic action. The reactions that can take place between the substances in cells are usually slow; for example, it would take days for even a small amount of starch to be hydrolysed to maltose (p. 16) by simply mixing the starch with water. In the laboratory, the reaction can be speeded up by adding acid and raising the temperature of the mixture to boiling point. High temperatures and acids are harmful to living cells, and one of the distinctive features of enzymes is that they accelerate reactions at low temperatures and without extreme chemical conditions. The enzyme in saliva will convert starch to sugar at room temperature in a minute or two; a reaction which would otherwise need fifteen minutes or more of boiling with hydrochloric acid.

Specificity. Any one enzyme will act as a catalyst for only one kind of reaction. An enzyme that builds proteins out of amino acids (p. 17) will not catalyse the hydrolysis of maltose. Thus for each type of reaction there is one specific enzyme, and they are often given names related to the reaction in which they participate, the name usually ending in *-ase*. An enzyme that catalyses the removal of hydrogen from a compound is called a *dehydrogenase*. Enzymes that break down proteins are *proteases*, and those that hydrolyse fats (sometimes called *lipids*) are *lipases*. Starch is a mixture of two substances, *amylose* and *amylopectin*, so enzymes that act on starch are called *amylases*.

Optimum temperature and pH. Chemical reactions are speeded up by an increase in temperature; a rise of 10 °C will double the rate of most reactions. The reactions in cells also are accelerated by temperature rise, but because enzymes are proteins they are adversely affected by high temperatures;

above 45 °C they are probably denatured (*see* p. 18). As the temperature of a cell is raised the reactions go faster, but as the temperature approaches 50 °C the enzymes are progressively inactivated so that they can no longer catalyse the reaction. The highest temperature at which reactions are speeded up without at the same time inactivating the enzyme is called the *optimum* temperature. Temperatures above or below the optimum will slow down the reaction. In man, the optimum temperature for most of the enzymes in his cells is between 30 and 40 °C (Experiment 1).

The structure and reactions of proteins, including enzymes, are affected by the acidity or alkalinity (pH) of the medium in which they are working. Just as there is an optimum temperature for enzymes there is also an optimum degree of acidity, but for somewhat different reasons. The acidity and alkalinity of the cytoplasm in cells varies very little but the optimum conditions for different digestive enzymes range from neutral to strongly acid (Experiment 2).

Extracellular enzymes. The majority of enzymes are *intracellular*, that is, they catalyse reactions taking place inside the cell. A few enzymes, however, are made in cells but released from the cells to do their work. The digestive enzymes are extracellular enzymes of this kind. They are made in gland cells but secreted (released) into the digestive tract before they become active, and here they start to break down the food. The digestive enzymes are considered in more detail on p. 62.

Respiration

The chemical reactions in the cell involve building up large molecules from small ones, or breaking down large molecules to smaller ones and reassembling them in a different way. There may also be other molecular changes in specialized cells; for instance, when a muscle cell shortens to produce muscle contraction there is a temporary rearrangement of its molecules. The movements of substances into and out of a cell may also involve chemical reactions. Many of these reactions involving enzymes need a supply of energy to make them take place. This energy is obtained from food substances such as sugars and fats. The molecules of the food substance are broken down to smaller molecules and the energy that was in their chemical bonds is transferred to other molecules in the cell. The food molecules are broken down in stages by enzymes (e.g. dehydrogenases) removing hydrogen and carbon atoms one at a time and eventually combining these atoms with oxygen to form water (the oxide of hydrogen, H_2O) and carbon dioxide (an oxide of carbon, CO_2). The carbon dioxide and water are eventually eliminated from the cell (Experiments 3 and 4). This transfer of energy from food to other chemicals in the cell is called *respiration*. In its simplest terms, respiration is the breakdown of carbohydrates and fats to form carbon dioxide and water with a corresponding release of energy for other reactions in the cell. It is sometimes expressed in the form of an equation

$$C_6H_{12}O_6 + 6O_2 = 6CO_2 + 6H_2O + 2\ 830\ \text{kilojoules}$$

glucose   oxygen   carbon dioxide   water   energy

but this represents only the beginning and the end of the process, because the glucose is actually broken down in small steps involving many intermediate compounds, with energy being produced at each step. The 2 830 kilojoules (kJ) represent the maximum energy to be obtained from one gram molecule (180 g) of glucose if it is completely oxidized to water and carbon dioxide.

A distinction is usually made between two forms of or stages in respiration called *aerobic* and *anaerobic*. Aerobic respiration involves the use of oxygen in the breakdown of carbohydrates or fats which are eventually oxidized completely to carbon dioxide and water. Anaerobic respiration is the breakdown of carbohydrates to release energy without the use of oxygen (*see* below). Each step in the chemistry of respiration is catalyzed by a specific enzyme.

The term 'respiration' is also often used loosely in reference to breathing, as in 'artificial respiration', 'pulse and respiration rate', or in connection with gaseous exchange as in 'the respiratory surface of the lungs', 'organs of respiration'. For this reason, the respiration described in this chapter is sometimes called *tissue respiration* or *internal respiration* to distinguish it from either the breathing movements (ventilation)

During vigorous activity, the oxygen supply may not be sufficient to completely oxidize the food required to meet the energy demands of the body, so that the products of the initial, anaerobic, stages (e.g. lactic acid) accumulate in the cell. These products have to be oxidized or converted back to carbohydrate so that even after the vigorous activity has ceased the uptake and use of oxygen continues at a high rate. The organism is said to have incurred an '*oxygen debt*' as a result of its excess of anaerobic respiration.

Some bacteria and fungi derive all or most of their energy from anaerobic respiration, and the end products are frequently alcohol and carbon dioxide; the process in this case is called *fermentation* (Experiment 5).

Adenosine triphosphate, ATP. The energy in the chemical bonds of carbohydrate and fat molecules is largely associated with hydrogen atoms. As the molecules are broken down in respiration, the hydrogen atoms and their energy are passed to a series of chemicals called *hydrogen acceptors*. As the hydrogen atom is passed from one hydrogen acceptor to the next, it releases a proportion of its energy and this is trapped by a substance called *adenosine diphosphate* (ADP). The chemical structure of ADP need not concern us except for the fact that it contains two phosphate groups, i.e. adenosine—phosphate—phosphate. The energy from the transferred hydrogen atom allows ADP to combine with a third phosphate group to make adenosine triphosphate (ATP), i.e. adenosine—phosphate—phosphate ~ phosphate. The chemical bond between the second and third phosphate is more easily broken than the bond between the first and second. When the third phosphate bond is broken it releases energy which can be used for other reactions (*see* Fig. 5.1).

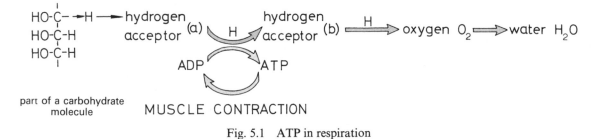

Fig. 5.1   ATP in respiration

or the intake of oxygen and the output of carbon dioxide (gaseous exchange).

Anaerobic respiration. This is the release of energy from food material by a process of chemical breakdown that does not require oxygen. The food, e.g. carbohydrate, is not broken down completely to carbon dioxide and water but to intermediate compounds such as lactic acid or alcohol.

$$C_6H_{12}O_6 = 6CO_2 + 2C_2H_5OH + 118\ \text{kJ}$$

glucose   carbon dioxide   alcohol   energy

The incomplete breakdown of the food means that less energy is released in anaerobic respiration than in aerobic respiration.

Both processes may take place in cells at the same time. Indeed, the first steps in the breakdown of glucose in respiration are anaerobic.

glucose $\xrightarrow[\text{anaerobic}]{}$ lactic acid $\xrightarrow[\text{aerobic}]{}$ carbon dioxide and water

ATP is a kind of universal and readily available 'energy currency'. It is used to drive a wide variety of chemical reactions in the cell, from the conversion of glycogen to glucose to the contraction of a muscle cell. In suitable chemical conditions, ATP breaks down to ADP and phosphate, releasing energy for some vital reaction. The ADP will eventually be used to rebuild ATP once more.

The energy from food molecules cannot be used directly for cell reactions but must first be transferred to ATP; the ATP is then available as an energy source, acceptable to a wide variety of different reactions. Moreover, the transfer of energy from food is a relatively slow process requiring many steps and is therefore unlikely to meet the demand for sudden and continued energy expenditure. The release of energy from ATP, however, is a rapid, single step.

ATP thus acts as a kind of energy store. Food is broken down steadily in the cell and a reserve of ATP molecules built up from ADP. One molecule of glucose has enough energy to build 38 molecules of ATP. When the cell needs energy it takes it from the ATP stock which is subsequently replenished by respiration of more food.

Protein synthesis

Protein synthesis has been described briefly in Chapter 3. On the ribosomes amino acids are assembled in a certain order to make particular proteins. The sequence of amino acids is dictated by molecules of a substance called *ribonucleic acid* (RNA) which is made in the nucleus but released into the cytoplasm where it combines temporarily with a ribosome. This 'messenger' ribonucleic acid 'calls up' amino acids which are present in the cytoplasm and, with the aid of enzymes, joins them together in a chain to make a protein. In this way the cell makes enzymes and all the proteins necessary for the structures in its protoplasm. Various stages in this process need energy which is supplied by ATP.

Transport

If a cell is to carry out the processes of respiration and protein synthesis it must obtain supplies of sugar, oxygen, amino acids and other substances, and it must be able to get rid of the waste products such as carbon dioxide and water which accumulate as a result of respiration and other chemical changes. Cells in the bodies of animals are bathed in a fluid, *tissue fluid*, which is derived from the blood. The blood keeps the tissue fluid supplied with food molecules and oxygen in ways described in more detail on p. 83. The cells extract the substances they need from the tissue fluid and release into it the substances they do not want. The methods by which cells take up substances through the cell membrane are not well understood but can be divided into two main processes, active and passive transport.

Passive transport includes processes such as diffusion and osmosis which are described more fully on p. 22. Diffusion occurs when molecules of a gas or a dissolved substance are unevenly distributed. The molecules are moving at random but eventually they will be evenly distributed (Fig. 5.2).

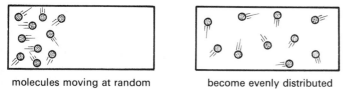

molecules moving at random   become evenly distributed

Fig. 5.2   Diffusion

If the cell membrane is permeable to the molecules (i.e. will let them through) the concentrations on each side of the membrane will eventually become equal whatever the inequality of the initial distribution (Fig. 5.3).

Diffusion could thus account for the movement of oxygen, glucose and amino acids into a cell and carbon dioxide and water out. If rapid respiration is taking place inside a cell, the concentrations of glucose and oxygen will fall as these substances are used up. The concentrations of glucose and oxygen in the tissue fluid outside the cell will be greater than the concentration inside and so these two substances will diffuse into the cell to restore the balance. Similarly, carbon dioxide

and water will accumulate inside the cell during respiration and diffuse out. Such a difference in concentration of a particular substance with respect to two locations is called a *diffusion gradient*.

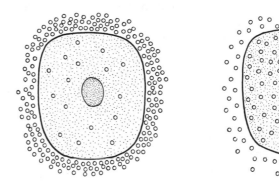

(a) *Greater concentration outside cell.*

(b) *Concentrations equal on both sides of cell membrane.*

Fig. 5.3   Molecules entering a cell by diffusion

Although diffusion *can* account for the movement of substances into and out of a cell, it is doubtful whether it is the only or even the most important method. It has been shown experimentally that cells can take up substances from the surrounding medium against a diffusion gradient, i.e. although the substance is more concentrated inside the cell than outside, the cell can still take it in. To explain this phenomenon it is supposed that there is a system of active transport.

Active transport. There is only limited experimental evidence to explain the mechanism of active transport, but the theory supposes that there is a carrier substance which can pass back and forth across the cell membrane. At the outside edge of the membrane it combines with a substance which the cell needs and then travels back, perhaps by diffusion, to the inside edge of the cell membrane where it breaks down, releasing the substance into the cytoplasm. The carrier molecule is then recharged with energy from ATP in the cytoplasm and returns across the membrane, again by diffusion, ready to collect the next molecule (Fig. 5.4). This consumption of energy is the one certain, measurable feature of active transport. Unless cells can respire there is no active transport.

Since the balance of chemicals in a cell is so critical it seems more likely that the uptake of substances by cells is under some kind of positive control like active transport, rather than merely dependent on a passive process such as diffusion.

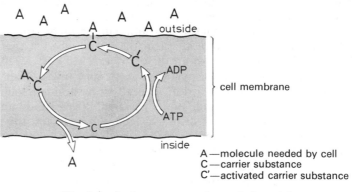
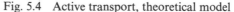

A —molecule needed by cell
C —carrier substance
C' —activated carrier substance

Fig. 5.4   Active transport, theoretical model

Metabolism

All the chemical activities which take place in cells and therefore in the organisms to which they contribute are described by the collective term *metabolism*. Metabolism is subdivided into *anabolism* and *katabolism*. Anabolism refers to the chemical reactions that build up molecules, e.g. protein synthesis, and katabolism to the breakdown reactions such as respiration.

Practical Work

Experiment 1   **Effect of temperature on enzymes**

Diastase is an enzyme extracted from germinating cereal grains. It acts on starch and hydrolyses it to maltose.

Place 5 cm^3 of 1 per cent starch solution in each of three test-tubes, and 5 cm^3 of 5 per cent diastase solution in each of three others. Prepare three water baths from beakers or cans containing (a) cold water and ice at about 10 °C, (b) cool water from the tap at about 20 °C, and (c) warm water at about 35 °C. Place a tube of starch solution and a tube of diastase solution in each water bath and leave them for five minutes to acquire the temperature of the water. Meanwhile, use a dropping pipette to place several rows of drops of dilute iodine solution on a tile or dish. When the five minutes is up, note the time and pour the diastase into the corresponding tube of starch solution, starting with the cold one. Wash the pipette in the warm water and use it to take a small sample from the test-tube in the warm water bath. Place this sample on the first iodine drop, which will probably go blue indicating the presence of starch. Rinse the pipette again and use it to take a sample from the tube in the cool water and place it on another iodine drop. Repeat the procedure for the tube in the ice water.

Continue taking samples in this way at intervals of about one minute. When a sample ceases to give a blue colour with the iodine the reaction is complete, i.e. all the starch has been changed by the enzyme to maltose. Note the time and take no more samples from this tube. Continue sampling from the other two tubes until they fail to produce a blue colour with iodine. In each case note the time for the reaction to reach completion, and take the temperature of the water bath.

Result. The reaction is most rapid at 35 °C and slowest at 10 °C.

Interpretation. An increase in temperature accelerates the action of diastase on starch, at least up to 35 °C.

Experiment 2   **The effect of pH on enzymes**

Human saliva contains an enzyme, amylase, which hydrolyses cooked starch to maltose (*see* Experiment 1, p. 69).

Place 5 cm^3 of 1 per cent starch solution in each of five tubes, labelled 1 to 5. Add acid or alkali as follows: to tube 1, 1 cm^3 M/20 sodium carbonate solution; to tube 2, 0.5 cm^3 M/20 sodium carbonate; tube 4, 2 cm^3 M/10 acetic acid; tube 5, 4 cm^3 M/10 acetic acid. Tube 3 is left without either acid or alkali. Using a dropping pipette, place rows of drops of dilute iodine solution on a tile or dish. Collect about half a test-tube full of saliva; note the time, then add 1 cm^3 saliva to each tube and shake them to mix the contents.

With a clean pipette take up a little of the mixture from tube 1 and place a drop or two on the first iodine spot. The blue colour indicates the presence of starch. Rinse the pipette in clean water and test a sample from each tube in turn, rinsing the pipette between each test. Test samples from each tube at approximately one-minute intervals. Eventually one of the samples will not go blue with iodine, which means that the reaction in that tube is complete and all the starch has been changed to maltose. Note the time and take no more samples from that tube. Continue sampling the other tubes, noting the time in each case when the starch has disappeared. After about fifteen minutes from the start of the experiment, stop testing and find the pH in each tube by placing a drop of liquid from each on a piece of pH paper and comparing its colour with that on the colour chart supplied.

The pH values will be approximately as follows.

Tube	1	2	3	4	5
pH	9	7	6–7	6	3

Result. Starch will disappear first from tube 3, more slowly from tubes 2 and 1, and more slowly still from tube 4. In tube 5, starch may still be present after fifteen minutes or more.

Interpretation. The optimum pH for salivary amylase is between 6 and 7. Acid conditions (pH 3) slow down the reaction very markedly. Alkaline conditions also retard the reaction but to a lesser extent.

Experiment 3   **Uptake of oxygen by living organisms**

About 20 g of seeds are soaked for twenty-four hours, the water poured away and the seeds left for two or three days in a closed container so that they start to germinate. Half of the seedlings are then killed by boiling them for five minutes followed by cooling in tap water.

Assemble the apparatus shown in Fig. 5.5. The manometers are made by fitting 2 cm^3 plastic syringe barrels to the capillary tube by means of rubber tubing. The test-tubes are 25 mm × 150 mm. The liquid in the manometer is water with a little colouring and detergent.

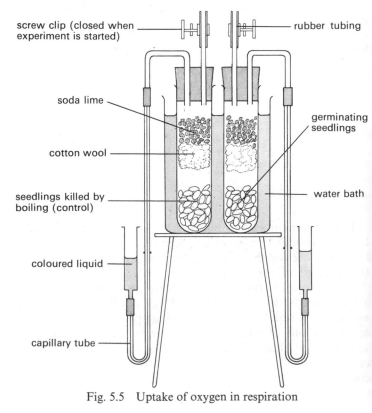

Fig. 5.5   Uptake of oxygen in respiration

Place 5 g sodalime in each test-tube and cover it with a layer of glass wool or cotton wool. Put 10 g live seedlings into one tube and 10 g dead seedlings into the other. Place both tubes, with screw clips open, in the water bath and leave them for five minutes to acquire the temperature of the water. Close both clips and after ten to fifteen minutes note any change in the level of liquid in the capillary tubes.

Result. The level of liquid should rise in the manometer connected to the living seeds and remain the same in the manometer connected to the dead seeds.

Interpretation. If the seeds are respiring they will be taking in oxygen and giving out, probably, almost an equal volume of carbon dioxide so that there would be no change in volume of the gas in the tube. Since the sodalime, however, absorbs all the carbon dioxide given out, the reduction in volume leading to the rise in liquid level is therefore most likely due to uptake of oxygen by the living seeds.

By surrounding both tubes with water, temperature fluctuations are reduced to a minimum and any temperature change that does occur will affect both tubes equally, so that a *difference* in level between the two manometers can be attributed to the presence of the living seeds.

Experiment 4   **Production of carbon dioxide by seedlings**

Some small seeds which will germinate rapidly are soaked for twenty-four hours and then allowed to germinate on moist cotton wool in a closed container. When they show signs of germinating, half of them are killed by boiling for five minutes. Two large test-tubes are prepared as in Fig. 5.6a. One tube is half filled with the living seedlings and the other tube with the dead ones. The mouth of each tube is covered with aluminium

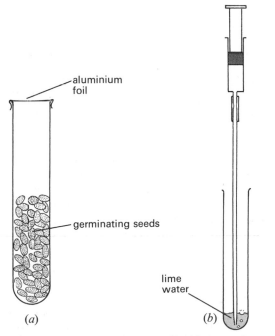

Fig. 5.6   Production of carbon dioxide by seeds

foil and they are left upright in a rack for thirty minutes. A length of glass tubing is fitted to a 10 cm³ syringe and a sample of air is taken from the seeds by pushing the tube through the foil and withdrawing the plunger. The air is slowly expelled through a small quantity of lime water in a test-tube (Fig. 5.6b). A sample of air from the second tube is tested in the same way.

Result. The air from the living seeds should turn lime water milky indicating the presence of carbon dioxide. The air from the dead seeds should not affect the lime water.

Interpretation. The living seeds have produced carbon dioxide. This is reasonable evidence that respiration is taking place.

Experiment 5   **Anaerobic respiration in yeast**

Some water is boiled to expel all the dissolved oxygen and when cool is used to make a 5 per cent solution of glucose and a 10 per cent suspension of dried yeast. 5 cm³ of the glucose solution and 1 cm³ of the yeast suspension are placed in a test-tube and covered with a thin layer of liquid paraffin to exclude atmospheric oxygen from the mixture. A delivery tube is fitted as shown in Fig. 5.7 and allowed to dip into clear lime

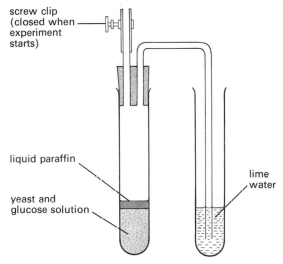

Fig. 5.7   Anaerobic respiration in yeast

water. A control experiment is set up in the same way but with a yeast suspension that has been boiled to kill the yeast cells.

In 10 to 15 minutes there should be signs of fermentation in the living yeast–glucose mixture and bubbles should be escaping through the lime water. If this does not happen, both tubes with the yeast should be warmed by placing them in a beaker or jar of warm water, up to 30 °C.

Result. The bubbles of gas from the tube with living yeast will turn the lime water milky showing that carbon dioxide is being produced. The dead yeast should not produce any gas.

Interpretation. The fact that the yeast is producing carbon dioxide is evidence that respiration is taking place. Since air was both expelled and excluded from the mixture, this respiration is going on in the absence of oxygen and must therefore be anaerobic.

Questions

1 (a) Where does respiration occur? (b) What is the importance of respiration? (c) What materials are used up during respiration, and what are the products?

2 What methods do organisms have for storing energy?

3 List the differences between aerobic and anaerobic respiration. Are these two forms of respiration mutually exclusive? Explain.

4 Which aspects of respiration can readily be measured or demonstrated?

5 In the mammal, which classes of food can be used to provide energy? Which ones provide the most energy? (*See* p. 33.)

6 If a biologist wants to demonstrate that a reaction is controlled by enzymes and will not take place without these enzymes, how, in principle, does he design his experiment?

7 What evidence would you look for in deciding whether a substance was entering a cell by active transport or passive diffusion?

6
Nutrition

The food taken in by man is used in three principal ways, namely for energy, growth and replacement.

(a) It is broken down in cells during respiration (p. 27) to provide energy for movement and essential chemical reactions.

(b) It provides the raw materials for making protoplasm and so contributes (i) to the growth of cells and tissues, (ii) to the replacement of cells which die, e.g. red blood cells and the cells of the epidermis, and (iii) to the repair of wounds and other damage to body structures.

The substances that can meet all these requirements are chemical materials with food value, namely proteins, fats and carbohydrates. In addition to these, the diet must contain water, salts, vitamins and roughage because although these substances have no energy value they do participate in chemical reactions or bodily functions.

Energy value of food

All three classes of food can be used to provide energy by respiration, and the total food taken in each day must be sufficient to provide energy to keep the cells alive and the systems working, to meet the demands of any activity the body undertakes, and to produce sufficient heat to maintain the body temperature and compensate for heat lost to the environment. It follows that the quantity of energy obtained from food that is needed by any one individual will depend on his environment, his age, size and activity as well as more subtle features such as sex and general metabolic rate.

For scientific purposes, the units in which energy is measured are called *joules* or *kilojoules*, one kilojoule being equivalent to 1 000 joules. The energy value of food is calculated by burning a known weight of it completely to carbon dioxide and water. The burning takes place in a special apparatus, a bomb calorimeter, designed to ensure that all the heat given out during the combustion is transmitted to a known weight of water whose temperature rise is measured. Since 4.2 joules of heat energy raise the temperature of 1 g water by 1 °C, the number of joules given out by the burning food can be calculated (Experiment 2). Whether the body can obtain the same quantity of energy from each gram of food depends on the efficiency of digestion, absorption and the chemical processes undergone by the food.

The energy requirements of man are found experimentally by measuring the amount of oxygen he uses up in different circumstances. If all the oxygen is used to obtain energy from food, the amount of energy produced can be calculated.

Because people differ so widely in their energy requirements, it is not possible to indicate the maximum or minimum number of joules required by man in general. Nevertheless, the table below gives some idea of energy needs based on measurements of a large number of adult European males.

	kilojoules (kJ)
8 hours asleep	2 500
8 hours awake and physically inactive	3 000
8 hours awake and physically active	6 500
Total	12 000

In tropical countries, the heat lost from the body to the surroundings is less than that lost in temperate or cold climates. The energy requirements in tropical countries are therefore less than those given above, but because of the wide individual differences and the shortage of reliable experimental evidence, scientists are reluctant to offer exact figures.

The figures for the 8 hours asleep, given above, show that merely to stay alive, i.e. to maintain *basal metabolism*, requires $3 \times 2\,500 = 7\,500$ kJ per day. The energy needed for 8 hours' work will depend very much on the nature of that work. Sitting at a desk requires little more energy than basal metabolism, but a person doing heavy manual work, for example a coal miner or a man felling trees, may need up to 16 500 kJ per day. Children need fewer joules than adults: an American 5-year-old might need only 6 700 kJ and an 11-year-old 10 500 kJ.

Any type of food can be used by the body to provide energy, but proteins are used firstly for body building and replacement so that carbohydrates and fats are the main sources of energy. If the daily intake of food does not provide sufficient joules, a human being will lose weight as the existing food stores and tissues of the body are oxidized to release energy, and the capacity for work will fall off. An intake of less than 6 000 kJ per day, if maintained for a long period, would produce wasting and death, although so inadequate a diet would probably give rise to malnutrition through lack of certain vitamins in the first instance. Reduction of total food taken in, even to two thirds of what is indicated as adequate, leads to less effective working of the mind and body and a greater susceptibility to such diseases as tuberculosis. If the carbohydrate eaten is in excess of the energy requirements of the body, it is converted to fat and stored under the skin and elsewhere so that the person becomes 'fat'.

Carbohydrates

Carbohydrates contain the elements carbon, hydrogen and oxygen; their chemistry is outlined on p. 15. The principal forms of carbohydrate in man's diet are starch, sugar and cellulose. Foods relatively rich in starch are the cereals such as wheat, barley, maize, oats, rice, millet and their products (e.g. bread), and peas, beans and certain 'root' crops (e.g. potatoes and cassava). Sugar is abundant in confectionery, cakes and jam. Cellulose occurs in all the whole plant material eaten, but is of no food value to man since he has no enzymes with which to digest it, though it has a mechanical function in the diet as roughage.

Carbohydrates are principally of value as energy-giving food, providing on average 17 kJ per gram. They are usually the cheapest and most abundant foods and therefore the main source of energy. In man, excess carbohydrate is stored as glycogen in the liver and the muscles, or converted to fat and stored beneath the skin and in other fat depots. Although the fat depots are a valuable reserve of energy, persistent eating of carbohydrates in excess of the body's energy requirements leads to obesity (fatness). Apart from the fact that obesity is usually considered unattractive and restricts normal activities, it is known that very fat people are, on average, less healthy in many respects than are slimmer people. The only sure way to get rid of excessive fat is to eat less food while taking care to maintain an adequate intake of proteins, vitamins and salts. A fat person wishing to become slimmer will need to stop eating before his hunger is satisfied.

Proteins

Proteins contain the elements carbon, hydrogen, oxygen, nitrogen and usually sulphur (*see* p. 17 for their chemistry). Examples of foods containing protein are lean meat, egg-white, beans, fish, milk and milk products such as cheese.

Proteins are broken down by digestion to amino acids (*see* p. 64) which are absorbed into the blood stream and eventually reach the cells of the body. In the cells, the amino acids are assembled to form the structural proteins of the protoplasm and its constituent enzymes (p. 27). There are only about 20 different kinds of amino acids but there are millions of different proteins. The difference between one protein and another depends on which amino acids are used to build it, how many of each there are, their sequence and their arrangement (Fig. 6.1).

Plants can build all the amino acids they need from carbohydrates and nitrates but animals cannot. They must therefore obtain their amino acids from proteins already made by plants

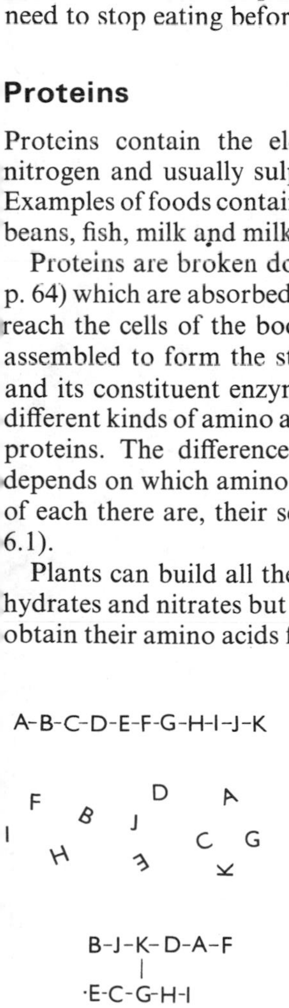

(a) *Representation of a small protein molecule. The letters are the amino acids.*

(b) *The protein is digested and the amino acids are set free.*

(c) *The same amino acids are built up into a different protein.*

Fig. 6.1 Amino acids and proteins

or present in the flesh of other animals, and so the diet must include a minimum quantity of protein of one sort or another. A diet with a sufficient energy content of fats and carbohydrates and rich in vitamins and salts but lacking protein will lead eventually to illness and death. Proteins are particularly important during periods of pregnancy and growth when new protoplasm, cells and tissues are being made. Growing children and pregnant women need more than average supplies of protein; manual workers, contrary to popular belief, probably do not.

Although animals cannot make amino acids they can, in some cases, convert one amino acid into another. There are, however, ten or more amino acids which animals cannot produce in this way and these *essential amino acids* must be obtained directly from proteins in the diet. Proteins which contain the essential amino acids in the right proportions are sometimes called *first class proteins*. Most animal proteins come into this category. Vegetable proteins often lack one or more of the essential amino acids (they are second class proteins) or contain them in the wrong proportions. To obtain the essential amino acids from plant protein alone, a very mixed vegetable diet in large quantities is needed. Vegetarians who include milk, cheese and eggs in their diet will not lack essential amino acids since these contain the highest proportion of all.

If proteins are eaten in excess, there will be more amino acids in the body than are needed to produce or replace cells. The excess amino acids are converted in the liver to carbohydrates, which are then oxidized for energy or converted to glycogen and stored. The energy value of protein when oxidized is 17 kJ per gram. Amino acids cannot be stored.

Estimates of the daily quantity of protein needed by man have been changing in recent years but it seems to be no more than about 0.6 g per kg body weight, i.e. an 80 kg man needs about 48 g protein each day assuming that the protein contains all the essential amino acids. Thus on average, a man needs about 40 g and a woman 30 g good quality protein per day. A pregnant woman will need at least 40 g to supply herself and her embryo which is building up its tissues, and a woman breast-feeding a baby should take in 60 g protein per day to compensate for the loss of protein in the milk. Babies need 1.5 g, young children 1 g and adolescents about 0.7 g per kg body weight.

Kwashiorkor. This is a Ghanaian term meaning 'the sickness the old baby gets when the new baby comes', and it is a protein deficiency disease which occurs all over the world, though it is known by thirty-eight different names.

The condition shows itself as the mother's milk falls off in quality and quantity after the first six months of breast-feeding, and the child's diet is supplemented by starchy, protein-deficient yam and cassava. Its occurrence is often most severe when breast-feeding stops altogether in order to make way for the next baby. The child becomes irritable and listless; the skin cracks and scales (Fig. 6.2); the liver is damaged and the child may die before the age of five. Amongst the Masai, however, who eat meat and drink milk, the disease is unknown.

It was known before the Second World War that the disease was due to a protein deficiency arising from a change to a vegetable diet after the more nutritious milk. Feeding with sufficient protein both cures and prevents the disease. The problem, however, is to find a protein-rich diet that can be provided and afforded in localities where animal protein,

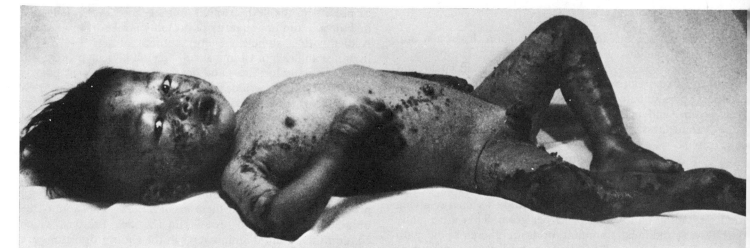

(a) On admission to hospital. (WHO)

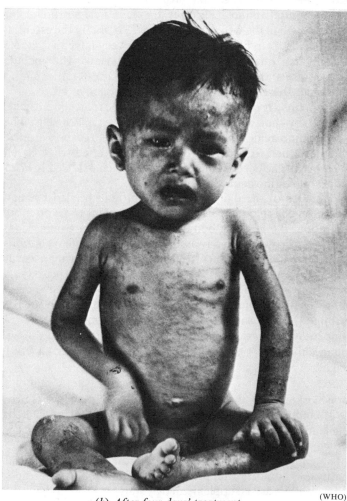

(b) After four days' treatment. (WHO)

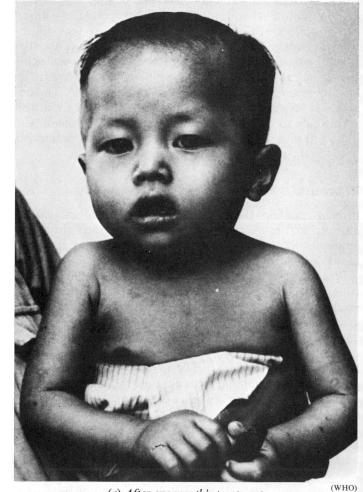

(c) After one month's treatment. (WHO)

Fig. 6.2   Child suffering from kwashiorkor

including milk, is very scarce. Soya beans are one source, and dietitians have evolved a mixture of corn, cotton seed, yeast and leaf meal which is both palatable and effective in curing the disease.

In Nigeria, a mixture of groundnut flour, dried yeast, milk protein, sugar, five minerals and seven vitamins is marketed under the name 'Amama'. It is inexpensive and, if added to the food at the rate of 30 grams per day, prevents kwashiorkor in children up to six or seven years old.

Fats

Like carbohydrates, fats contain only carbon, hydrogen and oxygen but in different proportions (p. 16). They are present in foods such as animal fat, butter, margarine, cheese, milk and groundnuts. Although fats are less easily digested and absorbed than carbohydrates, they have more than double the energy value, providing 39 kJ per gram. They can be stored in the body and thus provide an important way of storing energy.

About 25 per cent of the individual's energy requirements should be supplied by fats. Europeans eat 80–150 g per day, people in tropical countries somewhat less; Eskimos eat up to 300 g.

Although man can convert carbohydrates to fatty acids there are probably one or two that he cannot make, and it is necessary to take in some fat with the diet in order to supply these *essential fatty acids*. Fat, particularly animal fat, is needed for the fat-soluble vitamins A, D, E and K which it contains. In addition the use of fat and oil in the process of cooking usually makes the food more palatable.

Mineral salts and elements

In addition to the carbon, hydrogen, oxygen, nitrogen and sulphur present in carbohydrates, proteins and fats, a variety of other elements is needed for the chemical activities of the body and for the construction of certain tissues. These elements are obtained from food where they are usually combined in organic molecules.

Sodium, potassium, magnesium and phosphates are normally present in adequate quantities in the diet. Sodium and chlorine are taken in mostly as sodium chloride, which is used in cooking or added to the food. It is important in maintaining the osmotic concentration of the blood (pp. 23 and 72), in providing sodium ions for the transport of carbon dioxide as sodium hydrogencarbonate (bicarbonate) and chloride ions for the production of hydrochloric acid in the stomach. Potassium is present in most living cells, particularly red blood cells and muscles, and is important in growth. Cereals contain good supplies of potassium. Magnesium is a component of bone and is found in a wide variety of vegetable material. Phosphates are obtained in sufficient quantities from the protein part of the diet, if this is adequate. They are needed in the body for the formation of bone, nucleic acids (p. 166), ATP (p. 28) and enzymes, and they form part of most membranes. The elements mentioned above are most unlikely to be missing from any diet. On the other hand, calcium, iron and iodine are frequently in short supply.

Calcium. This element enters into the composition of bones as calcium phosphate and into the dentine of teeth. It also plays a part in the clotting of blood (p. 73), contraction of muscles, permeability of cells and conduction of nerve impulses. It is abundant in cheese and milk and in the latter form is most readily absorbed. Beans and soya flour contain appreciable quantities. In districts where the water supply comes from chalk or limestone areas, it will contain quantities of calcium hydrogencarbonate (bicarbonate). The absorption of calcium in the ileum depends on the presence of bile salts and adequate supplies of vitamin D.

Adults need about 800 mg calcium each day, children about 1 400 mg and pregnant or nursing mothers 1 600–2 000 mg. The demand of the growing foetus for calcium which is contributing to its skeleton depletes the mother's blood of its calcium ions. The milk secreted after birth also drains the maternal calcium resources. If there is insufficient calcium in the diet it will be withdrawn from the mother's bones and teeth to meet the requirements of the foetus.

Iron. Iron is another element likely to be deficient in the diet. It is essential for the formation of haemoglobin in the red blood cells and the hydrogen acceptor system (p. 28) in nearly all living cells. Adults need about 15 mg per day. Red meat, particularly liver, is the best source of iron, but eggs, spinach and other vegetables contain appreciable quantities. Iron is conserved in the body, very little being excreted. The liver is mainly responsible for the storage of iron from disintegrated red cells. Shortage of iron in the diet leads to one form of anaemia.

Anaemia is a shortage of red cells or haemoglobin in the blood. It may result from the failure of the red bone marrow to make enough cells or pigment, from an excessive rate of destruction of red cells, or simply from a shortage of iron in the diet. In the latter case, called iron-deficiency anaemia, the condition can be cured by eating meat, liver or green vegetables such as the leaves of spinach, cocoyam or groundnuts, all of which contain iron, or by taking tablets containing suitable compounds of iron.

Iodine. This is needed in small quantities, 0.05–0.1 mg per day, for the synthesis of thyroxine, the hormone of the thyroid gland (p. 157). A deficiency of iodine results in *'simple' goitre*, a gross swelling of the thyroid gland in the neck. This is most likely to occur in regions where iodides are absent from drinking water, such as Switzerland and parts of North and South America. Five million people in India are thought to suffer from iodine deficiency to the extent of goitre or cretinism (p. 157). The disease can be prevented by adding minute traces of iodides to drinking water or to table salt (iodized salt). After a certain age, goitre cannot be cured by administration of iodine. Seafood such as fish is the best source of natural iodine.

Other 'trace' elements. Very small quantities of cobalt, manganese, zinc, copper and fluoride are known to be essential but are far less likely to be missing from the diet than calcium, iron and iodine. Cobalt is involved in the formation of vitamin B_{12}, zinc in insulin, and fluorides in the teeth.

It is important to realize that although certain foods and salts may be rich in essential elements, they may not be in a form which the body is able to use or absorb. The phosphates in cereals cannot be utilized in the body; calcium taken in with fats or an excess of phosphates or alkalis is not likely to be efficiently absorbed. Doses of essential elements in organic or inorganic compounds will not cure a deficiency if absorption or metabolism of that element is faulty.

Vitamins

Vitamins are complex chemical compounds which, although they have no energy value, are essential in small quantities for the normal chemical activities of the body. It was not until about 1900 that their importance was realized by Gowland Hopkins and other workers.

If a diet is deficient in one or more vitamins it results in a breakdown of normal bodily activities and produces some symptoms of disease. Such diseases can usually be effectively remedied by including the necessary vitamins in the diet.

Plants can build up their vitamins from simple substances but animals must obtain them 'ready-made' directly or indirectly from plants.

Fifteen or more vitamins have been isolated and most of

them seem to act as catalysts in essential chemical changes in the body, each one influencing a number of vital processes; e.g. some of the B group vitamins form the hydrogen acceptors involved in respiration (p. 28).

Vitamins A, D, E and K are the *fat-soluble vitamins*, occurring mainly in animal fats and oils and absorbed along with the products of fat digestion. Vitamins B and C are the *water-soluble vitamins*.

Some of the important vitamins are set out in the table below, together with their properties. It must be emphasized that nearly all mixed diets will include adequate amounts of vitamins, and deficiency diseases are only likely to occur where the bulk of the diet consists of one or two kinds of food such as rice or maize.

Apart from ascorbic acid, vitamins are not seriously affected by cooking or canning processes. Vitamin C is not so much affected by boiling as by oxidation when exposed to the air. If vegetables are plunged into boiling water, the enzymes that help to oxidize the ascorbic acid are destroyed and its loss is minimized. Also, if only small quantities of water are used for boiling vegetables, relatively little ascorbic acid is dissolved out. Canning destroys only a small proportion of vitamin C, but prolonged storage of fruit and vegetables reduces the quantity of the vitamin quite markedly.

Vitamins and their characteristics

NAME AND SOURCE OF VITAMIN	DISEASES AND SYMPTOMS CAUSED BY LACK OF VITAMIN	NOTES
Vitamin A; retinol (fat-soluble) Milk, butter, cheese, liver, cod-liver oil. Fresh green vegetables for *carotene* (water soluble).	Reduced resistance to disease, particularly those which gain access through the skin. Poor night vision. Skin and cornea of eyes become dry leading to *xerophthalmia*.	The yellow pigment, carotene, present in green leaves and carrots, is oxidized in the body to make retinol. Retinol contributes to a light-sensitive pigment in the retina. Retinol is stored in the liver.
Vitamin B complex Ten or more water-soluble vitamins usually occurring together. Three are described here.	Since the B vitamins are present in most unprocessed food, deficiency diseases usually arise only in populations living on restricted diets.	Many B vitamins act as catalysts (co-enzymes) in the normal oxidation of carbohydrates during respiration. Absence of these catalysts leads to metabolic disturbances.
Thiamine (B_1) Whole grains of cereals, lean meat, yeast.	Wasting and partial paralysis, or water-logging of the tissues and heart failure; symptoms of two forms of *beriberi*.	Rice husks contain both thiamine and niacin, so highly milled rice is deficient in both. Maize is deficient in niacin. Populations living largely on milled rice or maize are very prone to the deficiency diseases of beriberi and pellagra.
Niacin (B_2, nicotinic acid, nicotinamide). Whole grains of cereals, lean meat, liver, yeast.	Skin eczema on exposure to sunlight, diarrhoea, wasting and mental degeneration; all symptoms of *pellagra*.	White flour (72% extraction) is deficient in thiamine which must be added to white flour used in bread-making.
Riboflavin Whole cereal grains, peas and beans, liver, kidney, milk.	Rarely the cause of deficiency disease. Degenerative condition of the skin, particularly round the mouth.	Badly planned slimming diets may be deficient in thiamine.
Vitamin C; ascorbic acid (water soluble) Oranges, lemons, grapefruit, blackcurrants, tomatoes, fresh vegetables, potatoes.	Bleeding under the skin, particularly at the joints. Swollen, bleeding gums, poor healing of wounds. These are all symptoms of *scurvy*.	Possibly acts as a catalyst in cell respiration. Scurvy is only likely to occur when fresh food is not available. Milk contains very little ascorbic acid, so babies need additional sources such as rosehip syrup.
Vitamin D; calciferol (fat-soluble) Fish-liver oil, butter, milk, cheese, egg yolk, liver.	Inadequate deposition of calcium in the bones causing *rickets* in young children because the bones remain soft and are deformed by the child's weight. Deficiency in adults causes *osteomalacia*; the vertebrae are compressed and the legs bowed.	Calciferol helps the absorption of calcium from the intestine and the deposition of calcium salts in the bones. Natural fats beneath the skin are converted to a form of calciferol by the action of sunlight or ultra-violet radiation. Impaired absorption of fats in the intestine leads to rickets or osteomalacia.
Vitamin E; tocopherol (fat-soluble) Wheat germ (embryo), e.g. in wholemeal bread; dairy products, meat).	Few deficiency effects apparent in man. Severe deficiency in infants may lead to high rates of destruction of red blood cells and hence to anaemia.	Experimentally induced deficiencies in pregnant rats leads to reabsorption of embryos and in males to degeneration of testes. Other pathological symptoms have been demonstrated in guinea pigs, rabbits and monkeys.
Vitamin K; phylloquinone, menaquinone (fat-soluble) Green vegetables contain phylloquinone.	In its absence, blood takes longer to clot and may result in bleeding diseases. Dietary deficiency unlikely to cause disease because intestinal bacteria can synthesize menaquinone.	Vitamin K is needed for the manufacture of a blood-clotting factor in the liver. Anything which impairs absorption of fats, e.g. bile deficiency, may lead to symptoms of fat-soluble vitamin deficiency disease irrespective of diet.

Water

Water makes up 70 per cent by weight of the body tissues and is a fundamental constituent of protoplasm. Man can live for two or three weeks without food, if relatively inactive, but may die in two or three days if deprived of water. Water plays an important part in the chemistry of digestion (p. 62) and transports digested food and many other substances in solution to all parts of the body. All the chemical reactions in the body take place in solution. Excretion of urine, elimination of faeces and evaporation from the skin and lungs result in a loss of 2–3 litres per day. About 1.5 litres of this is replaced by drinking liquids, and the remainder comes from the food.

Roughage

This consists largely of the cellulose in the cell walls of plants and cannot be digested by man. When present in sufficient quantities, these undigested residues add bulk to the other materials such as dead bacteria and epithelial cells which collect in the colon. This bulk is important since the physical stretching of the walls of the colon stimulates reflex peristalsis (p. 62) so moving the residues along the colon and initiating defaecation. One cause of constipation and its attendant disorders is insufficient roughage in the diet.

Milk

Milk is the sole article of diet during the first weeks or months of a mammal's life. It is an almost ideal food since it contains proteins, fats, carbohydrates, mineral salts, particularly those of calcium and magnesium, and vitamins. For adults, however, it is less satisfactory because of its high water content and lack of iron. Large volumes would have to be consumed if it were the principal article of diet for an adult, and serious blood deficiencies would result from the lack of iron. In the body of the embryo mammal, iron is stored while the embryo develops inside the body of its mother, and this supply must suffice until the young mammal begins to eat solid food.

Balanced diet

A balanced diet must contain
    (a) a sufficient number of joules of energy
    (b) proteins, fats and carbohydrates in the correct proportions
    (c) vitamins
    (d) mineral salts
    (e) water
    (f) roughage.
Tropical diets are often unbalanced for the following reasons.
    (i) They contain too much yam, cassava, banana and maize. These foods are easy to grow but deficient in protein. In pregnant mothers, babies and young children a protein shortage can lead to serious malnutrition such as kwashiorkor. Rice, millet, guinea corn and beans are a far better source of vegetable protein than cassava and yams. Maize contains some protein but does not provide all the amino acids needed by the body and, moreover, one of the B vitamins, nicotinic acid, cannot be adequately obtained from maize.
    (ii) They contain too little vitamin A. Special care needs to be taken to include green vegetables or red palm oil in the diet, in addition to tomatoes and other sources of carotene. Alternatively the vitamin A in the diet may be supplemented with fish-liver oil.
    (iii) In areas where the diet is mainly rice or maize, there is likely to be a shortage of vitamin B. Different methods of milling and cooking rice could reduce this deficiency, while a maize diet needs to be supplemented with other cereals to avoid pellagra (see table on p. 36).
    (iv) Insufficient joules, or in other words, not enough food. About half the people in the world, principally in Asia, South America and Indonesia, have an average daily intake of less than 9 240 kJ. Even allowing for children whose needs may be less than this, these figures suggest that many people have only enough food to stay alive and not enough to do a day's work. There appears to be no general food shortage in tropical Africa; the problems arise from eating the wrong kind of food rather than not eating enough.

Diets in the industrialized countries are often the subject of controversy and strongly held views, sometimes based on unfounded beliefs or, at best, on circumstantial and statistical evidence. There are schools of thought which believe that the amount of meat and other animal protein in the diet is unhealthy. There is circumstantial evidence associating a high level of animal fat in the diet with coronary heart disease. Similar evidence points to the high intake of sucrose as a contributory factor in this disease of industrial society. Surveys in large cities have sometimes revealed that inadequate quantities of vitamins A, D and C are being included in the diet. Two shortcomings of the diets in industrialized countries are, however, generally recognized. One is that too much carbohydrate is eaten, resulting in a large number of obese people (p. 69), and the other is the harmful effect of refined sugar on the teeth (p. 126).

If the food value, mineral and vitamin content of an article of diet is known it is possible to plan a diet which contains sufficient energy and the right proportion of the other constituents. The table on p. 39 gives an analysis of twenty-two common foods, with which a balanced diet could be planned. In using the table it should be remembered that
    (a) the weights quoted are for 10 g of the edible parts of the natural food;
    (b) the difference between the total weight of the components and the 10 g sample is made up by water and indigestible matter;
    (c) the food values will vary with the species of plant or animal material, their age, the season, the length of storage, etc.
    (d) tea and coffee have no food value apart from the milk and sugar which may be added;
    (f) fried food will have about 1 g extra fat and an extra 40 kJ for every 10 g food cooked.

Cooking. Cooking makes food easier to chew and swallow, easier to digest and generally more appetizing to eat. Heating softens or breaks open the cell walls of plant material and makes their contents available for digestion. Similarly the protein of meat and eggs and the starch from cereals and root crops is converted by heat to a more easily digestible form. The high temperatures used in cooking destroy many of the bacteria likely to be present in food and so improve its keeping properties and make it safer to eat. The most important disadvantage of cooking is the destruction of 50 per cent or more of the ascorbic acid in green vegetables, but this loss can be minimized by careful cooking as mentioned on p. 36.

Practical Work

Experiment 1   Determination of balanced diet

Draw up a table such as that given below and, using the foods listed on p. 39 (note that all the values in the table are for 10 g of food), fill in the details of what you consider a reasonable

thermometer, find the temperature of the water and make a note of it. In the nickel crucible or tin lid place 1 g sugar and heat it with the bunsen flame until it begins to burn. As soon as it starts burning, slide the crucible under the can so that the flames heat the water. If the flame goes out, *do not* apply the bunsen burner to the crucible while it is under the can, but return the crucible to the bunsen flame to start the sugar burning again and replace the crucible beneath the can as soon as the sugar catches light. When the sugar has finished burning and cannot be ignited again, gently stir the water in the can with the thermometer and record its new temperature. Calculate the rise in temperature by subtracting the first from the

Meal	Menus	Weight (in grams)	Kilojoules	Vitamins	Protein (in grams)
Breakfast	1 fried egg	65	$6.5 \times 67 = 435$	A, B, D	$6.5 \times 1.2 = 8$
	(cooking fat)	6	$0.6 \times 334 = 200$	A, D	
	1 slice bread	35	$3.5 \times 97 = 339$	B	$3.5 \times 0.8 = 28$
	(butter)	5	$0.5 \times 334 = 167$	A, D	
	1 cup coffee		0		
	($\frac{1}{4}$ cup milk)	60	$6 \times 28 = 168$	A, B, C, D	$6 \times 0.3 = 1.8$
	(teaspoon sugar)	7	$0.7 \times 162 = 113$		
Totals					

series of meals for one day. Work out the total energy value of the day's food intake and compare it with the figures given on p. 32. Also calculate the total protein content and indicate which vitamins are present.

The table is completed for one meal to show how to work out the values, but it will be necessary to weigh samples of the food selected in order to complete the calculations for the rest of the day. If your results do not conform to the criteria given on p. 37 for a balanced diet, suggest ways in which your day's menus could be adjusted.

Experiment 2   Energy from food

Arrange the apparatus as shown in Fig. 6.3. Use a measuring cylinder to place 100 cm³ cold water in the can. With the

second temperature. Work out the quantity of energy transferred to the water from the burning sugar as follows.

4.2 joules raise 1 g water 1 °C
100 cm³ cold water weighs 100 g
Let the rise in temperature be T °C

To raise 1 g water 1 °C needs 4.2 joules
∴ To raise 100 g water 1 °C needs 100×4.2 joules
∴ To raise 100 g water T °C needs $T \times 100 \times 4.2$ joules
∴ 1 g burning sugar produced $420 \times T$ joules

The experiment may now be repeated using 1 g vegetable oil instead of sugar and replacing the warm water in the can with 100 cm³ cold water.

(*Note.* The experiment is very inaccurate because much of the heat from the burning food escapes into the air without reaching the water, but since the errors are about the same for both samples, the results can at least be used to compare the energy released from sugar and oil.)

Experiment 3   Food tests

(a) *Starch.* A little starch powder is shaken in a test-tube with some cold water and then boiled to make a clear solution. When the solution is cold, 3 or 4 drops of iodine solution are added. The dark blue colour that results is characteristic of the reaction between starch and iodine.

(b) *Glucose.* A little glucose is heated to boiling point with some Benedict's solution in a test-tube. The solution will change from clear blue to opaque green, yellow and finally a brick-red precipitate of cuprous oxide will appear. If the liquid is allowed to boil, the mouth of the test-tube should be

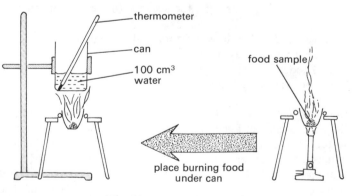

Fig. 6.3   Energy from food

Table of food values

Food	Energy value	Protein	Fat	Carbo-hydrate	Calcium	Iron	Vitamin A	Thiamine (B₁)	Ascorbic acid (C)	Vitamin D
10 grams	kilojoules	grams	grams	grams	milligrams	milligrams	micrograms	micrograms	micrograms	micrograms
Bread, wholemeal	101	0.96	0.3	4.7	2.8	0.3	0	24	0	0
Potato	32	0.2	0	1.8	0.8	0.07	0	11	2000	0
Rice	150	0.6	0.1	8.7	0.4	0.04	0	8	0	0
Beans	107	2.1	0	4.5	18.0	0.67	0	45	0	0
Groundnuts	245	2.8	4.9	0.8	6.1	0.2	0	23	0	0
Soya flour	181	4.0	2.4	1.3	21.0	0.7	0	74	0	0
Beef	131	1.5	2.8	0	1.0	0.4	0	7	0	0
Pork	171	1.2	4.0	0	1.0	0.1	0	100	0	0
Liver	58	1.7	0.8	0	0.8	1.4	600	30	2000	0.07
Chicken	60	2.1	0.7	0	1.1	0.15	0	4	0	0
White fish	30	1.6	0.05	0	2.5	0.1	0	6	0	0
Herring	80	1.6	1.4	0	10.0	0.15	4.5	3	0	2.2
Milk, whole	27	0.3	0.4	0.5	12.0	0.01	4.4	4	130	0.005
Dried milk, whole	206	2.7	2.8	3.8	81.0	0.07	24.6	31	1100	0.03
Butter	312	0.05	8.3	0	1.5	0.02	99.5	0	0	0.125
Cheese	173	2.5	3.5	0	81.0	0.06	42.0	4	0	0.04
Eggs	66	1.2	1.2	0	5.6	0.25	30.0	10	0	0.15
Sugar	165	0	0	10.0	0.1	0	0	0	0	0
Carrots	9	0.07	0	0.5	4.8	0.06	200	6	600	0
Spinach	9	0.3	0	0.3	7.0	0.3	100	12	6000	0
Orange	15	0.08	0	0.8	4.1	0.03	0.8	10	5000	0
Banana	32	0.1	0	1.9	0.7	0.04	3.3	4	1000	0

Some of these figures differ from those in the first printing of this book, as the latest data and most accurate conversion to SI units have been used. From McCance and Widdowson, *The Composition of Foods*, by permission of the Controller of Her Majesty's Stationery Office.

directed away from people as the solution is likely to 'bump' out of the tube. Sucrose is recognized by its failure to react with Benedict's solution until after it has been boiled with dilute hydrochloric acid and neutralized with sodium hydrogencarbonate.

(c) *Protein.* To a 1% albumen solution is added 5 cm³ dilute sodium hydroxide (CARE: this solution is caustic) and 5 cm³ 1% copper sulphate solution. A purple colour indicates protein.

(d) *Fats.* To a little water in a test-tube, containing four drops of Sudan Black, are added a few drops of liquid fat e.g. cooking oil. The tube is shaken to make an emulsion and left to stand. The fat droplets will coalesce at the surface carrying the dye with them.

(e) *Application of the food tests to food samples.* The tests above can be applied to samples of food such as milk, potato or yam, onion, groundnuts, egg-yolk and cheese, to find out what materials are present in them. The materials should be crushed, if they are solid, and shaken with water in a test-tube before applying the tests, in turn, to separate samples.

Experiment 4 Comparison of the vitamin C content of fruit juices

A blue dye, phenolindo-2-6-dichlorophenol (P.I.P. for short), is turned colourless by vitamin C (ascorbic acid). Place 1 cm³ of a 0.1 per cent solution of P.I.P. in a test-tube. Draw up exactly 2 cm³ fresh orange juice in a syringe (without the needle). Add the juice one drop at a time to the P.I.P. solution until it goes colourless. Note the volume of juice added (i.e. the difference between the volume left in the syringe and the original 2 cm³). Repeat the experiment with lemon juice and grapefruit juice and one of these juices that has been boiled.

Bottled or canned fruit squashes or cordials can also be tested.

Draw up a table to show the juices in order of vitamin C content on the assumption that the more vitamin C is present, the less juice is needed to decolourize the blue dye.

If syringes are not available, the juice can be added to the dye by means of a dropping pipette. The number of drops needed to decolourize the P.I.P. is counted. The pipette must be held vertically to ensure that the drop size does not vary too much.

(*Note.* (a) The acid in some fruit juices may turn the P.I.P. from blue to red but it is the point at which the dye becomes *colourless* which matters. (b) Vitamin C is not the only chemical which decolourizes P.I.P.)

See p. 268 for the formulae for the reagents needed for these experiments. All these experiments and many others are described in much greater detail in the laboratory manual *Food Tests* (*see* p. 269).

Questions

1 What principles must be observed when working out a diet designed to produce a reduction in body weight (a slimming diet)? What dangers are there if such diets are not scientifically planned?

2 Kwashiorkor is a protein deficiency disease which affects young children with unbalanced diets. Its onset is usually most severe when the child is weaned from its mother's milk to starchy plant foods such as yam and cassava which are eaten by the adults. Why does weaning mark the onset of the disease?

3 It is commonly believed that manual workers need much more protein than sedentary workers. Suggest why this idea is false.

4 Eating a large amount of protein at one meal is wasteful. It is better to take in a little protein at each meal. Why do you think this is the case?

5 What nutritional problems are likely to be experienced by (a) people living mainly on rice or maize, (b) strict vegetarians?

7

Sources of Food

Man obtains his food from plants and their products, and from animals which feed on plants. The food substances that provide him with energy or body-building materials are made, in the first instance, by plants. Obvious plant products in the diet are seeds, fruits, leaves and roots; but equally, flour and bread are derived from cereal grains, and sugar from stems and roots. Beef, milk, butter and cheese all come from cattle, but the raw materials for their manufacture were in the grass eaten by the cattle. No matter what article of diet is considered, the source of its matter and energy can be traced back to green plants. It is therefore of considerable practical and theoretical importance to understand the process by which green plants obtain their food. This process is called *photosynthesis*.

Photosynthesis

Green plants *make* their food. Although they need and use proteins, fats, carbohydrates and vitamins in the same way as do animals, they have to build up these complex organic food substances from simple inorganic materials which they obtain from the air and the soil (Experiment 1). Carbohydrates and fats are built up from carbon dioxide in the air and water from the soil (Experiment 2). Amino acids and proteins are made by combining the carbohydrates with nitrogen obtained in the form of nitrate ions in solution from the soil. The chemical reactions that build up all these molecules need a supply of energy, and this energy comes in the first instance from sunlight.

In the cells of the green parts of plants, particularly in the leaves, there are organelles called *chloroplasts* (Fig. 7.2). The chloroplasts contain a green chemical called *chlorophyll*. When light strikes a chlorophyll molecule some of the energy from the light is absorbed by the chlorophyll, making it temporarily unstable. The energy thus trapped in the chlorophyll molecule is used to split a water molecule into hydrogen and oxygen ions, and the chlorophyll molecule reverts to its stable condition.

The oxygen ions combine to make oxygen molecules, O_2, and consequently oxygen gas is produced by a green plant when photosynthesis is going on (Experiment 3). The hydrogen ions now contain the energy that was trapped by the chlorophyll and they are passed to a series of hydrogen acceptors, giving up their energy and forming ATP from ADP and phosphate in the same way as described on p. 28. The store of energy-rich ATP so produced is used firstly to make molecules of carbon dioxide and hydrogen combine to produce glucose and then to build up other molecules such as starch, cellulose and protein from the glucose molecules as indicated on pp. 15 and 16.

A simple definition of photosynthesis is the production of food by a green plant from carbon dioxide and water using the energy from sunlight which is trapped by chlorophyll. An equation is often given which sums up the process,

$$6CO_2 + 6H_2O \xrightarrow{\text{energy from sunlight}} C_6H_{12}O_6 + 6O_2$$

carbon dioxide   water   glucose   oxygen

but it is not a very accurate representation of the many chemical steps which actually take place.

A consideration of our dependence on plants for our food and the plants' dependence on sunlight for the energy to make their food, leads to the conclusion that man and all other living organisms obtain the energy for their living processes indirectly from the sun. When a molecule of glucose in the body is broken down by respiration, the energy released from it is the same energy that the plant put into making it and that energy came from sunlight.

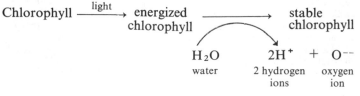

Chlorophyll $\xrightarrow{\text{light}}$ energized chlorophyll $\longrightarrow$ stable chlorophyll

H_2O $2H^+$ + O^{--}
water   2 hydrogen ions   oxygen ion

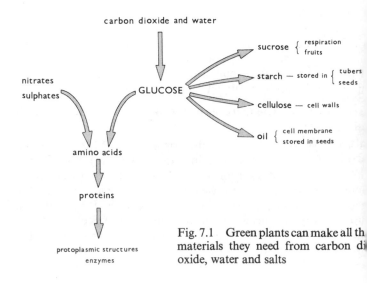

Fig. 7.1 Green plants can make all the materials they need from carbon dioxide, water and salts

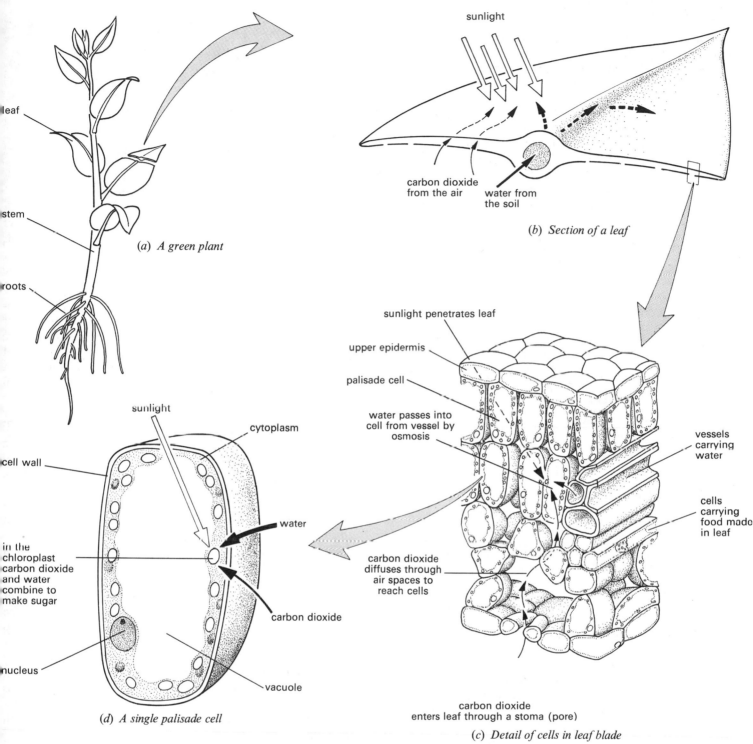

sunlight

carbon dioxide
from the air   water from
the soil

(b) *Section of a leaf*

leaf

stem

(a) *A green plant*

roots

sunlight penetrates leaf

upper epidermis

palisade cell

water passes into
cell from vessel by
osmosis

vessels
carrying
water

cells
carrying
food made
in leaf

carbon dioxide
diffuses through
air spaces to
reach cells

sunlight

cytoplasm

cell wall

water

in the
chloroplast
carbon dioxide
and water
combine to
make sugar

carbon dioxide

nucleus

vacuole

carbon dioxide
enters leaf through a stoma (pore)

(d) *A single palisade cell*

(c) *Detail of cells in leaf blade*

Fig. 7.2   Photosynthesis in a leaf

Synthesis of other materials by plants (Fig. 7.1). The plant can produce sucrose by combining two $C_6H_{12}O_6$ molecules (p. 16). Starch and cellulose are made by joining hundreds of glucose molecules in long chains *(polymerization)*. Energy from ATP is needed for this process, in addition to enzymes. The production of amino acids and proteins also needs ATP and enzymes as well as the elements nitrogen and sulphur. Other materials synthesized require metallic elements; for instance the chlorophyll molecule includes the element magnesium, the hydrogen acceptors need iron, the material between the cell walls incorporates calcium, while ATP contains phosphorus. These elements are obtained by the green

plant from the soil, where they occur as ions (p. 21) in solution in soil water (Experiment 4). Nitrogen, phosphorus and sulphur occur as nitrates, —NO_3, phosphates, —PO_4, and sulphates, —SO_4, respectively. These inorganic ions in the soil came originally from the rocks which gave rise to the soil but as the plants use them up, or as they are washed out of the soil by rain, they are replaced by the decay of plant and animal remains as described on p. 50. In agricultural practice, the supply of essential elements in the soil is increased by adding artificial 'fertilizers', such as ammonium sulphate which contains nitrogen and sulphur.

Agriculture

Origins. Some 10 000 years ago, man derived his food by collecting the edible parts of naturally growing plants and also, probably, small animals. More advanced groups took to organized hunting, when large animals were trapped and killed by bands of men working together. Today, Eskimos are an example of a specialized food-collecting and hunting community, their techniques being closely adapted to their environment, for instance their methods of catching fish.

Ten thousand years ago, the first attempts at food production were probably made in the Fertile Crescent of the Middle East (Fig. 7.3), although one authority believes South East Asia to have been a more likely starting point. Later, and probably independently, agriculture started in China, S.E. Asia and the New World, possibly the Andes. The uplands of the Fertile Crescent were grassy and forested, winter and spring rainfall was ample and the local food collectors

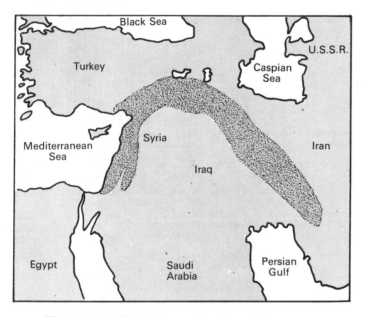

Fig. 7.3   The Fertile Crescent, ten thousand years ago

had acquired a great deal of knowledge about the local varieties of wild wheat, barley and other food plants. They would also have been familiar with wild horses, cattle, pigs, sheep and goats. The exact course of the beginnings of agriculture and the detailed steps by which it occurred are not known but the circumstances described above produce a picture, backed by archaeological evidence, in which a combination of a people with an advanced food-collecting culture and an extremely suitable environment, was an ideal situation for the change over from food-collection to food-production.

Picturesque stories can be constructed to explain how cultivation and animal husbandry could have come about: such as bringing home and rearing baby animals found on a hunting expedition, observing the germination of collected grains which had been dropped on to the soil or left in damp storage conditions, and so on; but the genuine evidence is too sparse and incomplete to make such reconstruction more valuable than speculation.

Principles of agriculture. 1 *Arable farming.* The principles of arable farming involve the removal of the natural vegetation from the soil in the first place. Then (a) the soil is planted

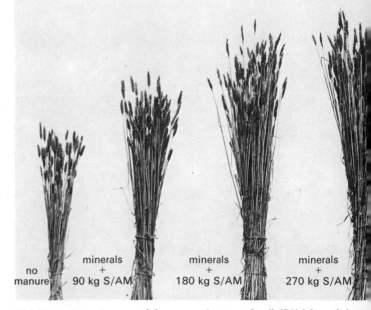

Fig. 7.4   Wheat harvested from equal areas of soil (S/AM=sulphate of ammonia)

with seeds of a single plant species, (b) their growth is encouraged by improving the soil fertility, e.g. adding water and mineral salts, and (c) plant competitors and parasites are eliminated by hoeing or spraying. In this way, a limited area of soil is made to produce a much larger quantity of edible plant material than if it were left to develop its natural vegetation such as grass or forest trees.

(a) The plant species cultivated today must have had their origins in wild plants, but by careful selection and cross-breeding over many hundreds of years they have become plants with large seeds (e.g. maize), edible fruits (e.g. pineapple) or substantial root or stem tubers (e.g. yam and potato). The process of breeding and selection continue even more intensively today on a scientific basis to try and find plants that yield more food, are resistant to disease or can survive in adverse conditions such as drought.

The agricultural practice of growing large colonies of a single species of plant is called *monoculture.*

(b) The soil used for agriculture is 'improved' mechanically by ploughing. This loosens the soil, admits air, allows water to drain and makes penetration by plant roots easier. The nutritive value of the soil is increased by adding natural fertilizers such as farmyard manure, or artificial fertilizers such as ammonium sulphate (Fig. 7.4). Soil structure and fertility are both improved by the practice of crop rotation (p. 53). If water is scarce it can be added to the soil by various methods of irrigation, and if the soil holds too much water it can be drained by digging ditches or placing pipes beneath the soil.

(c) In the favourable conditions provided by cultivation, plants other than the crop plants will grow and compete with them for water, root space, nutrients and light. Such plants are collectively called weeds. The weeds are kept in check firstly by ploughing the soil before planting and then by hoeing between the rows as the crops grow. Certain chemicals, *herbicides,* can be used to reduce weeds both before and after planting.

Fungus diseases of the crop plants are suppressed by selecting resistant strains of plant and by spraying chemical *fungicides* on the crop. Insect pests which eat or damage crop plants or their seeds are reduced by spraying the crops with *insecticides* and by dipping the seeds in similar chemicals before planting.

2 *Animal husbandry*. Animal protein contains more essential amino acids than does plant protein (p. 33) and man, generally, finds animal products particularly palatable. In consequence, man uses some of his crops to feed animals and then eats the animals or their produce such as milk and eggs.

The principles of animal husbandry are much the same as those applied in growing crops. A limited number of species is used. One such is the cow, which after years of selective breeding has high milk yield, produces much meat or is resistant to disease or adverse conditions. The animals are allowed to grow in as near ideal conditions as possible and pests and competitors are eliminated. Only about 10 per cent of the food given to animals appears as flesh, or eggs or milk. The rest is used for energy to keep the animal alive, maintain its temperature and enable it to move about. The logical step in modern animal husbandry is therefore to reduce the energy losses to a minimum. In 'factory' farming, the animals are kept indoors at a constant temperature to reduce heat losses, and their movements are restricted so that the food they eat is used for making flesh rather than being used for energy production. If the world population continues to increase at its present rate, it will become necessary to use more plant products directly for food instead of losing 90 per cent of their energy value by feeding them to animals.

weeds, fungal diseases and insect pests is a cause for concern because the chemicals used are often harmful to man and other animals (*see* p. 58).

Fishing

After animal husbandry, fishing is the only other important method of obtaining animal protein, and apart from fish farming, it is still at the stage of organized hunting. The principal large-scale methods of catching fish are trawling, drifting and lining.

Lining. The Newfoundland cod fishery uses lines bearing several thousands of baited hooks at 2-metre intervals, which are suspended at a suitable depth in the water, and examined and rebaited at regular intervals.

Drifting. To catch fish such as herring and mackerel which swim near the surface to feed on the zooplankton (p. 56), drift nets are used. These are about 15 metres deep and 3 or 4 kilometres long. They are thrown over the side of the boat and left floating at night, just below the surface of the water, in the path of migrating shoals or in a region where the fish are known to rise into the surface waters to feed (Fig. 7.5). The fish swim into the nets, which they cannot see in the dark-

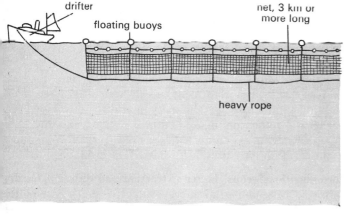

Fig. 7.5   Drifting

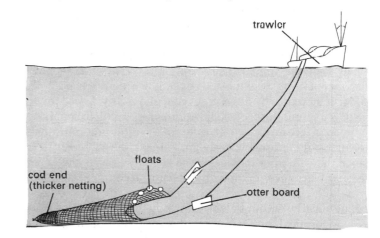

Fig. 7.6   Trawling

Hazards of agriculture. Agricultural practice is essential for feeding the present population of the world. If man were to revert to collecting and hunting his food, only a tiny fraction of the present world population could survive. Some authorities suggest that for each family of hunters and gatherers, five square kilometres of hunting territory is needed. The world population in this case could be about 10 million instead of its present 3 000 million.

Although agriculture is so essential to our continued survival, its widespread use and increased intensity carry certain dangers. Removal of natural vegetation and ploughing in some areas make the soil much more liable to be washed away by heavy rain or blown away by high winds (*see* Erosion, p. 53). Excessive use of some artificial fertilizers has led to streams and rivers becoming polluted with the chemicals which are washed out of the soil (*see* p. 52). The practice of growing plants of the same species very close to each other enables the diseases of these species to spread easily and rapidly from one plant to the next so that whole fields of crops can be infected and destroyed. The use of chemicals to control

ness, and become trapped in the meshes by the operculum, the bony gill cover. The nets are then hauled in and the fish shaken out into compartments on the deck.

This method is profitable only when large numbers of fish are known to be migrating; and at the moment, knowledge of the time and place of fish migrations depends more on the experience acquired by fishermen than on a scientific understanding of the causes.

Trawling. Fish which feed near the bottom of the sea on worms, molluscs and small fish, are called *demersal*. Examples are plaice, skate, sole, haddock and whiting. These are caught by a trawl net, a large, bag-like net which is drawn slowly by a trawler across the sea bottom (Fig. 7.6). The net is kept open by two otter boards attached one on each side of the net mouth in such a way that they tend to act as hydroplanes and move apart as the net is drawn along. After an hour or so of trawling, the net is hauled aboard, the 'cod end' opened and the fish released on the deck. The profitable limit for trawling is in water of not more than about 650 metres depth, with a sandy bottom and at temperatures above 0 °C.

Japan, Great Britain and the U.S.A. are the principal fish-catching countries and a conservative estimate of the weight of fish caught each year in the world is 20 million tonnes. As the intensity of fishing has increased in the last fifty years the question arises of whether we are depleting the stocks of fish in the sea. If the numbers taken were so great that only a few were left to breed and produce new stocks, the situation might be serious, but the evidence so far suggests that (a) a relatively small number of breeding adults are able to maintain a stable population of fish, despite intensive fishing, (b) the total weight of fish from the fishing grounds does not seem to be decreasing, and (c) the annual catch has not shown a steady decline but the fish of which it is composed are becoming smaller and the time and cost of catching them is consequently increasing.

The variety of figures available from the past fifty years suggests, by circumstantial evidence, a particular pattern of events. In an unfished area, many fish grow to a large size and take most of the available food, so restricting the growth of smaller fish. When such an area is first fished, the large fish are caught and a good haul is achieved in a short time and with minimum effort and expenditure. Subsequent catches are of smaller fish which take longer to make up an adequate haul and therefore increase the cost of fishing. This can go on until the balance between the cost of trawling and sale of fish becomes uneconomical.

The increase in the proportion of small fish is not in itself a bad thing, since when larger competitors are removed it seems likely that the smaller fish grow more rapidly. A 4-year-old fish increases its weight by 50 per cent in a year, while a 6-year-old fish increases by only 35 per cent and a 20-year-old by 1 per cent. A population of rapidly growing small fish may well convert food into flesh at a far more economic rate than a smaller population of slowly growing large fish. Nevertheless, since the catch per day's absence steadily falls as the average fish size declines, commercial fishing becomes less and less profitable. An optimum rate of fishing, which removes fish economically without depleting growing or breeding stock, is a theoretical possibility but has not yet been determined practically except perhaps in fish farming where more control can be exercised over the population and data are easy to obtain.

Fish farming. Fish farms introduce young fish into lakes and ponds, provide them with food so that they grow at a maximum rate and, at intervals, harvest and sell the fish over a certain size. The species of fish, the growth rate and the size of the population can thus all be controlled.

World food production

The world population is increasing at the rate of about 50 million people per year. Whether this rate of increase will continue is impossible to say but at the moment, the rate of increase is itself accelerating. United Nations experts suggest that by A.D. 2000 the world population may have increased from its present 3 300 million to 7 000 million. Such a rate of increase introduces many problems but one of the most urgent is the supply of food. Whether increase in food production can match this increase in numbers is another controversial matter, both in theory and in practice. Theoretically a ten- or twenty-fold increase in world food production seems possible, and yet in the ten years from 1960–70 the Food and Agriculture Organization of the United Nations (FAO) estimated that although food production increased by 2.7 per cent per year, the demand for food by an increasing population rose by 3.9 per cent per year. In Africa and the Near East, food production had not kept up with population growth and in Latin America it had barely kept pace. Clearly, a large proportion of the world population receives inadequate food, though often this is not so much a shortage in quantity as a lack of a small number of essential amino acids and vitamins. The situation gives little cause for complacency, but fatalistic gloom is of no value. The following paragraphs outline some of the ways in which food production can be increased.

Intensification of agriculture. The scientific principles of agriculture are mentioned on p. 42 and some of the consequences of bad agricultural practices discussed on p. 43. Not all land is suited to conventional agriculture, but land that is should be made to yield greater quantities of food while conserving its productive capacity.

In some areas, more intensive agriculture has been very effective. New varieties of wheat and rice in India, Pakistan and Sri Lanka, for example, with the aid of fertilizers and irrigation, have doubled or trebled the yields of grain. Crop varieties can be bred not only to raise their yields but to increase resistance to disease and adverse conditions. In this way, plants resistant to frost could be developed and grown in winter and spring in temperate zones so that the soil is productive all year round. Any land without green cover wastes valuable energy from sunlight.

Human sewage, often discharged wastefully into the sea, could be used, after treatment, as an agricultural fertilizer. Irrigation can increase productivity in arid regions. However, intensified production in agricultural regions and the conversion of new areas to agriculture need to be accompanied by conservation measures, as discussed on p. 53.

More nutritious crops, better extraction and different feeding habits. To raise the total energy value of man's diet to the arbitrary minimum of 12 000 kilojoules per day, though essential, is not enough. The most acute shortage is of proteins containing essential amino acids (p. 33). Peas, beans, groundnuts and green leaves contain a higher proportion of protein than many grains and far more than most roots such as yam and cassava. A great deal of work has to be done to find protein-rich crops which grow well in particular localities. European and North American garden vegetables do not grow well in tropical conditions, but new varieties of vegetable could be bred from existing wild types, increasing the leaf protein available in these regions.

Some methods of harvesting and extraction waste useful parts of plants. For example, extraction of oil from groundnuts, soya beans, coconuts and cotton seed tends to waste their high protein content when the residues are fed to animals. The world demand may be for oil but the need is for protein, and more efficient methods need to be devised for its extraction. The quantities of protein involved in these plants could supply an estimated third of the world's needs. In addition, methods of extracting protein from poisonous or unpalatable leaves could be sought.

As explained on p. 43 there is considerable loss of energy (up to 90 per cent) in the conversion of plant material to

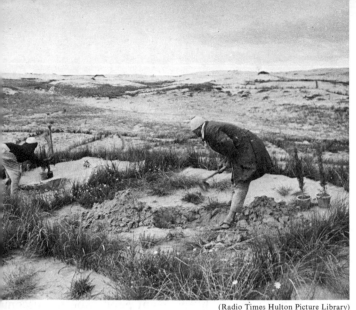
(Radio Times Hulton Picture Library)

Fig. 7.7 Dunes being stablilized by planting grass in 5 m squares in the desert in Tripolitania

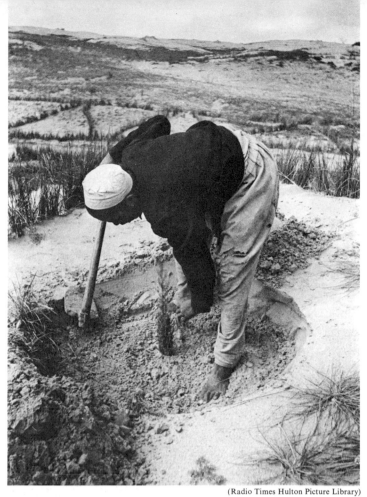
(Radio Times Hulton Picture Library)

Fig. 7.8 Trees are planted in the squares

animal products, and the most efficient use man can make of food plants is to eat them directly. A suitable combination of plant material can supply all the essential amino acids and it may be that we shall have to forgo, to some extent, the more palatable animal protein in order to make the best use of available food. We can afford to feed to animals only those plant products or residues that cannot be used directly by man.

Reclamation of land. Thoughtless conversion of marginal land to conventional agriculture may lead to severe erosion, but new farming methods may enable areas which now support only vegetation (such as tropical rain forest) to produce food. Unproductive areas may be reclaimed, as is happening in North Africa and Israel today. Although some areas of natural desert may never be productive in the conventional agricultural sense, there is abundant evidence that many desert margins were once far more productive than they are today. On the northern border of the Sahara and in the Negev and Kara Kum deserts of Israel and Russia, reclamation is being carried out with encouraging results.

The methods adopted fall roughly into two categories: (a) supplying water, and (b) establishing vegetation.

(a) *Water supply.* The water supply can be increased and controlled by replanting forests in the catchment areas and by carrying water in pipes from regions of high rainfall to arid regions. Dams are constructed to conserve water from winter floods which previously poured down the wadis and into the sea from the Kara Kum and Negev, or over the desert in the Sahara. Attempts have been made to remove the salt from sea water and brackish desert water. In Israel this has been carried out experimentally by distillation using the sun's energy, by deionization using chemical methods, or by using condensed water from power stations. In many cases, irrigation is all that is needed to make the soil productive.

(b) *Recolonization of arid areas by plants.* Firstly, coarse grasses are planted in rectangular grids. Their roots bind the soil and their foliage reduces wind erosion. In the squares of the grid are planted trees such as acacia, which can survive in conditions of water shortage. The roots and foliage of the trees enhance the soil-holding properties of the grasses. Finally, olive trees and date palms can be established and what was once shifting sand can be converted to stable, productive soil (Figs. 7.7–7.9).

All these measures must be introduced with due consideration for the indigenous human population. It is one thing to see the solution to a problem but another to enlist the support of people who are reluctant to change their way of life. The nomads' goats are a menace to the recolonization schemes, but employing the nomads themselves to guard the plantations from wandering herds is more likely to achieve success than repressive measures.

Successful desert reclamation has its attendant problems. Irrigation increases the chances of locust infestation by making conditions suitable for their breeding, and also helps to spread the snails that carry bilharziasis (p. 220). Similarly, fungus diseases which were suppressed by the hot, dry desert climate may flourish in irrigated areas. One thing is certain: the plants

Fig. 7.9 Aerial photograph showing desert reclamation
(Hulton Educational Publications)

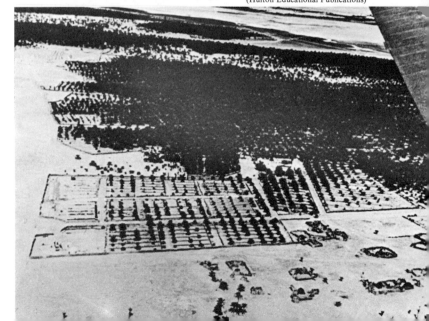

and animals and even the people who farm them must be well adapted to the environment. It is useless to introduce European pedigree cattle into tropical areas where they are unlikely to do well. The farm animals and plants must be bred from existing types that are already well adapted to arid conditions.

In some cases the large sums of money which might be spent on reclaiming desert areas, where the final yield may be small, would be better spent in improving productive or partially productive land.

Apart from the reclamation of eroded land, it may be possible to make areas such as the African swamps productive. Straightforward drainage seems to increase the hazards of malaria, although if the eradication programme succeeds this will cease to be an obstacle. The swamps may, however, be better suited to rice growing or fish farming than to conventional agriculture.

Marine husbandry. Even in well-fished areas, only a tiny fraction of the surface-feeding fish are caught and many areas such as the Pacific and Indian Oceans are under-exploited. Some biologists look forward to the day when man farms the sea rather than goes hunting in it.

Pest control. 10 000 million kilograms of produce are lost each year to pests and diseases. Eradication or control of these pests and diseases would make this food available for human consumption. Modern pesticides have played an enormous part in reducing such losses but they are not without their hazards (*see* p. 58).

New methods of obtaining food. Most of the methods described below are in the experimental stages and are not in themselves likely to solve a world food shortage. Nevertheless, in certain regions they may make an important contribution.

Fig. 7.10 Hydroponic culture. In this experimental situation tomato plants are growing in a nutrient solution circulating through the black plastic tubing. No sand or other material is used for rooting the plants, which are supported by taut strings. Since soil is not used, water losses by surface evaporation are greatly reduced

(Dr A. J. Cooper, Glasshouse Crops Research Institute)

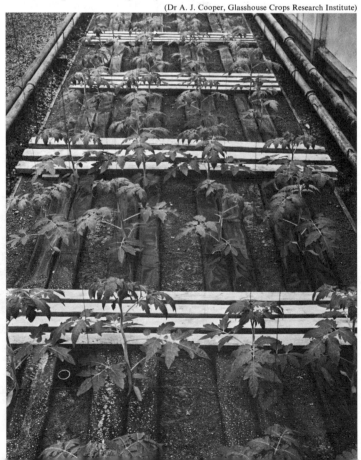

(a) *Game cropping.* As a result of work carried out in parts of Africa, it seems that the natural communities of wild animals, 'game', could if efficiently controlled or mixed with cattle provide more meat than cattle alone and with less damaging effects on the environment. The reasons for this are as follows:

(i) Game animals are resistant to the trypanosomes carried by tsetse flies, which bring the disease ngana to domestic cattle.

(ii) Game use a wide range of vegetation, from the browsing of leaves by giraffes to the grazing of grass by the antelope. Cattle, however, feed almost exclusively on grass and are less interested in other vegetation.

(iii) The equilibrium established between the various wild mammals and the diverse plant population has become stable over millions of years of evolution. Some farming communities are more concerned with the numbers of cattle than with their quality and so tend to overstock and overgraze, thus destroying the habitat and its food resources.

Judicious protection of game and its habitat, with controlled slaughter, can be made to yield meat in valuable quantities. For example, hippos in Uganda provide 3 000 tonnes of meat per annum. Game cropping has also a psychological value in offering an outlet for 'hunting' other than indiscriminate poaching which often involves cruelty and destruction when the brush is burned to drive out game, killing many other species and ruining the habitat.

(b) *Culture of algae.* Agricultural crops make efficient use of only 0.3 per cent of incident sunlight. Many microscopic algae use as much as 2 per cent. One such unicellular alga, *Chlorella,* can be grown in solutions containing salts, if suitably exposed to sunlight. No soil is needed and less water than rooted plants since transpiration does not occur. At 26 °C, *Chlorella* divides every 14 hours and its cells contain 30 to 50 per cent protein, including most of the essential amino acids, and vitamins, particularly carotene, the precursor of vitamin A. Chickens have been shown to digest *Chlorella* powder and thrive on it, though rats are unable to do so. *Chlorella* thus seems to be an unlikely source of food for man but may be of value as fodder for cattle or chickens.

In Israel, an experimental station produces about 550 grams of *Chlorella* per square metre per day using tanks of nutrient solutions exposed to sunlight. Other systems have been tried to avoid overcrowding, shading and overheating. In America the culture solution has been circulated in transparent tubes with good results so far. Theoretically 1 250 kilograms per hectare of *Chlorella* could be produced each day. This is no better than the rate of production under conventional agriculture in good conditions, but these culture methods may have something to offer in arid zones with little prospect of irrigation and very little cloud cover throughout the year.

(c) *Hydroponics.* Experiments were started in 1957 in the Sahara where nutrient solutions were fed to plants in otherwise infertile desert sand. The technique adopted is similar to that described for solution 1 of Experiment 4, p. 48, but the plants are rooted in sand or other inert material (Fig. 7.10). The water requirements are much less and the yield per square metre much greater than that of conventional palm-grove oasis cultivation.

(d) *'Synthetic' food.* Factory synthesis of food from materials such as coal or petroleum, even if possible, is unlikely to equal the efficiency of green plants, but the synthesis of proteins from sugars and inorganic salts by micro-organisms is theoretically possible on a large scale. For example, to quote a leading research worker in this field, 'In 24 hours half a tonne of bullock will make 500 grams of protein; half a tonne of yeast will make 50 tonnes and needs only a few square yards to do it on.' Urea, glycine, ethanoic (acetic) acid, succinic and malic acids can all be synthesized, and might be used by animals as energy sources. 'Amama' is a mixture of groundnut flour, dried yeast, milk casein, sugar, five minerals and seven vitamins. As such it is hardly a synthetic food, but it is sold in Nigeria at a low cost, and if added at the rate of 30 grams per day to the food of 6- or 7-year-old children helps to reduce the incidence of kwashiorkor (p. 33). Similar concentrated mixtures of amino acids and vitamins might help to reduce the incidence of other deficiency diseases, without any vast increase in the demand on agricultural productivity.

(e) *Education.* Before any progress can be made in applying new ideas, governments and people must be made aware of the problems and prospects, the dangers and the hopes of intensified or novel agricultural practices. Farming methods and feeding habits may have to undergo drastic changes, and the sooner the facts are presented to the people, the sooner they will become acclimatized to the new ideas. In this way, opposition of the conservative and traditional variety, if not exactly eliminated, might at least become informed and constructive.

Practical Work

Experiment 1   **The production of starch by a green plant**

A potted plant is watered and placed in a dark cupboard for 48 hours during which time any starch present in its leaves is removed. After two days, the plant is taken from its cupboard and one of its leaves tested for starch as described below. If the test leaf proves to contain no starch, one or more of the leaves on the plant are partly covered with a strip of aluminium foil (Fig. 7.11) and the whole plant left in sunlight or strong artificial light for three hours or more. After this time the leaf with the foil strip is detached, the foil removed and the leaf tested for starch.

Result. Only those parts of the leaf that received light will go blue with iodine.

Interpretation. The blue colour indicates that starch has been made in the leaf which was previously free from starch. The fact that the area under the foil strip has produced no starch suggests that light is essential for starch production by photosynthesis.

Starch test. Prepare a beaker or can of boiling water. Hold the leaf in forceps and dip it momentarily in the water. Place the leaf in a test-tube and cover it with ethanol (industrial methylated spirit). Make sure all bunsen burners or spirit lamps are extinguished and place the test-tube in the boiling water (Fig. 7.12). The alcohol will boil and extract the chlorophyll from the leaf. When the alcohol is green and the leaf is white or very pale green pour off the alcohol, take out the leaf, dip it once again in the hot water to soften it and spread it flat on a tile or dish. Cover the leaf with iodine solution and if any starch is present in it, a blue colour will appear.

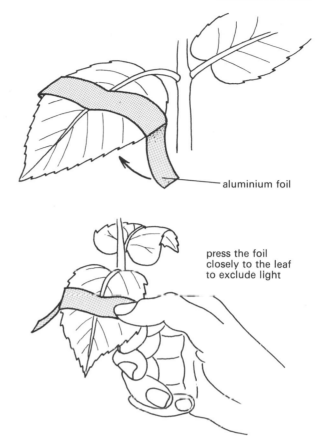

aluminium foil

press the foil closely to the leaf to exclude light

Fig. 7.11   Starch production in leaves

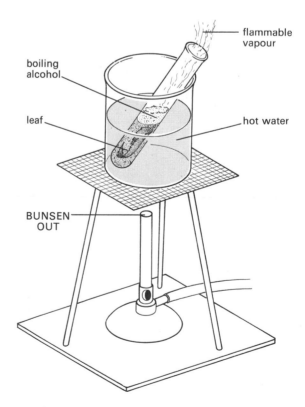

flammable vapour

boiling alcohol

leaf

hot water

BUNSEN OUT

Fig. 7.12   Extracting chlorophyll from a leaf

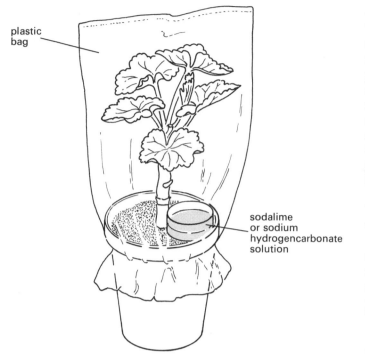

Fig. 7.13   The need for carbon dioxide

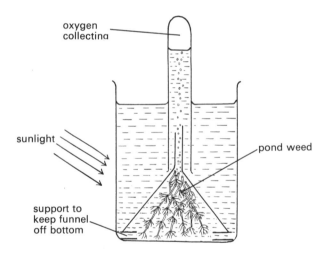

Fig. 7.14   Collecting oxygen from pond weed

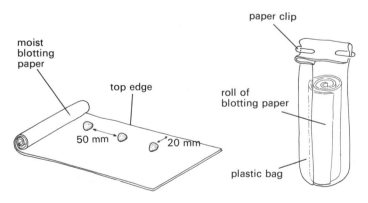

Fig. 7.15   Growing seedlings

Experiment 2   **The plant's need for carbon dioxide**

Two potted plants are watered and left in a dark cupboard for 48 hours so that all starch is removed from their leaves. After this period, one of the leaves from each plant is removed and tested for starch as described above. There should be no blue colour with iodine. Both plants are then watered and enclosed in clear plastic bags, as shown in Fig. 7.13, but one contains a dish of sodalime which absorbs all the carbon dioxide in the enclosed area, while the other has a dish of sodium hydrogencarbonate solution which will release carbon dioxide into the air. Both plants are placed in sunlight for three hours or more after which a leaf from each is detached and tested for starch.

Result. The leaf deprived of carbon dioxide will not turn blue, while that from the carbon dioxide-enriched atmosphere will turn blue.

Interpretation. The fact that no starch is made in the leaf deprived of carbon dioxide suggests that the latter must be necessary for photosynthesis and starch production. The control (the plant with added carbon dioxide) rules out the possibility that high humidity or temperature in the plastic bag prevents normal photosynthesis.

Experiment 3   **Oxygen from pond weed**

A short-stemmed funnel is placed over some pond weed (*Elodea* or *Ceratophyllum*) in a beaker of water, preferably pond water, and a test-tube filled with water is inverted over the funnel stem (Fig. 7.14). The funnel is raised above the bottom of the beaker to allow free circulation of water. The apparatus is placed in sunlight and bubbles of gas soon appear from the cut stems, rise and collect in the test-tube. When sufficient gas has collected, the test-tube is removed and a glowing splint inserted in it. A control experiment should be set up in a similar way but placed in a dark cupboard. Little or no gas should collect.

Result. The glowing splint bursts into flame.

Interpretation. The relighting of a glowing splint does not prove that the gas collected is *pure* oxygen but it does show that, in the light, this particular plant has given off a gas which is considerably richer in oxygen than is atmospheric air.

(*Note*. Pond weed is used for this experiment because it is easier to collect the gas given off than from a land plant. It is however, possible to demonstrate that all green plants give off oxygen in the light and it is this which replenishes the oxygen used up by combustion and respiration.)

Experiment 4   **The plant's need for mineral elements**

Some small seeds (e.g. wheat, sorghum, vigna) are soaked in water for 24 hours and then rolled up in moist newsprint or blotting paper. The paper rolls are stood on end in polythene bags (Fig. 7.15) for a few days until the seeds have germinated. Four seedlings at about the same stage of development are selected and each is wrapped in cotton wool and placed in the mouth of a test-tube, its roots dipping into one of four solutions (Fig. 7.16). Solution 1 contains all the elements thought to be necessary for the production of proteins, chlorophyll, enzymes, etc.; solution 2 contains the same elements except for calcium; solution 3 lacks only nitrates, and 'solution' 4 lacks all salts, i.e. it is distilled water. The plants are allowed to grow for two or three weeks in the light, the solutions being topped up with distilled water when the level drops. After this time the seedlings are compared for colour, size, number of leaves, length of roots, etc.

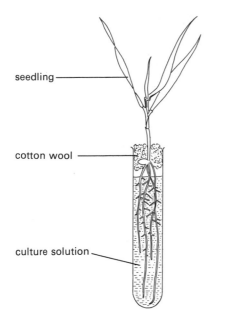

seedling

cotton wool

culture solution

Fig. 7.16   Seedling in water culture

Result. When nitrates are absent, the plant lacks the nitrogen needed to make proteins, so it is likely that the plant in solution 3 will be small and pale in colour. Calcium is needed for proper development of cell walls and its absence will have a bad effect on the growth of the seedling in solution 2. The

seedling in distilled water is deprived of all mineral salts though it is still able to make carbohydrates by photosynthesis. When it has exhausted the food reserves in its seed, it may cease growing and die. The reason for using small seeds in this experiment is that they quickly use up their own food reserves and become dependent on the solutions.

The formulae for the reagents and solutions for these experiments are given on p. 268. These experiments and many others are described more fully in the laboratory manual *Photosynthesis* (*see* p. 269).

Questions

1   A group of explorers is stranded on a barren island where there is no soil and no vegetation. From their stores they have salvaged some living hens and some wheat. To make these resources last as long as possible should they
   (a) eat the wheat and when it is finished, kill and eat the hens, or
   (b) feed the wheat to the hens, collect and eat the eggs laid and when the wheat is gone, kill and eat the hens, or
   (c) kill and eat the hens first and when they are finished, eat the wheat? Justify your answer.
2   What are the requirements for photosynthesis? How are these requirements met in (a) a land plant, (b) an aquatic plant?
3   It can be claimed that the sun's energy is used indirectly to produce a muscle contraction in your arm. Trace the steps in the transfer of energy which would justify this claim.
4   Proteins contain carbon, hydrogen, oxygen, nitrogen and often sulphur. Name the source from which a green plant obtains each of these elements.
5   What factors do you think will limit the quantity of food that can be produced from a given area of soil? Suggest ways in which these limits could be raised by artificial means.

8

Soil

Components

Soil consists of a mixture of (a) mineral particles such as sand and clay, (b) humus, (c) water, (d) air, (e) dissolved salts, and (f) bacteria and fungi.

(a) **Inorganic particles** are formed from rocks which have been weathered and broken down. Particles from 2 to 0.02 mm diameter are classified as sand, 0.02 to 0.002 mm as silt and less than 0.002 mm as clay (Experiment 1). Chemically, sand is silicon oxide while clay may be various complexes of aluminium and silicon oxides. Iron oxide may give a red or brown coating to the particles.

Aggregates of these inorganic particles together with humus produce *crumbs* up to about 3 mm in diameter, which form the 'skeleton' of the soil. The crumb structure of a soil depends on the proportion of clay, sand and humus and the activities of plant roots; a good crumb structure is one of the most important attributes of a soil.

(b) **Humus** is the finely divided organic matter incorporated into the crumbs; it originates mainly from decaying plant remains (Experiment 2). The presence of humus in the crumbs affects the colour and physical properties of the soil. Humus is black, structureless, often forms a coating around sand particles, and may be important in glueing particles together to form soil crumbs. A sandy soil deficient in humus tends to have a poor crumb structure and is easily blown away if exposed by ploughing. The exclusive use of chemical fertilizers on certain soils in dry climates may lead to the formation of dust bowls or the advance of desert margins.

The bacterial decay of humus and the organic matter from which it originates produces the nitrates and other mineral salts needed for plant growth.

(c) **Water** is spread over the sand particles or clay aggregates as a thin film which adheres by capillary attraction. It may also penetrate the aggregates and be held to the clay particles by chemical forces. When a soil contains as much water as it can hold by capillary and chemical attraction (i.e. any more would drain away by the force of gravity), it is said to be at *field capacity*. Capillary attraction will tend to distribute water from regions above field capacity to drier regions. The forces holding water in the soil also set up considerable opposition to the 'suction' of plant roots when the soil begins to dry out.

(d) **Air** occurs in the spaces between the aggregates or sand particles unless the soil is waterlogged, in which case the air spaces are blocked up. A supply of oxygen is essential for the respiration of roots and some soil organisms, e.g. bacteria.

(e) **Salts.** Salts in the soil water are dissolved out from either the surrounding rock or from humus and organic matter in the soil. They make a very dilute solution in the soil water but are vital for plant growth, as explained on p. 41.

(f) **Bacteria.** Many microscopic plants, fungi and animals live in the soil, but among the most important to plant life are the bacteria which break down the organic matter and humus to form soluble salts which can be taken up in solution by roots. Other bacteria convert atmospheric nitrogen to organic compounds of nitrogen (*see* p. 51).

Types of soil

Heavy soils. A soil in which clay particles predominate and which has a poor crumb structure will be sticky and difficult to plough or dig. This results partly from chemical and capillary forces acting on the very large surface area of the minute clay particles, making them difficult to separate. When dry, the soil forms hard clods which do not break up readily during cultivation.

The small distances between particles (Fig. 8.1*a*) tend to produce poor aeration and drainage, but the large surface presented by the particles retains a high proportion of water in conditions of drought. There is also less tendency for soluble minerals to be washed away because they are held chemically to the clay particles.

A heavy soil can be made lighter, more workable and permeable to water and air by adding lime or organic matter, e.g. farmyard manure. The lime makes the particles clump together or *flocculate,* the clumps of particles behaving like the larger particles of a light soil. The crumb structure of a clay soil can be improved by growing grass on it for a year or two.

Light soils. The large, inorganic particles of a light soil give it its sandy texture (Fig. 8.1*b*). The wider separation of the particles leads to better aeration and drainage but there is a smaller surface for the water film. Such a reduced surface lessens the surface forces (surface tension) of the water and makes it easier to separate the particles in ploughing and digging, and the clumps break up easily when dry.

The mineral salts are more liable to be washed out from a lighter soil and it loses water rapidly in dry conditions. Its water-holding properties and nitrogen content can be improved by adding farmyard manure or compost (rotted vegetable matter).

Loam. A soil with a balanced mixture of particle sizes, a good humus content and stable crumb structure is called a loam. Loams are the most productive soils in agriculture.

Laterite soils. A laterite soil is formed in tropical conditions, where high temperatures cause very rapid decomposition of organic matter and the heavy rain washes out many of the minerals including much of the silica. The soil consists mainly of alumina particles coloured red with iron oxide, and is deficient in humus and mineral nutrients. When it dries, the alumina and iron oxide particles stick together forming a hard layer which is poorly aerated and difficult to plough or dig.

Soil pH (acidity). The pH of soils varies. A soil on limestone or chalk may be alkaline, up to pH 8. Some clay soils and soils containing much organic matter may be acid, down to pH 4.5. Acid conditions in the soil often lead to a deficiency of minerals by making them more soluble and easily washed out by rain. Alkaline conditions, on the other hand, may make some minerals so insoluble that they cannot be taken up in solution by the plant.

A pH of about 6.5 is considered favourable for most crops and cultivation methods can be used to adjust the pH. For example, application of lime (calcium hydroxide) will raise the pH of an acid soil, while addition of ammonium sulphate will lower the pH of an alkaline soil.

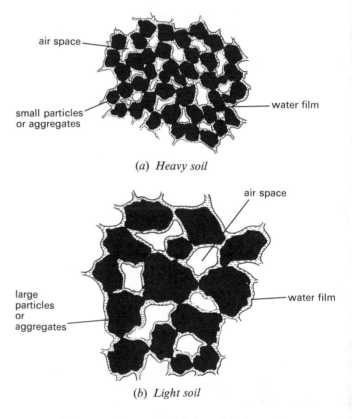

(a) Heavy soil

(b) Light soil

Fig. 8.1　Structure of light and heavy soils

Soil fertility

In natural conditions soil fertility is maintained by the activity of the organisms living on it or in it. For example, the plant roots maintain the soil's crumb structure and the burrows of earthworms enhance its drainage. Although plants remove mineral salts they are replaced by the death and decomposition of plant and animal bodies. This cycle of uptake and return of minerals from the soil applies to all the mineral elements in the soil but can be studied in detail by reference to nitrogen, the element needed by plants to make their proteins.

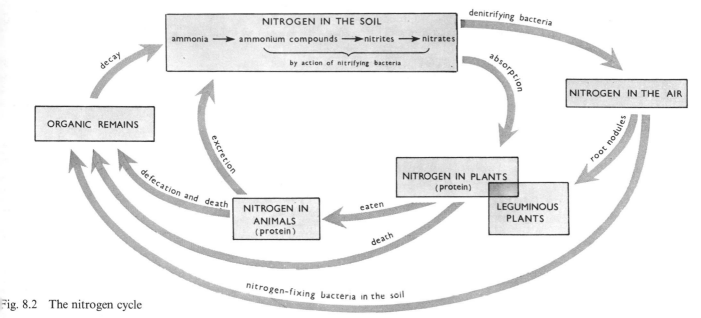

Fig. 8.2 The nitrogen cycle

The nitrogen cycle. When a plant or animal dies its tissues decompose, largely as a result of the action of enzymes and bacteria. One of the important products of this decomposition is ammonia, which is washed into the soil where it forms ammonium compounds (Fig. 8.2).

Nitrifying bacteria. In the soil there are many bacteria and certain of these, the *nitrite bacteria,* oxidize the ammonium compounds to nitrites. Others, the *nitrate bacteria,* further oxidize nitrites to nitrates, which are taken up in solution by plants. The faeces of animals contain organic matter which is similarly broken down, and their urine is rich in nitrogenous waste products such as ammonia, which can be oxidized to nitrates by soil bacteria.

$$NH_3 \longrightarrow -NO_2 \longrightarrow -NO_3$$
ammonia   nitrite   nitrate
           ion   ion

Each step involves an increase in the proportion of oxygen in the molecule. Such reactions are called oxidations, and need well-aerated soil with a good supply of oxygen if they are to proceed effectively.

The bacteria derive energy from these oxidative processes in much the same way as plants and animals derive energy from respiration by oxidizing carbohydrates to form carbon dioxide and water (p. 27).

Nitrogen-fixing bacteria. Although green plants cannot utilize the nitrogen in the atmosphere, there are bacteria in the soil which absorb and combine it with other elements, so making nitrogen compounds such as amino acids. This is called the *fixation of nitrogen.* Such nitrogen-fixing bacteria, as well as existing free in the soil, are found in special root swellings or *nodules* (*see* Fig. 8.3) in plants of the pea family such as soya bean, groundnuts and lucerne, and these plants, if part of their vegetation is ploughed back into the soil, increase its nitrogen content. For this reason they are included in the system of crop rotation used in agricultural practice (*see* p. 53).

Denitrifying bacteria. Also present in the soil are bacteria that obtain energy by breaking down compounds of nitrogen to gaseous nitrogen which consequently escapes to the atmosphere.

Lightning. The high temperature of lightning discharge through the atmosphere causes nitrogen and oxygen to combine, forming the gases nitrous and nitric oxide. These dissolve in the rain making weak nitrous and nitric acids which, when washed into the soil, combine with other elements there to form nitrites and nitrates. This is said to add some millions of tonnes of nitrogen to the soil every year.

To sum up, the processes that remove nitrates from the soil are dissolving out by rain, absorption by plant roots and denitrification by bacteria. Processes that increase the nitrate content of the soil are the activities of nitrifying and nitrogen-fixing bacteria and lightning. When these two sets of processes are in balance, the nitrate content of the soil remains more or less constant.

Fertilizers. The practice of agriculture interrupts natural cycles by removing the crops at harvest but not returning to the soil the dead remains of either the plants or the animals which eat

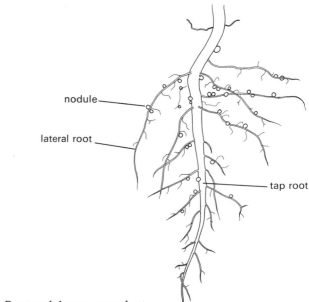

Fig. 8.3 Root nodules on groundnut

them. If this practice is continued, the soil's supply of mineral salts will be greatly reduced and the yield from the crops will fall off drastically.

Wheat has been grown and harvested on an experimental strip at Rothamsted Experimental Station in England for over one hundred years without anything being added to the soil. In this time, the yield has dropped from 14.7 kg to 6.9 kg per 100 m². The soil nitrogen, however, has remained at a steady concentration over the last eighty years, and this is probably attributable to the nitrogen-fixing bacteria and other micro-organisms present in the soil (Fig. 8.4). Similar results have been obtained in Kenya, where the yield of maize from an experimental plot dropped from 5 800 kg per hectare to 2 240 kg per hectare in only three years.

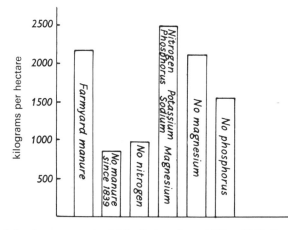

Fig. 8.4   Average yearly yields of wheat from 1852 to 1925, Rothamsted Experimental Station

To make good the losses from the soil, the farmer adds either farmyard manure or artificial fertilizers (Fig. 8.5).

Manure. Manure is the collected faeces of farm animals, usually mixed with straw or other litter and allowed to decay for several months. When it is ploughed into the soil it provides organic matter which (a) decays to give the nutrient salts needed by plants and (b) provides the material needed to form humus. Untreated human sewage, although it would help to complete the nitrogen cycle, is not used on crops because of the dangers of spreading intestinal diseases such as cholera, typhoid and dysentery, but treated sewage and sewage sludge which has been fermented at a high temperature can be a safe and useful fertilizer for the soil.

Artificial fertilizers. Although small mixed farms may produce enough manure to maintain soil fertility, large-scale arable farms do not and the minerals must be replaced by more direct chemical means. The artificial fertilizers are made in factories from sulphuric acid, ammonia, lime, slag from steel processing, and other industrial wastes.

(i) *Sulphate of ammonia* (ammonium sulphate) is made from ammonia and sulphuric acid. It provides nitrogen and sulphur.

(ii) *Basic slag* is made by grinding the slag from steel-making furnaces. It contains lime and phosphorus.

(iii) *Superphosphate.* Basic slag or natural rock, rich in phosphates, is crushed and treated with sulphuric acid. It supplies phosphorus.

Hazards of using chemical fertilizers. Long-term experiments show that by applying to the soil a programme of crop rotation

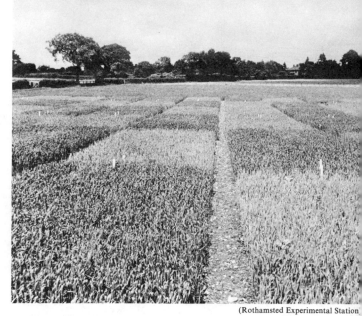

(Rothamsted Experimental Station)

Fig. 8.5   Experimental plots of wheat. The rectangular plots have been treated with different fertilizers

and using farmyard manure, the yield of crops can be increased over a fifty-year period. The long-term effects of using chemical fertilizers, in particular the soluble salts of nitrogen, are far less satisfactory. Whereas organic manure contributes to the humus content of the soil, helping to maintain its crumb structure and hence its porosity and permeability to air, the continued exclusive use of chemicals leads to a loss of the organic humus, a deterioration of crumb structure and a decrease in porosity. As a consequence, in these poorly aerated soils the plant roots are deprived of oxygen and cannot absorb the salts effectively (*see* p. 29, Active transport). The unabsorbed nitrates are washed by rain from the soil and eventually drain into rivers and lakes. Here they stimulate excessive growth of microscopic plants, algae. The algae grow quickly, die and decompose. The bacterial decomposition of their cells requires a supply of oxygen from the dissolved gases in the water. Eventually the oxygen supply is so depleted that fish and other aquatic animals are suffocated and die, and the semi-decomposed organic remains of the algae form a foul mud. This over-fertilization or *eutrophication* of lakes and rivers results not only from the excess of nitrates added to the soil but from the sewage effluents of cities and intensive animal-rearing units.

Lake Erie in America receives water draining from 75 000 square kilometres of farmland and the effluents of large cities such as Detroit and Cleveland. In its waters eutrophication has produced an organic mud with a phenomenal oxygen deficit. At the moment, a tenuous layer of iron oxide separates the organic mud from the water above but further removal of oxygen will dissolve this layer and allow the organic matter to mix with the water and produce anaerobic conditions.

Another harmful long-term effect of the exclusive use of chemical fertilizers, particularly on light soils, is that with destruction of the crumb structure the soil is much more likely to become dry and powdery and be blown away by the wind when it is not protected by a plant cover. This leads to loss of valuable topsoil, and in extreme cases to dust-bowls and deserts.

In the short term, heavy application of nitrates to crops can raise the level of free nitrates in the food plants to a point where the plants are poisonous to eat.

In order to feed the population of the world, it is essential to use chemical fertilizers but it is also essential that their use is carefully controlled. Two possible solutions to the problems outlined above are (a) the development of chemical fertilizers that are less soluble and release their nitrogen slowly into the soil at a rate to suit the demands of the plants, and (b) more efficient and extensive use of organic manure to help conserve the humus and maintain the soil structure.

Crop rotation. Different crops make differing demands on the soil; e.g. maize takes more than average amounts of phosphate from the soil. By changing the crop grown on a certain field from year to year the soil is not depleted of one particular group of minerals. Leguminous crops such as beans and groundnuts may help to restore the nitrogen content of the soil with their root nodules containing nitrogen-fixing bacteria, provided some of their vegetation is ploughed back into the soil as 'green manure'. A year or two of grass greatly improves the soil's crumb structure.

Rotating the crops also reduces the competition from weeds and the hazards of insect or fungus infestations that are characteristic of one kind of crop. For example, successive crops of potatoes on a soil will increase the population of the fungus causing the disease 'potato blight'. A field freed for a few years from potatoes will show a reduced incidence of this disease.

Other methods of improving fertility. As well as controlling the mineral content of the soil, the processes of ploughing, draining, and irrigating the land regulate its air and water content as mentioned on p. 42.

Erosion

Erosion means the removal of topsoil, usually by the action of wind and rain (Fig. 8.7a and Experiment 3).

(a) **Deforestation.** The soil cover on steep slopes is usually fairly thin but can support the growth of trees. If the forests are cut down to make way for agriculture, the soil is no longer protected by a leafy canopy from the driving rain. Consequently some of the soil is washed away into the rivers, which become choked with silt and are liable to overflow their banks.

(b) **Poor farming methods.** Ploughing loosens the soil and destroys its natural structure. Failure to replace humus after successive crops, and burning the stubble or weeds, reduces the water-holding properties so that the soil dries easily and may be blown away as dust. On sloping ground, such soil may be eroded by water.

(i) *Sheet* erosion is the imperceptible removal of thin layers of soil; it usually leads to:

(ii) *Rill* erosion, in which the water cuts channels. The channels deepen as the volume of run-off increases and so become gulleys.

(iii) *Gulley* erosion. The gulleys so formed reach enormous proportions (Fig. 8.6) so that thousands of hectares of topsoil are carried off. Gulley erosion is often accentuated by careless ploughing and may follow the tracks made by vehicles, goats, cattle and other farm animals.

(c) **Overgrazing.** Too large a population of animals on a given area will not make economic use of the food they eat, since its scarcity will make their growth rate too slow. In addition,

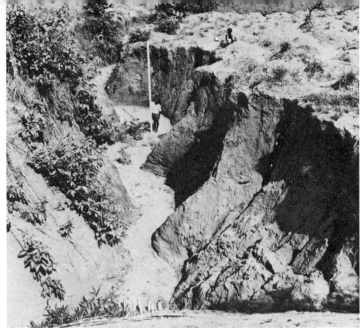

(Agricultural Information Section, Ministry of Agriculture, Enugu, Eastern Nigeria)

Fig. 8.6   Gulley erosion in Eastern Nigeria

sheep and goats graze the vegetation very closely, leaving little plant cover on the soil, while their hooves trample and compact the soil into a hard layer. Consequently there is less absorption of rain; the soil dries out quickly and may eventually be blown away.

Methods of reducing erosion (Fig. 8.6b)

(a) **Terracing.** This is cultivation along the line of the contours, in horizontal strips supported by walls, so breaking up the steep downward rush of the surface run-off. Terracing is a useful temporary measure against water erosion, but is a rather costly and difficult method of farming.

(b) **Contour ploughing.** Ploughing at right angles to the slope, i.e. along the contours instead of up and down the hill, allows the furrows to trap water rather than channel it away to start gully erosion.

(c) **Correct crops for the soil.** Steep slopes which should not or cannot be ploughed are covered with pasture crops. The foliage reduces the run-off, and the roots hold the soil in place. The following table illustrates this point.

Indicated time necessary to remove 18 cm topsoil from a 10 per cent slope, sandy clay loam, Southern Piedmont

Type of ground cover	kg soil removed annually per 1 000 m²	Number of years needed to erode 18 cm topsoil at this rate
Virgin forest	5	500 000
Grass	775	3 225
Rotation	35 800	70
Cotton	79 000	32
Bare ground	166 000	15

(From Bennett, *Elements of soil conservation*, Table 5, McGraw Hill, 1947)

(d) **Reafforestation.** Mountainous areas that have suffered from erosion are replanted with trees, so reducing the run-off and controlling floods. Controlled thinning of forests, however, is also desirable, since thickly afforested areas may prevent too large a proportion of water from ever reaching the ground.

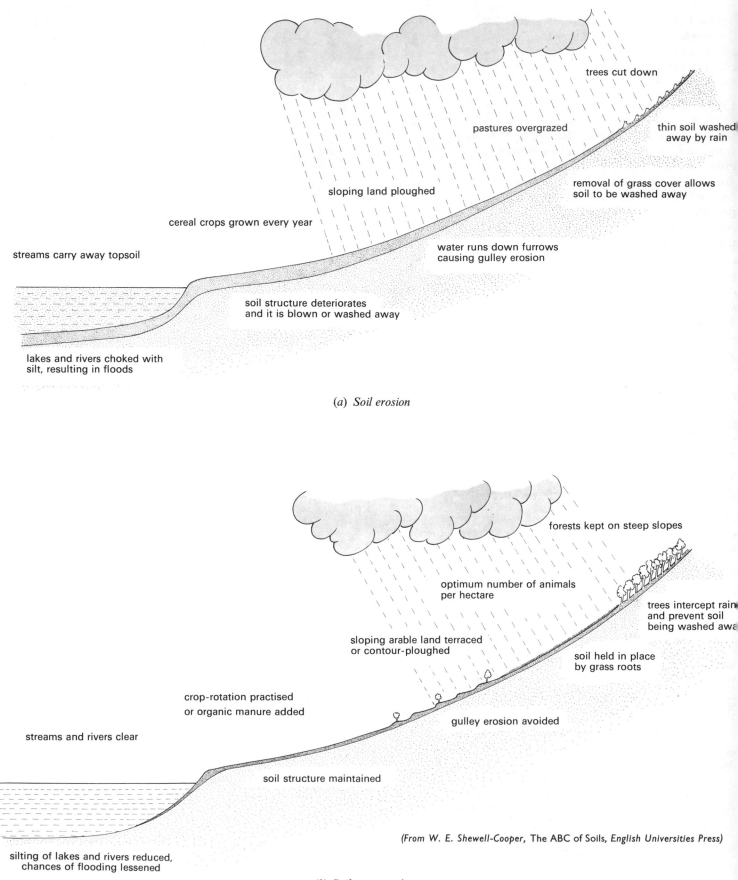

trees cut down

pastures overgrazed

thin soil washed
away by rain

sloping land ploughed

removal of grass cover allows
soil to be washed away

cereal crops grown every year

water runs down furrows
causing gulley erosion

streams carry away topsoil

soil structure deteriorates
and it is blown or washed away

lakes and rivers choked with
silt, resulting in floods

(a) *Soil erosion*

forests kept on steep slopes

optimum number of animals
per hectare

trees intercept rain
and prevent soil
being washed away

sloping arable land terraced
or contour-ploughed

soil held in place
by grass roots

crop-rotation practised
or organic manure added

gulley erosion avoided

streams and rivers clear

soil structure maintained

(From W. E. Shewell-Cooper, The ABC of Soils, *English Universities Press)*

silting of lakes and rivers reduced,
chances of flooding lessened

(b) *Soil conservation*

Fig. 8.7

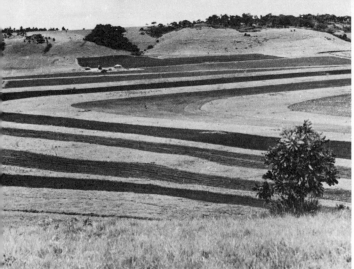

(Agricultural Information Section, Ministry of Agriculture, Enugu, Eastern Nigeria)

Fig. 8.8 Contour strip cropping in the University farm, Nsukka, Eastern Nigeria

e) **Strip cropping.** This consists of alternate bands of tilled and untilled soil following the contours (Fig. 8.8). Grass and cover-crop strips, between strips of ploughed land carrying grain, prevent the soil being washed away from the tilled portions. By alternating the grass and grain each year, the soil is allowed to rebuild its structure while under grass. Strip cropping is also effective against wind erosion if the strips are planted at right angles to the direction of the prevailing wind.

Practical Work

Experiment 1 **Observation of mineral particles in soil**

Some dry soil is sieved to remove stones and particles larger than about 3 mm. The soil is crushed lightly to break up aggregates of particles and 50 g is placed in a small, flat-sided bottle. The bottle is filled with water almost to the top, the cap screwed on and the bottle shaken for at least 30 seconds to disperse the soil throughout the water. The bottle is then allowed to stand for 10 to 15 minutes so that the soil settles down (Fig. 8.9). The large particles will fall most rapidly and

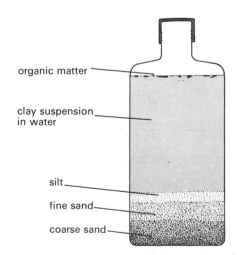

Fig. 8.9 Mineral particles in the soil

form the bottom layer. Smaller particles will contribute to successively higher layers and much of the clay will remain in suspension in the water. The larger particles of organic matter

will float to the top. If the layers are distinct enough to be measured, the results can be used to compare soils from different areas.

Experiment 2 **Organic matter in the soil**

A sample of soil is dried in an oven at 100 °C for 24 hours or alternatively spread out on newspaper to dry in the air. The soil is then sieved to remove stones and particles larger than about 3 mm, 50 g of it is placed in a metal tray or tin can and heated strongly from below with a bunsen flame for 15 minutes. If the soil blackens and smoke is given off, this is evidence for the presence of organic matter. When the soil is cool, it is weighed. The loss in weight will represent partly the quantity of organic matter burnt away and partly the evaporation of water that had not completely escaped from the soil during drying. The experiment should be repeated to compare, for example, a poor laterite soil with a fertile garden soil.

Experiment 3 **Demonstration of erosion**

Obtain two metal or plastic trays about 5 cm deep. Fill one with soil and press it down tightly. Pour water on it carefully till it is saturated and then leave the tray tilted on end to let the surplus water drain away. Cut a rectangle of turf to fit exactly into the second tray. Water this in the same way as the soil.

Place the tray with the turf at an angle of about 45° in a plastic bowl or similar container and water the soil from a watering can with a fine 'rose' fitted, for 30 seconds (Fig. 8.10). Empty the bowl and repeat the experiment with the soil.

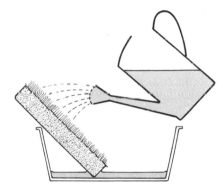

Fig. 8.10 Demonstration of erosion

Compare the quantity of soil washed into the bowl in each case. A further comparison can be made by cutting all the grass blades from the turf and watering it again. If a quantitative comparison is wanted, the soil washed into the basin can be collected by allowing it to settle, decanting the excess water, collecting, drying and weighing the soil.

Questions

1 What do you suppose is the biological significance of the following agricultural practices: (i) ploughing farmyard manure (animal faeces and straw) into the soil, (ii) adding lime to the soil, (iii) spreading sulphate of ammonia on the land?

2 Outline the ways in which careless agricultural practices can lead to rapid erosion of a light sandy soil.

3 Study the diagram of the nitrogen cycle (Fig. 8.2, p. 51) and suggest ways in which civilized man interferes with this natural chain of events.

4 List the ways in which soil fertility can be improved and indicate any disadvantages of these practices.

9
Food Chains and the Balance of Nature

All animals derive their food either directly or indirectly from plants. Carnivorous animals feed on other animals which themselves may feed on smaller animals, but sooner or later in such a series we come to an animal that feeds on vegetation. For example, guppies eat mosquito larvae, and mosquito larvae feed on microscopic plants in the pond or lake. This kind of relationship is called a *food chain*. The basis of food chains on land is vegetation in general, but particularly grass and other leaves. In water, the basis is *phytoplankton* (Fig. 9.1): the millions of microscopic plants living near the surface of the sea, ponds and lakes. These need only the water round them, the dissolved carbon dioxide, salts and sunlight to make all their vital substances (p. 40). Feeding on these microscopic plants are tiny animals, *zooplankton* (Fig. 9.2), such as the crustacea and the larvae of many kinds of animal. The small animals of the zooplankton are eaten by the surface-feeding fish; the fish, in turn, form part of the diet of other animals, including man.

This description of a food chain is inadequate in two respects, since it seems to suggest (a) that there are similar numbers of organisms at each stage in the chain, and (b) that one organism feeds exclusively on another. An alternative way of expressing the relationships of a food chain which overcomes the first objection, is by a pyramid of numbers, or pyramid of weight. Fig. 9.3 expresses this diagrammatically. At the beginning of a food chain, the organisms are usually small and very numerous. The plants of the phytoplankton are microscopic and very abundant. The animals of the zooplankton which feed on the phytoplankton, though still microscopic, are much larger than, for example, the diatoms. The fish

which eat the zooplankton are many times larger and far less numerous. Finally, it takes a large number of fish to feed one man.

These numerical relationships reflect the losses involved in the transference of energy and matter at each stage of a food chain. For every 100 kJ of energy present in the grass eaten by a cow, only about 5 kJ is used for making new flesh and bone. About 60 kJ is lost by not being wholly digested and utilized, and 35 kJ is used in respiration to meet the animal's energy needs. In food chains in general, about 10 per cent of the weight of food eaten is converted to new living matter, the other 90 per cent is undigested or used for energy. This shows why a large mass of living organisms at the beginning of a food chain will support only a small number of carnivorous animals at the end.

The second objection to the early description of the food chain is that any given animal, particularly a predator, does not usually live exclusively on one type of food. For example, lions may hunt gazelle, or zebra; young crocodiles eat water bugs, while older crocodiles eat fish. These more complex relationships can be shown as a *food web* (Fig. 9.4), but even this is greatly simplified and generalized.

If the population of one of the animals in a food web is altered, all the others are affected. In 1906 a game reserve was created in the Grand Canyon, U.S.A. Killing of deer was prohibited and hundreds of mountain lions, wolves and other predators of deer were killed. The deer multiplied rapidly in the absence of predators, so that by 1923 the population of deer had increased from 4 000 to 100 000. The range was depleted by overgrazing and thousands of deer were dying

Fig. 9.1 Phytoplankton. These microscopic plants are diatoms
(Dr D. P. Wilson)

Fig. 9.2 Zooplankton. Mostly adult and larval crustacea from the sea
(Dr D. P. Wilson)

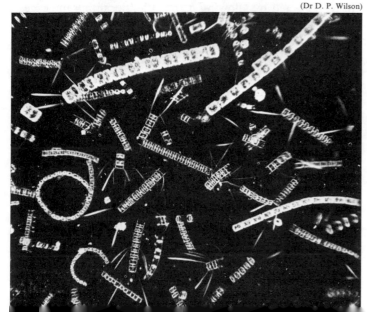

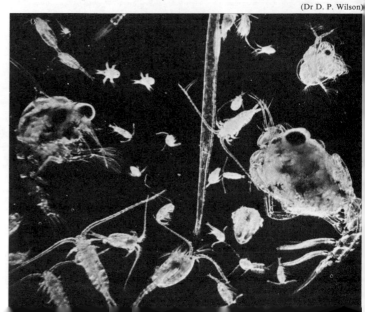

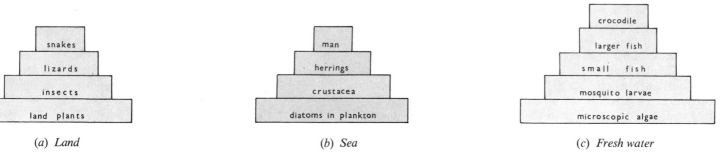

(a) *Land*   (b) *Sea*   (c) *Fresh water*

Fig. 9.3 Examples of food chains

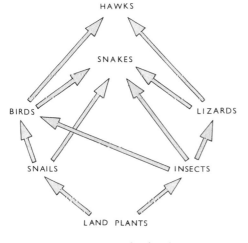

Fig. 9.4 A food web

from starvation. In 1954–5, when the rabbits in Britain were almost exterminated by the disease myxomatosis, the vegetation in what had been rabbit-infested areas changed, and sheep could graze where rabbits had previously eaten all the available grass; trees which had hitherto been nipped off as seedlings began to grow to maturity, with the result that what had once been grassland, e.g. chalk downs, started to become scrub and eventually woodland. Foxes ate more voles, beetles and blackberries than before and attacked more lambs and poultry.

Ultimate sources of energy

All the energy released on the Earth, apart from atomic energy and tidal power, comes from the sun, via food oxidized in animals and plants, coal from fossilized forests, petroleum from deposits of marine algae, or hydro-electric power from rainwater in lakes. There are ways of using the sun's energy directly and making it heat water to produce steam, but, at the moment, one of the best ways of trapping sunlight is to grow plants from which food and other energy-rich products can be collected.

Of the sunlight that reaches an area of grassland, only about 2 per cent is used for photosynthesis. The rest escapes the leaves, is reflected from their surface or is used to evaporate water from them in transpiration. When the vegetation is eaten by animals, only about 10 per cent of the food is converted to milk, meat or eggs; the other 90 per cent is used as a source of energy by the animal, or lost in faeces and urine. It follows that the most efficient use is made of plants when they are eaten directly by man and that their conversion to animal products is a wasteful process.

The carbon cycle

Food chains and food webs are but one link in the constant use and re-use of the Earth's chemical resources. The nitrogen cycle described on p. 51 is one example of this, and the carbon cycle described below is another. The carbon cycle consists, in essence, of the processes that increase or decrease the carbon dioxide in the environment (Fig. 9.5).

Removal of carbon dioxide from the atmosphere. Green plants, by their photosynthesis (p. 40), remove carbon dioxide from the atmosphere or water in which they grow (Experiment 3). The carbon of the carbon dioxide is incorporated at first into carbohydrates such as sugar or starch, and then eventually into the cellulose of cell walls and the proteins, pigments and other organic compounds comprised in living organisms. When the plants are eaten by animals the organic plant matter is digested, absorbed and built into compounds making the animals' tissues. Thus the carbon atoms from the plant become an integral part of the animal.

Addition of carbon dioxide to the atmosphere. (a) *Respiration.* Plants and animals obtain energy by oxidizing carbohydrates in their cells. breaking the compounds down to carbon dioxide and water (*see* p. 27). These products are excreted and the carbon dioxide returns once again to the environment (Experiment 2).

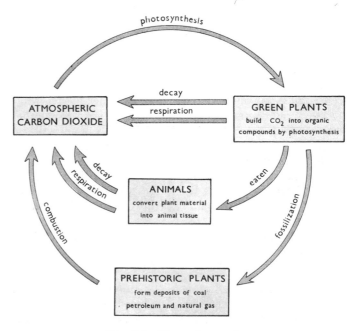

Fig. 9.5 The carbon cycle

(b) *Decay.* The organic matter of dead animals and plants is used by bacteria and fungi as a source of energy. The micro-organisms decompose the plant and animal material, converting the carbon compounds to carbon dioxide.

(c) *Combustion.* In the process of burning carbon-containing fuels such as wood, coal, petroleum and natural gas, the carbon is oxidized to carbon dioxide (Experiment 1). The hydrocarbon fuels originate from communities of plants, such as prehistoric forests or deposits of marine algae which have only partly decomposed over the millions of years since they were buried.

Thus, an atom of carbon which is today in a molecule of carbon dioxide in the air, may tomorrow be in a molecule of cellulose in the cell wall of a blade of grass. When the grass is eaten by a cow, the carbon atom may become one of many in a protein molecule in the cow's muscle. When the protein molecule is used for respiration, the carbon atom will enter the air once again as carbon dioxide. The same kind of cycling applies to nearly all the elements of the Earth. No new matter is created but it is repeatedly rearranged. A great proportion of the atoms of which you are composed will, at one time, have been an integral part of many other organisms.

Today, man's activities affect these cycles. For example, the nitrogen present in his excretory products is not usually re-cycled to the land producing his food; the carbon fuels are burned in ever-increasing quantities, depleting their sources and adding more carbon dioxide to the atmosphere.

The balance of nature

The 'balance' is a dynamic equilibrium and not a static state. For example, in one year in a given area there may be a population of 50 shrews which prey on a population of 10 000 beetles. Five years hence there may still be a 'balance' of 50 shrews and 10 000 beetles, but they will not be the same ones. The numbers will have been maintained against considerable pressures to change them. If each pair of shrews has three litters of six young per year and all the youngsters survived, the population of shrews after only one year would be 950. The beetles' reproductive capacity is greater still. There must therefore be a high mortality of both animals for the numbers to remain in balance from year to year.

In a natural environment the vegetation will support the herbivorous creatures which, in turn, will feed the carnivores; the natural cycles replenish the soil and nourish the plants. If the predators become too numerous, the herbivores will be eaten in greater numbers and their population will diminish; the vegetation, temporarily relieved from grazing, will grow more densely. Eventually the population of predators, having depleted the herbivores which constitute their food, will decline; the reduction of predators and the more luxuriant vegetation will permit the herbivores to flourish once more. Thus the populations remain basically constant with relatively minor fluctuations.

Civilized man, however, with his technology and agriculture, interrupts the natural cycles and disturbs the balance of nature to an extent which gives cause for concern.

(a) **Deforestation.** Trees may be cut down to make way for agriculture or to use the timber. If limited felling is done in the right areas and with provision for reafforestation, a balanced community can be maintained. The soil on sloping ground, however, is often thin and once the tree cover is removed is no longer protected by the leaf canopy from the forces of wind and rain. The topsoil is washed away, silting up rivers and lakes and causing floods (*see* p. 54).

(b) **Erosion.** Repeated ploughing of soils, exclusive use of artificial fertilizers and overgrazing of pastures can, in certain areas, lead to soil erosion as described on p. 53, ultimately making the land incapable of supporting life of any kind.

(c) **Eutrophication.** This is the overgrowth of aquatic plants resulting from an excess of nitrogenous salts reaching the rivers. The nitrates may come from farmland where heavy application of soluble nitrogenous fertilizers is taking place or from the effluent of treated sewage. Its effects are discussed more fully on p. 52.

(d) **Monoculture.** A natural environment usually has a wide variety of vegetation at different levels, flowering and fruiting at different times. This vegetation is exploited in different ways by the animals living there; e.g. deer browse on the leafy branches, rabbits crop the turf, squirrels take berries and nuts from the trees, and worms consume the leaves that fall from them. Agricultural practice involves removal of the natural plant and animal community and its replacement with large populations of a single species of plant or animal; arable fields given over to wheat, pastures supporting sheep exclusively. This practice obviously makes the environment unsuitable for the majority of its original inhabitants, indeed it is meant to; a mixed population of cereal and weeds is commercially undesirable. The practice of monoculture, however, has its disadvantages.

Parasites and pests, which in a mixed community find their hosts well spaced, can spread rapidly in a monoculture since suitable hosts are growing closely together. In many parts of Africa there is evidence to suggest that more protein could be obtained by harvesting the mixed populations of wild animals living in a natural environment than is derived from the herds of sickly cattle which replace them and destroy their habitat.

(e) **Pesticides.** To protect the plants in a monoculture from the depredations of insects the crops are often sprayed with insecticides such as the chlorinated hydrocarbon DDT. This prevents the loss of hundreds of tonnes of food but in some cases it upsets the dynamic balance of life in unexpected ways. For example, the chemicals affect harmful and beneficial insects alike, so that after spraying orchards to eliminate the codling moth whose larva burrows into apples, enormous numbers of red mites appeared because the spray had killed the spiders that normally preyed upon them.

For a few years after it had been discovered and developed, DDT seemed to be the perfect insecticide. Used to kill body lice and mosquitoes, it must have saved thousands of lives by eradicating typhus and malaria, spread respectively by these insects in certain areas and conditions. The concentrations used seemed harmless to man and other animals though, in higher concentrations, it was known to be poisonous, particularly to fish.

Unfortunately, however, when DDT is taken in with food and water it is not all eliminated from the body, a proportion being retained and accumulated in the fat deposits of the body. When, in some animals, the fat is mobilized for respiration, harmful quantities of DDT may be released into the blood.

The animals at the end of food chains are particularly vulnerable when DDT is used to kill insect pests on a large scale. In America, DDT was used to kill the beetle that transmits Dutch elm disease. The spray and the sprayed leaves reached the soil where the DDT was taken up by worms. When birds, notably the American robin, ate the worms, they accumulated lethal doses of DDT and whole populations of birds were wiped out.

A similar event occurred when an insecticide was used to kill gnat larvae in Clear Lake, California. At a concentration of 0.015 parts per million of insecticide in the lake water the fish were unharmed. After five years, however, the Western grebes on the lake were dying in large numbers. Although the water contained only 0.015 ppm the plankton living in the waters had accumulated the compound to a level of 5 ppm. The small fish which fed on the plankton contained 10 ppm and the predatory fish even higher concentrations. The grebes which fed on the larger fish had as much as 1 600 ppm in their body fat.

DDT is a stable compound and its effects last for a long time; a good property for an insecticide but potentially disastrous for the balance of nature. When applied to the crops, it reaches the soil and destroys the insect life there. Eventually it reaches the rivers, lakes and oceans where if sufficient accumulated, it could begin to poison the fish and other marine life.

There is no end to the examples of man's wilful or unwitting depredation of the Earth; the excessive killing of animals for food or profit, to a point where they are exterminated altogether; irrigation schemes which make dry areas more productive but spread the water snails that carry the disease bilharziasis; clearing tropical forests for agriculture and so providing conditions in which the tsetse fly can breed and spread sleeping sickness.

One is forced to the conclusion that the demands made on the biological systems of the world to support an ever-increasing human population and a rising standard of life will, unless stringently controlled, eventually destroy all natural resources and make the Earth's surface uninhabitable.

Practical Work

Experiment 1 Carbon dioxide from combustion of organic matter

Set up the apparatus as shown in Fig. 9.6a. Light the candle and start the filter pump (or aspirator) so that any gases from the candle flame are drawn through the test-tube.

Result. After a few minutes, water will condense in the stem of the funnel and the glass tubing and the lime water will go milky.

Interpretation. Candle wax is a hydrocarbon, containing carbon and hydrogen only. When it burns, the hydrogen combines with oxygen to make hydrogen oxide (water) which comes off as water vapour and condenses in the funnel stem. The carbon combines with oxygen to make carbon dioxide, which turns the lime water milky.

If the lime water in the tube is renewed, the experiment can be repeated by drawing the gases from a burning groundnut (peanut), or other suitable food sample, through the apparatus. The nut is stuck on the end of a mounted needle, ignited with a match or bunsen flame and held beneath the funnel.

To prove that the water vapour and carbon dioxide come from the burning substances and not from the atmosphere, the

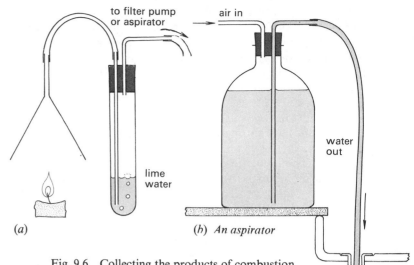

Fig. 9.6 Collecting the products of combustion

experiment should be repeated for the same length of time with nothing under the funnel, to show that there is no condensation in the funnel and that the lime water stays clear. (Although carbon dioxide *is* present in the atmosphere, there is so little of it (0.04 per cent) that it will not turn the lime water milky in this experiment.)

(*Note.* If a filter pump is not available, an aspirator can be set up as in Fig. 9.6b. A large jar is filled with water and fitted with a cork carrying two tubes as shown. The short glass tube is connected to the apparatus and by sucking through the long rubber tube, a siphon is started. As water runs out of the jar, air is drawn through the apparatus to replace it.)

Experiment 2 Production of carbon dioxide by living organisms

The apparatus and chemicals are assembled as in Fig. 9.7 The sodalime in A absorbs carbon dioxide from the atmosphere, and so the lime water in B should remain clear throughout the experiment. When the apparatus is connected to a filter pump or aspirator (*see* Experiment 1 and Fig. 9.6b) air is drawn through vessel C which contains one or more living organisms, e.g. toads or mice.

Result. The lime water in D goes milky, while that in B remains clear.

Interpretation. The organisms in C must be producing carbon dioxide.

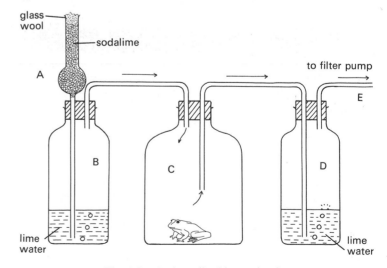

Fig. 9.7 Carbon dioxide production

Experiment 3   **Gaseous exchange in leaves**

Three test-tubes are washed with tap water, distilled water and hydrogencarbonate indicator in turn before placing 3 cm³ hydrogencarbonate indicator in each. A green leaf is placed in tubes 1 and 2 so that each leaf is held against the walls of the tube and does not touch the indicator (Fig. 9.8). The three tubes are closed with bungs, tube 1 is covered with aluminium foil, and all three are placed in a rack in direct sunlight or a few centimetres from a bench lamp for about forty minutes.

Result. The indicator (which was originally orange) should not change colour in tube 3, the control; that in tube 1, with the leaf in darkness, should turn yellow; and in tube 2, with the illuminated leaf, the indicator should be scarlet or purple.

Interpretation. Hydrogencarbonate indicator is a mixture of dilute sodium hydrogencarbonate solution with the dyes cresol red and thymol blue. It is a pH indicator in equilibrium with the atmospheric carbon dioxide, i.e. its original colour represents the acidity produced by the carbon dioxide in the air. Increase in atmospheric carbon dioxide makes it more acid and it changes colour from orange to yellow. Decrease in atmospheric carbon dioxide makes it less acid and causes a colour change to red or purple.

Thus the results provide evidence that in darkness (tube 1) leaves produce carbon dioxide (from respiration), while in light (tube 2) they use up more carbon dioxide in photosynthesis than they produce in respiration. Tube 3 is the control, showing that it is the presence of the leaf which causes a change in the atmosphere in the test-tube.

For experiments on gaseous exchange in man see p. 90. The formulae for hydrogencarbonate indicator and other reagents are given on p. 268.

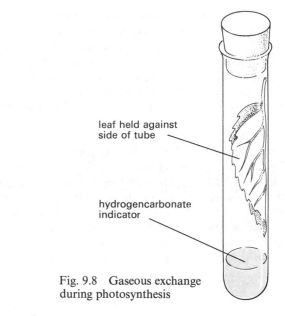

leaf held against side of tube

hydrogencarbonate indicator

Fig. 9.8   Gaseous exchange during photosynthesis

Questions

1   Trace the food chains involved in the production of the following articles o man's diet: eggs, cheese, bread, meat, wine. In each case show how the energy in the food originates from sunlight.
2   Discuss the advantages and disadvantages of man's attempting to exploi a food chain nearer to its source, e.g. the diatoms of Fig. 9.1.
3   Construct a diagram, on the lines of the carbon cycle (Fig. 9.5), to show the cycling process for hydrogen.
4   How do you think evidence is acquired in order to assign animals such a leopard and pigeon to their position in a food web?
5   What would be the desirable qualities of an insecticide to control an insec pest of a crop plant? What might be the disadvantages of total eradication o such an insect pest?
6   Why are the animals at the end of a food chain likely to be more seriously affected by a harmful pesticide than the animals at the beginning?

10

The Digestion, Absorption and Metabolism of Food

To be of any value to the body, the food taken in through the mouth must enter the blood stream and be distributed to all living tissues.

Digestion is the process by which insoluble food consisting of large molecules is broken down into soluble compounds with smaller molecules. These smaller molecules, in solution, pass through the walls of the intestine and eventually enter the blood stream. Digestion and absorption take place in the alimentary canal (Figs. 10.1 and 10.2), digestion being brought about by chemical compounds called enzymes (*see* p. 27). The alimentary canal is a muscular tube running from mouth to anus with a glandular lining called the *mucous membrane* or *mucosa*. In general, the alimentary canal has an outer tough coat over layers of longitudinal and circular unstriated muscle (p. 119) which themselves enclose a *submucosa* containing networks of blood capillaries and a plexus of nerve fibres. Lining the inside of the alimentary canal is the mucous membrane or mucosa, consisting of an epithelium beneath which is connective tissue and a thin layer of unstriated muscle (Fig. 10.5) The outer muscular layers propel the contents of the alimentary canal while the mucosa secretes (a) enzymes which digest the food and (b) mucus which lubricates and protects the internal surface of the gut.

Certain regions of the alimentary canal are specialized for particular functions and have differing structures. Digestive juices are secreted into the alimentary canal from glands in the

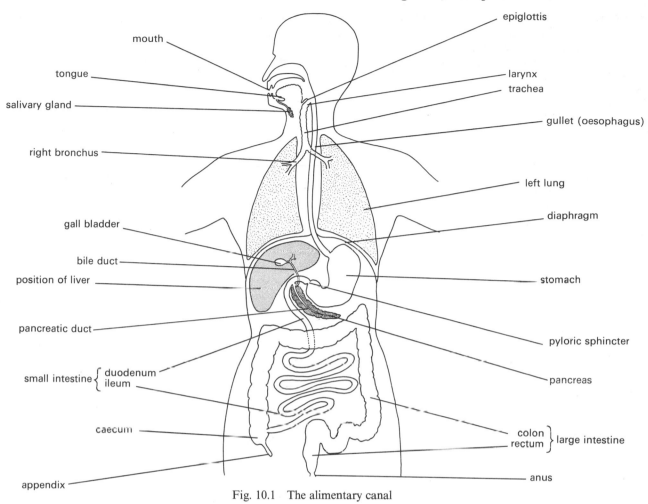

Fig. 10.1   The alimentary canal

Fig. 10.2   Alimentary canal of a rat unravelled

(Dissection by Gerrard & Haig Ltd)

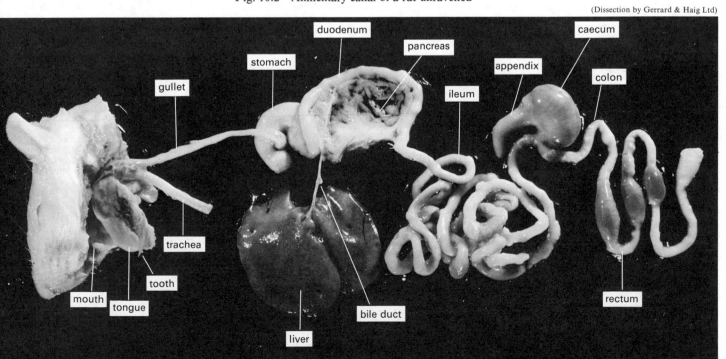

mucosa or through ducts from glandular organs outside it. The food is broken down in stages as it passes through the alimentary canal until the digestible material is dissolved and absorbed. The indigestible residue is expelled along with other products through the anus.

Enzymes are chemical compounds, protein in nature, made in the cells of living organisms. They act as catalysts and accelerate the rate of chemical changes in the organism without altering the end products. They occur in great numbers and varieties in all protoplasm and without them the chemical reactions would be too slow to maintain life. The vast majority of enzymes are *intracellular,* that is, they carry out their functions in the protoplasm of the cell in which they are made. Some enzymes, however, are secreted out of the cell in which they are made, to be used elsewhere. These are called *extracellular* enzymes. Bacteria (p. 195) and fungi secrete such extracellular enzymes into the medium in which they are growing. The higher organisms secrete extracellular enzymes into the alimentary tract to act on the food taken into it.

The chemical process of digestion is basically *hydrolysis,* in which the protein, carbohydrate and fat molecules have certain of their chemical bonds broken by adding the elements of water, –H and –OH, at these points. The process is discussed more fully on p. 16. Hydrolysis of food substances takes place on simply adding water, but the reactions are too slow to meet the needs of the body. The rates of the reactions are, however, greatly increased by enzymes, which speed up the hydrolysis and produce soluble products within minutes. Each type of food and each stage in its digestion needs a particular enzyme; those acting on starch are called *amylases,* those hydrolysing proteins are *proteinases,* and *lipases* accelerate the digestion of fats. The properties of enzymes are discussed more fully on p. 27, and the generalizations about them apply equally to digestive enzymes, namely (a) they speed up chemical reactions but cannot alter the end products, (b) they catalyse only one type of reaction, (c) their rate of working is influenced by temperature and pH, and (d) they are inactivated by temperatures above 45 °C.

Movement of food through the alimentary canal

Ingestion is the act of taking food into the alimentary canal through the mouth.

Swallowing (*see* Fig. 10.3). In swallowing, the following actions take place: (a) the tongue presses upwards and back against the roof of the mouth, forcing the pellet of food, called a *bolus,* to the back of the mouth or *pharynx*; (b) the soft palate closes the opening between the nasal cavity and the pharynx; (c) the laryngeal cartilage round the top of the trachea, or windpipe, is pulled upwards by muscles so that the opening of the larynx lies beneath the back of the tongue, and the opening of the trachea is constricted by the contraction of a ring of muscle; and (d) the *epiglottis,* a flap of cartilage, directs food over the laryngeal orifice. In this way food is able to pass over the trachea without entering it. The beginning of this action is voluntary, but once the bolus of food reaches the pharynx, swallowing becomes an automatic or reflex action. The food is forced into and down the *oesophagus,* or gullet, by *peristalsis* (*see* below). This takes about six seconds with relatively solid food and then the food is admitted to the stomach. Liquid travels more rapidly down the gullet. A small volume of air is inevitably swallowed with the food and accumulates in the upper part of the stomach.

Peristalsis (Fig. 10.4). The walls of the alimentary canal contain circular and longitudinal muscle fibres. The circular muscles, by contracting and relaxing alternately, urge the food in a wave-like motion through the various regions of the alimentary canal.

Egestion. The expulsion from the alimentary canal of the undigested remains of food is called *egestion.*

Digestion in the mouth

In the mouth the food is chewed and mixed with saliva. Chewing reduces the food to a suitable size for swallowing and

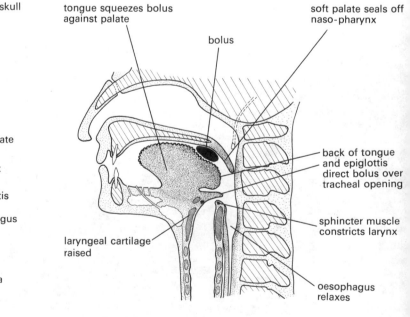

Fig. 10.3   Section through head to show swallowing action

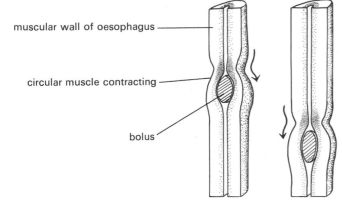

Fig. 10.4   Peristalsis

also increases the available surface for enzymes to act on. Saliva is a digestive juice secreted by three pairs of glands whose ducts lead into the mouth (Fig. 10.3). The glands include two types of cell, one of which produces mucus and the other an enzyme, salivary amylase. The resulting fluid, which may be secreted in quantities up to 1.5 litres per day by an adult, is watery and neutral or slightly acid. The mucus helps to lubricate the food and stick the particles together, while the amylase acts on cooked starch and begins to break it down to maltose (p. 16), a soluble sugar (see Experiment 1). The longer that food is retained in the mouth, the further this starch digestion proceeds and the more finely divided does the food become as a result of chewing; but the digestive action of the salivary amylase does not seem particularly important since even well-chewed food does not remain long enough in the mouth for much digestion of starch to take place, although saliva will continue to act for a time even when food is passed to the stomach.

Small quantities of saliva are secreted continually, so keeping the lining of the mouth moist and permitting clear speech. In addition, dissolving some of the food taken into the mouth enables the taste-sensitive cells of the tongue to be stimulated by the chemicals present (see p. 132).

Digestion in the stomach

This part of the alimentary canal has very elastic walls and so can be extended by the accumulation of a relatively large quantity of food, which is retained by the closure of the pyloric sphincter at the lower end of the stomach. These characteristics of the stomach enable the food from a particular meal to be stored for some time and released at intervals to the rest of the alimentary canal. If there were no stomach, food would have to be taken every twenty minutes or so.

There is no evidence to indicate that absorption, other than that of water, salts, alcohol and a little glucose, takes place in the stomach, but its mucosa produces gastric juice. There are numerous tube-like glands in the mucous membrane, which open in small groups into pits (Figs. 10.5 and 10.6). Lining the glandular tubes are three types of cell which produce *pepsinogen,* hydrochloric acid and mucus respectively, making up gastric juice which is secreted through the pits into the stomach. Gastric juice may also contain, in young children, an enzyme called *rennin.* When pepsinogen and hydrochloric acid meet in the stomach the former is activated to produce the enzyme *pepsin* which acts on the long chain molecules of

proteins and breaks them down to shorter chains of more soluble compounds called *peptides* (see p. 17 and Experiment 2). Rennin, if present, clots the protein in milk, but pepsin alone has a similar effect and it is thought that the acidity in an adult's stomach would be too great for the effective action of rennin. The hydrochloric acid makes a solution of about 0.5 per cent by weight in the gastric juice, providing the optimum pH (see p. 21) for pepsin to work in and also probably killing many of the bacteria taken in with the food. The salivary amylase swallowed with the food cannot digest starch in acid conditions, but it seems likely that it continues to act within the bolus of food until this is broken up and hydrochloric acid reaches all its contents.

The rhythmic peristaltic waves passing across the stomach from the oesophageal to the pyloric end, about once every twenty seconds, churn up the food and gastric juice to a creamy fluid called *chyme.* This reduction of a meal to a fluid consistency and its delivery in small quantities at a time to the rest of the alimentary canal is perhaps the most important function of the stomach.

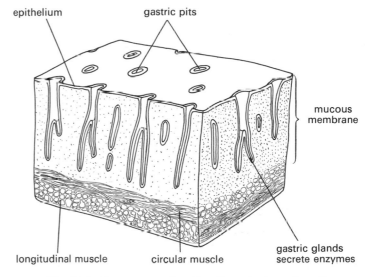

Fig. 10.5   Stereogram of section through stomach wall

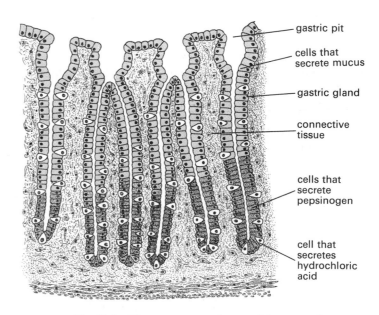

Fig. 10.6   The mucous membrane of the stomach

The length of time for which food is retained in the stomach depends to a large extent on the contents of the meal. Water may pass through in a few minutes, a meal of starch such as porridge may be retained less than an hour, one containing meat will be held longer while the presence of fat considerably retards the emptying of the stomach. Excitement may accelerate emptying, and fear may stop the gastric movements and cause the stomach to retain its contents up to twelve hours. When digestion in the stomach is complete, the pyloric sphincter relaxes from time to time allowing a little chyme to pass through into the first part of the small intestine, called the *duodenum*.

Digestion in the duodenum

An alkaline juice from the pancreas and bile from the liver are poured into the duodenum. The pancreas is a cream-coloured gland lying below the stomach (Fig. 10.7). Its cells

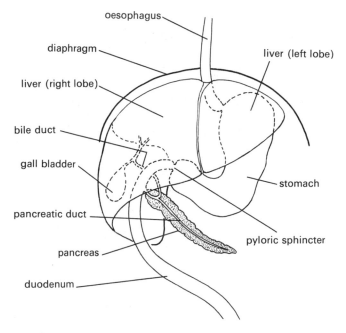

Fig. 10.7   Relationship of stomach, liver and pancreas

make about 1 500 cm^3 pancreatic juice per day, containing water, sodium hydrogencarbonate and three principal enzymes—an amylase, a lipase and *trypsinogen*—which act on starch, fats and proteins respectively. Trypsinogen is inactive until it meets a chemical activator called *enterokinase* secreted by the duodenal mucosa. The enterokinase activates the trypsinogen which becomes the enzyme *trypsin*; this enzyme breaks down proteins to peptides, which another enzyme converts to amino acids (*see* p. 17). Starch is broken down to maltose by the amylase, while fats are split into fatty acids and glycerol by the lipase (*see* p. 17 and Experiment 3). Glands in the duodenal mucosa produce mucus.

The sodium hydrogencarbonate in pancreatic juice partly neutralizes the acid chyme from the stomach and so creates a suitable pH for the pancreatic and intestinal enzymes.

Bile is a green, watery, alkaline fluid made continuously in the liver at the rate of about 500–1 000 cm^3 per day, stored in the gall bladder and conducted to the duodenum by the bile duct.

The gall bladder can hold about 30 cm^3 bile and concentrate it about ten times by absorbing water. When food enters the duodenum from the stomach, the gall bladder contracts and expels bile into the duodenum.

The colour of the bile is derived largely from the breakdown products of the red pigment *haemoglobin* from decomposing red blood cells. Bile also contains complex organic salts which assist the digestion and absorption of fats, principally by reducing the surface tension of the fat drops. This results in their forming an emulsion of tiny droplets whose increased surface area permits rapid digestion by lipase. Most of the bile salts are reabsorbed in the small intestine and returned by the circulatory system to the liver where they stimulate further secretion of bile. Any disorder which impairs the absorption of fats also reduces the uptake of the fat-soluble vitamins A, D and K.

Peristaltic waves pass down the duodenum and ileum at about 2 cm per second, moving the semidigested food along. In addition, there are muscular movements which churn the fluids back and forth.

Digestion in the ileum

The remaining three metres of small intestine after the duodenum are called the ileum. Mucus and several enzymes are secreted as intestinal juice by its mucosal lining. *Erepsin*, a mixture of proteinases, completes the digestion of protein by reducing peptides to amino acids; amylase converts unchanged starch into maltose and a lipase splits any remaining fats into fatty acids and glycerol or glycerides. In addition the disaccharide sugars, maltose, sucrose and lactose, are broken down into the monosaccharides, glucose, fructose and galactose, by enzymes specific for each sugar.

Cellulose cannot be digested by humans, but in the paunch (rumen) of cows and goats, the large intestine of the horse and the caecum of the rabbit live a vast number of bacteria and other micro-organisms which are able to break down cellulose and are themselves eventually digested.

Most of the digestible material by this stage is reduced to soluble compounds which can pass through the intestinal lining and into the blood stream.

Prevention of self-digestion. The glandular lining of the alimentary canal secretes mucus continually and independently of enzyme secretion. This mucus helps to lubricate the passage of food but also prevents the digestive juices from reaching and digesting the alimentary canal itself. The cells which make the protein-digesting enzymes would themselves be digested by these chemicals were it not for the fact that the enzymes are made in an inactive form and cannot work until they reach the cavity of the alimentary canal, where they are activated by the chemicals present. Trypsin, for example, is made and secreted as an inactive substance, trypsinogen. When trypsinogen is set free in the duodenum, the enterokinase present converts it to active trypsin. This trypsin cannot now digest the duodenal walls because of their protective coating of mucus.

Absorption in the ileum

Nearly all the absorption of digested food takes place in the ileum. The following characteristics of the ileum greatly facilitate its absorbing properties:

(a) it is very long, and so presents a large absorbing surface to the digested food;

(b) this surface is greatly increased by thousands of tiny, finger-like projections called *villi*, 20–40 to each square millimetre (Figs. 10.8 and 10.10);

(c) the lining epithelium is very thin and the fluids can pass rapidly through it;

(d) there is a dense network of blood capillaries in each villus (Fig. 10.9).

The molecules of amino acids and glucose pass through the epithelium and capillary walls to enter the blood plasma. They are then carried away in the capillaries, which unite to form veins and eventually join up to form one large vein, the

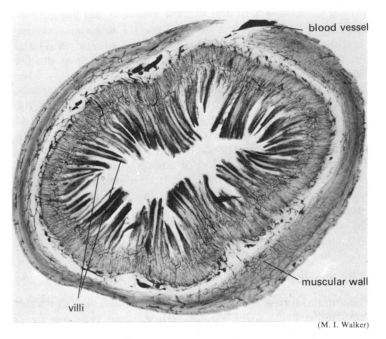

(M. I. Walker)

Fig. 10.10 Transverse section through ileum of cat showing villi

hepatic portal, which carries all the blood from the intestine to the liver. The liver may retain or alter some of the absorbed substances (*see* p. 69). After this, the digested food reaches the general circulation.

Glycerol, glycerides and fatty acids from the digestion of fats may also enter the capillaries of the villus, but for the most part the products of fat digestion are built up into fats again in the epithelium of the intestinal mucosa and then enter the *lacteals* to be carried away in the lymph. Large fatty acid molecules may enter the lacteals, while the smaller molecules are carried in the capillaries together with amino acids, glucose and related sugars. Total digestion of fats to fatty acids and glycerol is not essential for absorption, but the emulsification by bile

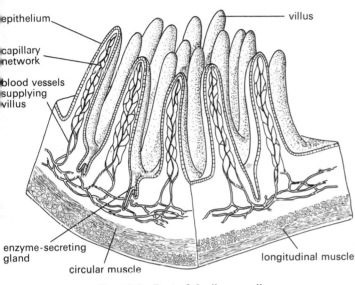

Fig. 10.8 Part of the ileum wall

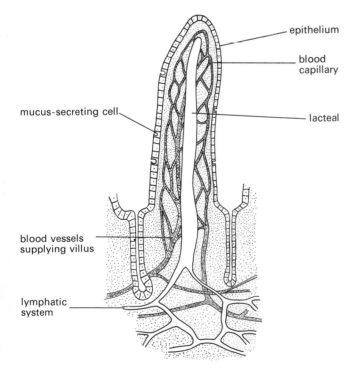

Fig. 10.9 Structure of villus

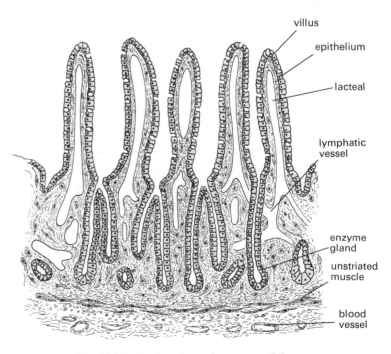

Fig. 10.11 Section through mucosa of ileum

salts is very important and there is evidence that partial production of fatty acids and glycerol greatly accelerates emulsification of undigested fats. The fat-soluble vitamins A, D and K are absorbed along with the fats. The lacteals open into the lymphatic system (p. 83) which forms a network all over the body and eventually empties its contents into the blood stream.

The movements of the dissolved substances through the intestinal wall cannot be explained by diffusion alone. The soluble molecules may enter into chemical combination with substances in the epithelial cells in the course of their journey, for example the combination of glucose with phosphate, but the detailed mechanisms have not been worked out.

The food may spend from three to four hours in the small intestine before it passes into the large intestine through the ileo-colic sphincter.

The large intestine (colon and rectum)

The material passing into the large intestine consists of water and undigested matter, largely cellulose and vegetable fibres (roughage), dead bacteria, mucus and dead cells from the lining of the alimentary canal. The colon secretes no enzymes and can absorb little or no digested food. It does, however, absorb much of the water from the undigested residues and other waste. The copious secretion of digestive juices extracts a great deal of water from the blood and pours it into the alimentary canal. If this water were not returned to the blood stream by the colon, the loss of fluid from the body would be excessive and lead to dehydration. This is one of the dangers of acute and prolonged diarrhoea (*see* p. 67). In normal conditions the partially dried and semi-solid wastes, the *faeces* are passed into the rectum by peristalsis and expelled at intervals through the anus.

The entry of the contents of the colon into the rectum distends it and sets off a sensory impulse which produces the urge to defaecate, i.e. expel the faeces. Habit and opportunity control this urge and defaecation may take place with a frequency varying from three times a day to every third day according to the individual, there being no special physiological value in any particular frequency.

The components of faeces are largely the product of the alimentary tract itself, e.g. dead cells from its mucosa, dead bacteria and mucus, and are therefore produced whether food is taken or not, though the composition will vary with the food. There is some indication that a large residue of undigested cellulose giving bulk to the contents of the colon is effective in setting off the peristaltic reflex, so that a diet containing roughage may prevent constipation in those prone to this disorder.

Digestive action

Region of alimentary canal	Digestive gland	Digestive juice produced	Enzymes in the juice	Class of food acted upon	Substances produced	Notes
MOUTH	Salivary glands	Saliva	Salivary amylase	Starch	Maltose	Slightly acid or neutral. Mucus helps form bolus. Water lubricates food.
STOMACH	Gastric glands (in stomach lining)	Gastric juice	Pepsin	Proteins	Peptides	0.5% hydrochloric acid also secreted, provides acid medium for pepsin and kills most bacteria. No absorption except of alcohol.
			(Rennin)	(Milk protein)	(Clots it)	
DUODENUM	Pancreas	Pancreatic juice	Trypsin	Proteins and peptides	Amino acids	Two other protein-digesting enzymes are present. Bile emulsifies fats and aids their absorption. Duodenum contents slightly acid.
			Amylase	Starch	Maltose	
	(Liver)	(Bile)	Lipase	Fats	Fatty acids and glycerol	
ILEUM	Glands in ileum lining between villi	Succus entericus	Erepsin	Peptides	Amino acids	Most absorption occurs in the ileum.
			Lipase	Fats	Fatty acids and glycerol	
			Maltase	Maltose	Glucose	
			Sucrase	Sucrose	Glucose and fructose	
			Lactase	Lactose	Glucose and galactose	
COLON						Absorption of water

Constipation. Retention of the contents of the lower colon for long periods may lead to constipation. The urge to defaecate is depressed and the faeces are difficult to expel. Constipation may accompany or cause other symptoms of ill-health, not on account of the toxic products of bacterial decay in the colon but because of the physical distension of the rectum. Laxatives are chemicals which act by irritating the lining of the colon and in this respect are harmful on account of the likelihood of developing a dependence on these chemicals to produce regular emptying of the colon.

Diarrhoea usually results from inflammation of the large or small intestine during bacterial or virus infection. The irritation brings about frequent and violent peristalsis which expels the contents of the colon before they have been retained long enough for adequate absorption of water. Normally the residues should spend from 12 to 24 hours in the large intestine, being moved on by vigorous waves of peristalsis three or four times a day.

Caecum and appendix. These are relatively small structures in man and their functions, if any, are not clear. In herbivores such as the rat and the horse, the caecum and appendix are much larger and it is here that most of the cellulose digestion takes place, largely as a result of bacterial activity. In man, bacteria invade the colon soon after birth and play a part in producing vitamin K and some vitamins of the B group.

Control of secretion

Digestive juices are only secreted when food is present in the appropriate part of the alimentary canal. In this way, wastage of enzymes is avoided. Secretion is co-ordinated by both the nervous and endocrine systems (p. 145).

Saliva is secreted continuously but the presence of food in the mouth sets off a nervous reflex, initiated in the sensory cells of the taste buds (p. 132), resulting in not only a greater volume of salivary secretion but also an increase in its enzyme content. Salivation is also subject to conditioned reflexes (p. 150).

Secretion in the stomach is initiated by a reflex set off by the presence of food in the mouth, and maintained by the presence of food, especially meat, in the stomach. A hormone, *gastrin*, is liberated by the pyloric end of the stomach and, on returning to the gastric glands in the blood circulation, stimulates the continued production of enzymes. The first reflex, as in salivation, is subject to conditioning and is inhibited by fear or disgust.

Pancreatic secretion takes place when the acid contents of the stomach reach the duodenum causing the production of two hormones, *secretin* and *pancreozymin*, which on being conveyed in the circulation to the pancreas stimulate it to produce enzymes. Secretin, however, is produced before food reaches the duodenum and its release is therefore likely to be initiated by nervous reflex. The pancreatic fluid resulting from stimulation by secretin is watery and alkaline, while that resulting from the effect of pancreozymin is rich in enzymes.

Intestinal secretion is likely to be the result of the mechanical stimulation of the intestinal wall by the presence of food and the effect of the digested products on its mucosa.

Hunger and thirst. The causes of the sensation of hunger are not understood but it is apparent that the sensation is an essential preliminary to adequate feeding. The depression of the sensation of hunger could lead to inadequate intake in respect of both dietetic balance (p. 37) and energy value. Smoking, chewing and the action of certain drugs will reduce hunger.

The empty stomach has been shown in some cases to contract slowly for periods of about 20 seconds over half an hour and may thus produce the 'pangs' of hunger, though it is more likely that there are centres of hunger and satiety in the brain. Hunger is a physiological need for food, whereas appetite is a psychological anticipation of food. It appears that appetite is an aid to digestion and that one's psychological state when eating can influence the course of digestion, probably by its effect on the muscular action of the alimentary canal and the secretion of enzymes. As has already been pointed out, fear and disgust can inhibit the secretion of saliva and gastric juice. Tension and disharmony at meal times therefore may produce indigestion.

Indigestion is the term applied in general to all sensations of discomfort in the stomach or duodenum. The causes vary from simple over-distension by eating too much or the accumulation of gases, to ulceration and excessive production of hydrochloric acid. 'Acid indigestion' is a fruitful source of profit for the manufacturers of patent alkalies, but only a doctor can diagnose whether the pain is the result of excessive hydrochloric acid in the stomach. Although in many cases antacids (alkalis) relieve the symptoms of indigestion by neutralization of hydrochloric acid, they can be harmful if taken over long periods. The sodium hydrogencarbonate (bicarbonate) mixtures can cause a disturbance in the salt balance in the body, and by suppressing the symptoms they may postpone a medical consultation by which a serious condition such as a stomach ulcer would be diagnosed.

Utilization of digested food

The products of digestion are carried round the body in solution in the blood. From the blood, most living cells are able to absorb and metabolize glucose, fats and amino acids.

(a) **Glucose.** During respiration in the protoplasm, glucose is oxidized to carbon dioxide and water (*see* p. 27). This reaction releases energy to drive the many chemical processes in the cell, and in specialized cells produces, for example, contraction (muscle cells) and electrical changes (nerve cells).

(b) **Fats.** Fats are incorporated into cell membranes and other structures in cells. The fats not used for growth and maintenance in this way are oxidized to carbon dioxide and water, releasing energy for the vital processes of the cells. Twice as much energy is obtained from fats as from glucose.

(c) **Amino acids** are absorbed by cells and reassembled to make proteins (p. 17). These proteins may form visible structures such as the cell membrane and other components of the protoplasm or the proteins may be enzymes which control and co-ordinate the chemical activity within the cell.

Amino acids not required for building proteins are deaminated in the liver, that is, their nitrogen is removed and the residue is used in the same way as carbohydrate, namely oxidized, or converted to glycogen and stored.

Storage of digested food

If the quantity of food taken in exceeds the energy requirements of the body or the demand for structural materials, it is stored in one of the following ways:

(a) **Glucose** (Fig. 10.13). The concentration of glucose in the blood of a person who has not eaten for eight hours is usually between 90 and 100 mg/100 cm^3 blood. After a meal containing carbohydrate, the blood sugar level may rise to 140 mg/100 cm^3 but two hours later, the level returns to about 95 mg.

The sugar not required immediately for the energy supply in the cells is converted in the liver and in the muscles to glycogen. The glycogen molecule is built up by combining many glucose molecules in a long branching chain rather similar to the starch molecule. About 100 g of this insoluble glycogen is stored in the liver and about 300 g in the muscles. When the blood sugar level falls below 80 mg/100 cm^3, the liver converts its glycogen back to glucose and releases it into the circulation. The muscle glycogen is not normally returned to the circulation but is used by active muscle as a source of energy in much the same way as glucose.

The glycogen in the liver is a 'short-term' store, sufficient for about only six hours if no other glucose supply is available. Excess glucose not stored as glycogen is converted to fat and stored in the fat cells of the fat depots. (*See* below.)

(b) **Fats.** Certain cells can accumulate drops of fat in their cytoplasm. As these drops increase in size and number, they join together to form one large globule of fat in the middle of the cell, pushing the cytoplasm into a thin layer and the nucleus to one side (Fig. 10.12). Groups of fat cells form *adipose tissue* beneath the skin and in the connective tissue of most organs (Fig. 14.3, p. 97).

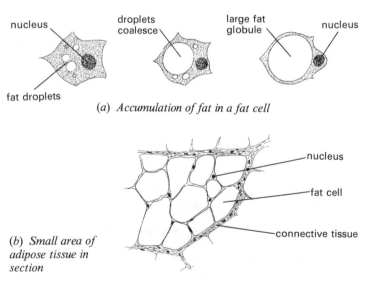

(*a*) *Accumulation of fat in a fat cell*

(*b*) *Small area of adipose tissue in section*

Fig. 10.12   Adipose tissue

Unlike glycogen, there is no limit to the amount of fat stored and because of its high energy value it is an important reserve of energy-giving food.

(c) **Amino acids** (Fig. 10.14). Amino acids are not stored in the body. Those not used in protein formation are deaminated. The protein of the liver and tissues can act as a kind of protein store to maintain the protein level in the blood, but absence of protein in the diet soon leads to serious disorders.

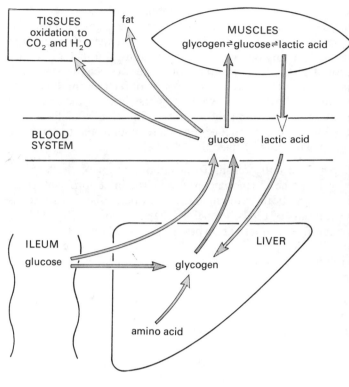

Fig. 10.13   Carbohydrate metabolism

(Figs. 10.13 and 10.14 by kind permission of Bell, G. H., Davidson, J. N., Scarborough, H., *Textbook of Physiology and Biochemistry*, 4th edn, Edinburgh, Livingstone, 1959)

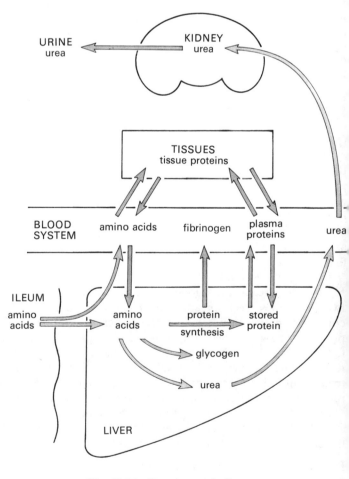

Fig. 10.14   Protein metabolism

The rate of oxidation of glucose and its conversion to glycogen or fat is controlled by hormones (p. 156). When intake of carbohydrate and fat exceeds the energy requirements of the body, the excess will be stored mainly as fat. Some people never seem to get fat no matter how much they eat, while others start to lay down fat when their intake only marginally exceeds their needs. Putting on weight is unquestionably the result of eating more food than the body needs but it is not clear why individuals should differ so much in their reaction. The explanation probably lies in the hormonal balance which, to some extent, is determined by heredity. A slimming diet designed to reduce calorific intake must, nevertheless, always include the essential amino acids, vitamins, mineral salts and certain essential fatty acids.

The liver

The liver is a large, reddish-brown organ which lies just below the diaphragm and partly overlaps the stomach (Fig. 10.7). In addition to a supply of oxygenated blood from the *hepatic artery*, it receives all the blood that leaves the alimentary canal. It has a great many important functions, some of which are described below. (*See* Figs. 10.13 and 10.14.)

1 **Regulation of blood sugar.** The liver is able to convert glucose, amino acids and other substances to an insoluble carbohydrate, *glycogen*. Some of the glucose so converted may be taken from the *hepatic portal* vein carrying blood rich in digested food from the ileum to the liver. About 100 g glycogen is stored in the liver of a healthy man. If the concentration of glucose in the blood falls below about 80 mg/100 cm^3 blood, some of the glycogen stored in the liver is converted by enzyme action into glucose and it enters the circulation. If the blood sugar level rises above 160 mg/100 cm^3, glucose is excreted by the kidneys. A blood glucose level below 40 mg/100 cm^3 affects the brain cells adversely, leading to convulsions and coma. By helping to keep the glucose concentration between 80 and 150 mg the liver prevents these undesirable effects and so contributes to the homeostasis (*see* below) of the body. (*See* Fig. 11.9 for circulatory supply to liver.)

2 **Formation of bile.** Green and yellow pigments are formed when the red blood cells break down. These pigments are removed from the blood by the liver and excreted in the bile. The liver also produces bile salts which play an important part in the emulsification and subsequent absorption of fats (p. 64).

Bile is produced continuously by the liver cells, but stored and concentrated in the gall bladder. It is discharged through the bile duct into the duodenum when the acid chyme arrives there. Bile is reabsorbed with the fats it emulsifies and eventually returns to the liver.

3 **Storage of iron.** Millions of red blood cells break up every day. In the liver their decomposition is completed and the iron from the haemoglobin is stored.

4 **Deamination.** Excess amino acids are not stored in the body. Amino acids that are not built up into proteins and used for growth and replacement are converted to carbohydrates by the removal from the molecule of the *amino group*, $-NH_2$, which contains the nitrogen. The residue can be converted to glycogen, being stored or oxidized to release energy. The nitrogen of the amino group is converted in the liver to *urea*, an excretory product that is constantly eliminated by the kidneys.

5 **Manufacture of plasma proteins.** The liver makes most of the proteins found in blood plasma, including fibrinogen which plays an important part in the clotting action of the blood (p. 73).

6 **Body heat.** The above list shows that a great many chemical changes go on in the liver and many of them release energy in the form of heat. This heat is distributed throughout the body by the circulatory system and helps to maintain the body temperature.

7 **Use of fats in the body.** When fats stored in the body are required for use in providing energy, they travel in the blood stream from the fat depots. When they reach the liver they are converted to substances which can be readily oxidized by other tissues to release energy.

8 **Detoxication.** Poisonous compounds, produced in the large intestine by the action of bacteria on amino acids, enter the blood, but on reaching the liver are converted to harmless substances, later excreted in the urine. Many other chemical substances normally present in the body or introduced as drugs are modified by the liver before being excreted by the kidneys. The hormones, for example, are converted to inactive compounds in the liver so limiting their period of activity in the body.

9 **Storage of vitamins.** The fat-soluble vitamins A and D are stored in the liver. This is the reason why animal liver is a valuable source of these vitamins in the diet. The liver also stores a product of the vitamin B_{12}. This product is necessary for the normal production of red cells in the bone marrow.

Homeostasis

A complete account of the functions of the liver would involve a very long list. It is most important, however, to realize that the one vital function of the liver, embodying all the details outlined above, is that it helps to maintain the concentration and composition of the body fluids, particularly the blood.

Within reason, a variation in the kind of food eaten will not produce changes in the composition of the blood.

If this *internal environment*, as it is called, were not so constant, the chemical changes that maintain life would become erratic and unpredictable so that with quite slight changes of diet or activity the whole organization might break down. The regulation of the internal environment is called *homeostasis* and is discussed again on pp. 72, 92 and 157.

Practical Work

Experiment 1 **The digestive action of saliva on starch**

Saliva is collected in a test-tube after rinsing the mouth to remove traces of food, and about 1 cm^3 is added to each of two test-tubes, A and B, containing approximately 2 cm^3 of 2 per cent starch solution. A control is set up by preparing two more tubes, C and D, with the same volume of starch solution but with boiled saliva. After 5 minutes, tube A is tested with iodine solution while tube B is boiled with Benedict's solution (*see* p. 38). The controls C and D are similarly tested.

Result. Failure to obtain a blue colour with iodine indicates that starch is no longer present, while a red precipitate with Benedict's reagent shows that a sugar has been produced. Control C should give a blue colour with iodine while D should not give a red precipitate with Benedict's solution.

Interpretation. The disappearance of starch and the appearance of sugar when unboiled saliva is present suggests that the latter contains an enzyme that promotes this change.

Experiment 2   The action of pepsin on egg-white (albumen)

The white of one egg is stirred into 500 cm³ tap water. The mixture is boiled and filtered through glass wool to remove large particles. About 2 cm depth of the cloudy suspension is poured into each of four tubes labelled A to D. To A is added 1 cm³ of 1 per cent pepsin solution; to B is added 3 drops of dilute hydrochloric acid; to C, 1 cm³ of pepsin solution and 3 drops of acid; and to D, 3 drops of acid and 1 cm³ boiled pepsin solution. All four test-tubes are placed in a beaker of water at 35–40 °C for 5–10 minutes.

Result. The contents of tube C only will become clear; the others will remain cloudy.

Interpretation. The change from a cloudy suspension to a clear solution suggests that the solid egg-white particles have been digested to soluble products. This result, and those of the controls A, B and D, support the idea that pepsin is an enzyme that digests albumen (a protein) in acid conditions.

Experiment 3   The action of lipase

5 cm³ milk and 7 cm³ dilute (M/20) sodium carbonate solution are placed in each of three test-tubes labelled 1 to 3, and six drops of phenolphthalein are added to each tube to colour the contents bright pink. To tubes 2 and 3 is added 1 cm³ of 3 per cent bile salts solution. To tubes 1 and 3 is added 1 cm³ of 5 per cent lipase solution, and to tube 2 an equal volume of boiled lipase solution.

Result. In 10 minutes or less, the colour of the liquids in tubes 1 and 3 will change to white, tube 3 changing first. The liquid in tube 2 will remain pink.

Interpretation. Lipase is an enzyme that hydrolyses fats to fatty acids and glycerol. When lipase acts on milk fats, the fatty acids so produced react with the alkaline sodium carbonate and make the solution more acid. In acid conditions the pH indicator, phenolphthalein, changes from pink to colourless. The presence of bile salts in tube 3 seems to accelerate the reaction, although bile salts with the denatured enzyme in tube 2 cannot bring about the change on their own.

For experiments investigating the effect of temperature and pH on enzyme action see p. 30.

(*Note:* these experiments and several others are fully detailed in the laboratory manual *Enzymes—see* p. 269.)

Questions

1 List the chemical changes undergone by (a) a molecule of starch from the time it is placed in the mouth to its ultimate use in providing energy; (b) a molecule of protein from the time it is swallowed to the time when its components are used in a cell (other than the liver).

In each case, state where the changes are taking place.

2 Write down the menu for your breakfast and lunch (or supper); indicate the principal food substances present in each component of the meal and state the final digestion product of each and the use your body is likely to have made of them.

3 Suggest reasons to explain why digestion takes place in stages, e.g. in the mouth, stomach and duodenum, rather than at the same time and in one place.

4 Study the chemistry of carbohydrates, proteins and fats (or any *one* of these) on pp. 16–17. Write the structural formula, as simply as possible, of starch, a protein and a fat and show how the molecule is broken down by digestive enzymes to the products which are absorbed in the ileum. Indicate the point at which the enzymes attack the food molecules.

11

Blood, its Composition, Function and Circulation

Composition

Blood consists of a suspension of red cells, white cells and platelets in a liquid called plasma. In an adult man there are five to six litres of blood in the body while a woman, on average, has one litre less.

Cells

Red cells (erythrocytes) (Figs. 11.1*a* and 11.2). The red cells are minute, biconcave discs consisting of spongy cytoplasm in an elastic cell membrane. During their formation they have nuclei, but these are lost before they enter the circulation. In the cytoplasm of the erythrocytes is a red pigment called *haemoglobin,* which constitutes about 95 per cent of the solids in the cell, the remaining 5 per cent consisting of enzymes, salts and proteins.

Haemoglobin is a protein with iron in its molecule. It has an affinity for oxygen and readily combines with it in conditions of high oxygen concentration and alkalinity. It forms an unstable compound called *oxyhaemoglobin,* which equally

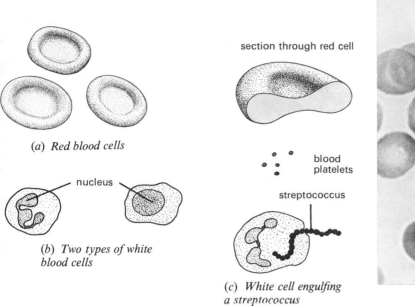

(a) *Red blood cells*

section through red cell

blood platelets

nucleus

streptococcus

(b) *Two types of white blood cells*

(c) *White cell engulfing a streptococcus*

Fig. 11.1   Blood cells

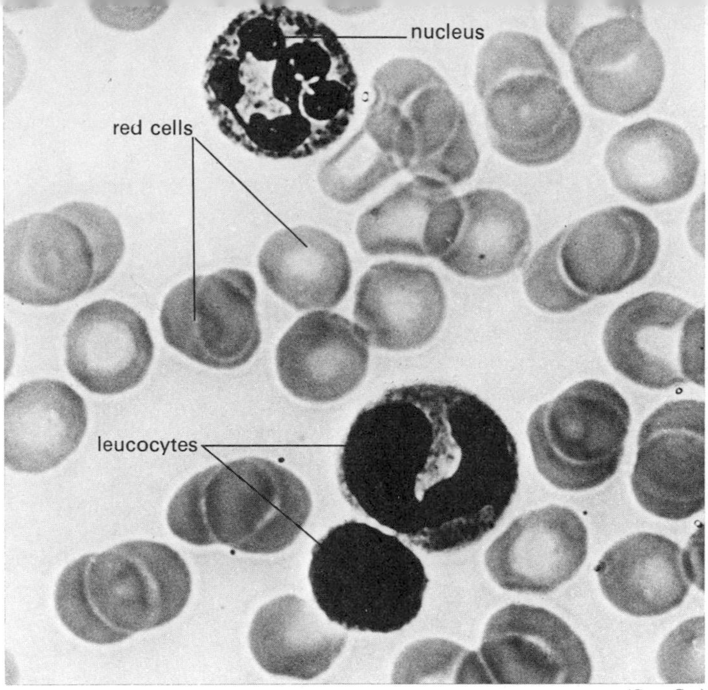

nucleus

red cells

leucocytes

(Gene Cox)

Fig. 11.2   Red and white cells in the human blood

readily breaks down and releases the oxygen in conditions of low oxygen concentration and raised acidity. This property makes it very efficient in transporting oxygen from the lungs, where the oxygen concentration is high, to the tissues, where it is lower. The total absorbing surface presented by the membranes of all the red cells is about 3 000 square metres.

The red cells are made principally in the red bone marrow of the short bones such as the sternum, ribs and vertebrae. The cells lining the blood vessels and blood spaces in the red marrow divide repeatedly, budding off new cells which themselves divide again. Red cell formation takes about seven days, after which the nucleus disappears, the haemoglobin is formed and the cell is released into the circulation.

There are about five and a half million cells in a cubic millimetre of blood. One cell survives for about four months after which it breaks down and is disintegrated in the liver and spleen, partly as a result of ingestion by phagocytes (*see* p. 72). Part of the haemoglobin from the spent red cells is changed to *bilirubin* and *biliverdin,* green pigments which eventually form part of the bile. The iron from the haemoglobin is retained in the liver and spleen cells and probably used again for new erythrocytes. About 200 000 million red cells are formed and destroyed each day, representing about one per cent of the total. To examine the condition of the cells in the blood-forming marrow, a sample is usually taken from the sternum (breastbone), a procedure called *sternal puncture.*

At high altitudes atmospheric pressure is low, making it more difficult for the lungs to extract oxygen from the air. In these conditions, the red marrow makes greater numbers of red cells. There is a steady increase in the numbers of red cells in the blood of mountain climbers who spend long periods at high altitudes. This *acclimatization* takes several weeks. People living permanently at high altitudes have more red cells in their blood than people at sea level but there are other long-term physiological changes as well, e.g. a rise in blood pressure in the pulmonary artery and a thickening of the right ventricle (p. 79).

Anaemia is a shortage of red cells in the blood which may arise through a large loss of blood, insufficient iron taken in with the diet, failure of the red marrow to make erythrocytes or excessive destruction of the cells. The anaemic person usually feels weak, breathless and tired.

Loss of blood as a result of injury can usually be made good by transfusion. In diseases like malaria, however, the red cells are destroyed by the disease organism and only by killing the parasites can the anaemia be stopped. Lack of iron in the diet can be corrected by increasing its meat and liver content or by taking iron-containing tablets, but if absorption of iron in the ileum is deficient the iron compounds may not be taken up or used. Increasing the intake of iron is also of little value if the formative chemistry of haemoglobin is out of order.

Extensive destruction of red cells follows an incompatible transfusion (p. 75) or occurs sometimes in newborn babies if the mother and father are not of the same Rhesus blood group (p. 76). The accumulated pigments from the rapidly destroyed red cells lead to a yellow discolouration of the skin called jaundice.

Pernicious anaemia occurs when the red marrow ceases to produce enough red cells. It was found that the symptoms of this disease could be arrested by feeding raw liver to the patients. Later an extract from the liver was made which had the same effect. It seems that normally there is made in the stomach and stored in the liver a substance which plays a vital part in stimulating the red cell production. A substance called vitamin B_{12}, a growth-promoting vitamin, has also been shown to have a stimulating effect on red cell production, possibly in conjunction with the substance made in the stomach.

Sickle-cell anaemia is an inherited condition. The haemoglobin molecules have a slightly different composition from normal which causes them to form rod-like structures at low oxygen concentrations. These structures distort and eventually destroy the red cells (*see* p. 168).

White cells (leucocytes) (Figs. 11.2 and 11.3). There is about one white cell to every six hundred erythrocytes, the actual numbers varying from 4 000 to 13 000 cells per cubic millimetre. Accurate estimation is made difficult by the fact that their distribution in different parts of the body is very variable.

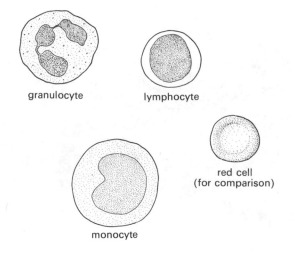

granulocyte   lymphocyte

red cell
(for comparison)

monocyte

Fig. 11.3   Three types of leucocyte

About 70 per cent of the white cells are of a type called *granulocytes*. They are larger than the red cells, irregular in shape and can change their form. They have a nucleus characteristically divided into two or three lobes, and there are many granules in their cytoplasm. These cells can move by a flowing action of their cytoplasm and, in certain situations, can pass out of the capillaries by squeezing between the cells of the capillary wall. They are made in the red marrow but outside the blood vessels. When mature they enter the circulation by passing through the capillary walls. They can ingest and destroy bacteria and dead tissue cells by flowing around, engulfing and digesting them. This action is called *phagocytosis* and these leucocytes are said to be *phagocytic*. The granulocytes accumulate at the site of an injury or infection and devour invading bacteria and damaged tissue, so preventing a spread of harmful bacteria as well as accelerating the healing of the infected region. Granulocytes survive for about a week.

Of the white cells, 23 per cent are *lymphocytes,* which are smaller than the granulocytes and have a round nucleus which occupies most of the cell. Lymphocytes are made in the lymph nodes and spleen (p. 84) and they make some of the chemicals called antibodies which are effective against foreign organisms and proteins in the blood. Lymphocytes survive on average for 100 days but some probably live for years. *Monocytes* are white cells with a simple or slightly lobed nucleus. They are made in the lymph nodes and spleen and are able to ingest almost any type of foreign particle. The life span for monocytes is not known for certain.

Platelets. These are pieces of special blood cells budded off in the bone marrow and they play an important part in the clotting action of the blood (p. 73). There are between 250 000 and 500 000 of them in each cubic millimetre of blood and they appear under a high-powered microscope as tiny oval structures.

Plasma

The liquid part of the blood is called plasma. It is a solution or suspension in water of many compounds. Some of the most important compounds are the plasma proteins, including albumin, globulin, fibrinogen and the antibodies. Other important constituents of plasma are the salts, or more strictly the ions, of sodium, potassium, calcium, chloride, phosphate and hydrogencarbonate. Varying in quantity with the area of the body and its activity, plasma will also contain food substances (e.g. amino acids, glucose and fats), hormones, pigments (e.g. bilirubin, a bile pigment), urea and other nitrogenous compounds.

The sodium hydrogencarbonate (bicarbonate) acts as a chemical 'buffer', that is, it allows the blood to absorb hydrogen ions without effectively increasing its acidity (*see* p. 21). This is important since the chemical reactions in living cells are very sensitive to the slightest change of pH.

Serum is the name given to blood plasma from which the fibrinogen has been removed.

Functions of the blood

It is convenient at this point to distinguish between the functions of (a) the blood, which provides and controls the internal fluid surrounding the cells, and (b) the circulation, which distributes food, oxygen, etc. to all parts of the body.

(a) **Blood and the internal environment.** All the living cells of the body are bathed by a fluid derived from blood plasma. This fluid, called *tissue fluid,* supplies them with the food and oxygen necessary for their living chemistry and removes the products of their activities which, if they accumulated, would poison the cells. The composition of the plasma is very precisely regulated by the liver and kidneys, so that the living cells are soaked in a liquid whose composition varies only within narrow limits. This provides them with the environment they need and enables them to live and grow in the most favourable conditions.

A single-celled animal living in a pond is able to adapt itself to variations of temperature, acidity, food and oxygen concentration, or move to a situation where these are favourable, but the cells of a complex organism have become specialized and unless the conditions are more or less right they will not work properly. The regulation of the composition of the tissue fluid is an aspect of *homeostasis* (*see* p. 92).

(b) **Circulation.** The movement of blood in the vessels around the body constantly changes the fluid surrounding the living cells so that fresh supplies of oxygen and food are brought in as fast as they are used up and poisonous end products are not allowed to accumulate. The following account is concerned principally with the circulation as a transport system rather than with the chemical properties of blood fluid as an internal environment.

On average, a red cell would complete the circulation of the body in 45 seconds.

1 **Transport of oxygen from the lungs to the tissues.** In the lungs, oxygen dissolves in the blood and is thus carried to all parts of the body. If the oxygen simply made a physical solution with the blood plasma, its solubility is such that it could not constitute more than 0.36 per cent by volume of the oxygenated blood. In fact there is 20 per cent by volume of oxygen present in the blood. This is because the combination of oxygen with haemoglobin in the red cells effectively takes up the oxygen from physical solution in the plasma and carries it in a chemically combined form.

As the blood passes through the lung capillaries it loses some of its carbon dioxide, so becoming more alkaline, and it is exposed to the relatively high concentration of oxygen in the air sacs of the lung. In these conditions, the haemoglobin combines with oxygen to make the unstable oxyhaemoglobin. Active tissues produce carbon dioxide and use oxygen. When blood reaches these tissues the conditions of raised acidity and low oxygen concentration cause the oxyhaemoglobin to break down, releasing its oxygen. The oxygen diffuses out of the cell membrane into the plasma, through the capillary wall and into the respiring cells.

Oxyhaemoglobin is bright red, while haemoglobin is a darker red colour.

2 Transport of carbon dioxide from the tissues to the lungs. Carbon dioxide produced from actively respiring cells diffuses through the capillary walls and dissolves in the plasma. As in the case of oxygen, a solution of carbon dioxide in blood would not exceed 2.7 per cent by volume and yet up to 60 per cent is found in the blood. Most of the carbon dioxide must therefore be carried in a combined form, usually as hydrogencarbonate (bicarbonate) ions ($-HCO_3^-$) which are transported in both the plasma and the red cells. The less oxygen there is present in the haemoglobin, the more carbon dioxide can the red cells carry. This favours the exchange of carbon dioxide and oxygen in the lungs and tissues. In the lungs, the hydrogencarbonates break down to carbon dioxide and water and the carbon dioxide diffuses through the capillary walls into the alveoli of the lungs (p. 87). Both the formation and breakdown of hydrogencarbonate are accelerated by an enzyme in the red cells called *carbonic anhydrase.*

3 Transport of excretory material from the tissues to the kidneys. Many of the chemical reactions involving proteins and amino acids form nitrogenous end-products which are poisonous, e.g. urea and uric acid. These substances enter the capillary or lymphatic systems and are carried off in the plasma or lymph. When they reach the kidneys a large proportion of them are removed and excreted (p. 94).

4 Transport of digested food from the ileum to the tissues. The soluble products of digestion enter the capillaries of the villi lining the ileum (p. 65). They are carried in solution by the plasma and after passing through the liver, enter the general circulation. Glucose and amino acids pass out of the capillaries and into the cells of the body. Glucose may be oxidized, in a muscle for example, and provide the energy for contraction; amino acids will be built up into new proteins and make new cells and tissues.

5 Distribution of hormones. Hormones are chemicals that affect the rate of vital processes in the body (p. 156). From the glands that make them, they are carried in the blood plasma all around the body. Each hormone has one or more 'target' organs and affects the rate at which the organ works.

6 Distribution of heat and temperature control. Muscular and chemical activity releases heat. These processes are going on far more rapidly in some parts of the body than in others, for example chemical activity in the liver and muscular action in the limbs. The heat produced locally is distributed all round the body by the blood, and in this way an even temperature is maintained in all regions.

The diversion of blood to or away from the skin also plays a part in keeping the temperature constant (*see* p. 98).

7 Formation of clots. When a blood vessel is cut open or its lining damaged, the platelets adhere to the damaged area. The protein, fibrinogen, in the plasma is converted to fibrin which appears to come out of solution as filaments radiating from the platelets. The network of fibres across the wound makes a plug which stops any more blood leaking out and prevents the entry of bacteria and poisons. Eventually the dried blood clot shrinks, hardens and forms a scab which protects the damaged area while new tissue is forming.

The details of the coagulation of the blood are very complicated and not all biologists agree about the different stages. It is very important that normal blood in undamaged vessels should not coagulate, and this may be the reason for the complex series of changes that must take place before clotting occurs.

The fibrinogen in the plasma is converted to fibrin by the enzyme-like action of *thrombin,* provided sufficient calcium ions are present in the plasma. In normal plasma, thrombin is in an inactive form known as *prothrombin.* In the region of the wound the damaged tissues and the platelets are thought to produce a substance called *thrombokinase* (thromboplastin) which converts prothrombin to thrombin.

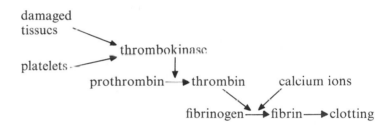

Prothrombin is made in the liver and a substance called vitamin K (p. 36) is essential for its production. Bile salts are necessary for the absorption of this fat-soluble vitamin, which is made by intestinal bacteria.

After coagulation, clot shrinkage pulls the tissues closer together and new cells made at the margins of the wound begin to spread over the inner surface of the scab, forming a new layer of skin at the rate of about 0.5 mm per day. New capillary branches grow from others in the area, and cut nerves grow out into the tissues. When the scab falls off a deep cut, a scar may be left due to the thinness of the epidermis and the extra white fibrous tissue in the dermis.

Haemophilia is an inheritable disease in which a person's blood clots only very slowly owing to the lack of a substance needed for the formation of thrombokinase, or perhaps insufficient platelets. Such people are liable to lose disproportionate quantities of blood from even minor wounds.

8 Prevention of infection. (a) *Infected wounds.* Normally the skin or the lining of the alimentary canal is a barrier to the entry of any bacteria. The layer of dead cells on the skin provides a mechanical barrier while the mucus and chemicals of the alimentary canal offer a chemical defence. If the skin is broken, however, and bacteria enter the cut, certain of the white cells migrate out of the capillaries in that region and begin to engulf and digest damaged tissues or any bacteria which have invaded the tissues. Sometimes large quantities of dead white cells together with digested and liquefied tissues accumulate at the site of the wound and form pus. The ingestion of bacteria by the white cells and the clot formation which prevents free circulation localize the site of infection, and most of the bacteria are destroyed before they can enter the general circulation. Those bacteria which do escape into the blood stream are trapped by stationary cells, like granulocytes, in the lymph nodes, spleen or liver. These stationary white cells are called *macrophages*.

Certain virulent strains of bacteria cannot be ingested by the white cells until they have been acted upon by chemicals called *antibodies* which are secreted into the blood. If these antibodies are not already present in the blood or are not made quickly enough, the virulent bacteria may invade the whole body and give rise to general disease symptoms.

Other defence mechanisms come into action in the region of a wound, which either facilitate those already described or directly increase the chances of successful healing.

(i) A chemical similar in its action to—if not identical with—*histamine* is set free by the damaged tissues and causes the capillaries in that region to expand. The arterioles supplying the skin in that region also dilate so that more blood reaches the surface of the skin and the rate of flow is increased. This gives rise to the redness and warmth in the vicinity of a wound and also increases the supply of antibodies and leucocytes.

(ii) Another chemical from the damaged tissues makes the capillaries more permeable. This allows the leucocytes to squeeze out of the capillaries more easily but in addition permits some proteins to escape into the tissues. The osmotic pressure exerted by these proteins extracts water from the blood vessels and the fluid accumulates in the region of the wound giving rise to the familiar swelling. The accumulated fluid drains into the lymphatics and this direction of flow may be effective in carrying bacteria away from the blood circulatory system and into the lymphatic system where the lymph nodes quickly remove bacteria. In fact, the clotting of blood and the clumping of groups of bacteria by antibodies often prevents bacteria from entering either the blood or the lymphatic system.

(iii) The pain-sensory endings in the wounded area become more sensitive and tend to reduce movement of or interference with a damaged area. This may have beneficial effects in healing.

Asepsis. Cleanliness in dealing with wounds reduces the chances of bacterial infection. The dressing of a wound should include first a thorough washing of the area to remove, mechanically, as much bacteria-containing material as possible, and finally a sterile dressing to cover the wound and prevent further bacteria from reaching it. It follows that the instruments, dressings and hands of any assistants must be as free from bacteria as possible (*see* p. 206).

Antitetanus. With deep flesh wounds, an antitetanus injection is often given since, if tetanus bacteria enter the wound, by the time typical symptoms appear the tetanus toxin is firmly attached to the nervous system and almost unassailable by antibodies. The injected antitetanus antibody inactivates the bacteria before they leave the blood stream.

(b) *Disease and immunity.* Many diseases are caused by the presence of bacteria or viruses in the body, and the symptoms may be due to one or more of the following: the foreign proteins of the bacteria themselves; the poisonous chemicals (usually proteins) called *toxins*, which are produced by the bacteria; and the breakdown products of the infected tissue. Recovery from the disease and the development of immunity to further attacks, in some cases, depend to a large extent on the production in the blood of antibodies. These antibodies are proteins, produced by cells such as lymphocytes and released into the plasma. They may affect bacteria or their products in a number of ways:

(i) *opsonins* adhere to the outer surface of bacteria and so make it easier for the phagocytic white cells to ingest them;

(ii) *agglutinins* cause bacteria to stick together in clumps; in this condition, the bacteria cannot invade the tissues;

(iii) *lysins* destroy the bacteria by dissolving their outer coats;

(iv) *antitoxins* combine with and so neutralize the poisonous toxins produced by the bacteria.

The foreign bodies that stimulate the blood to produce antibodies are called *antigens*. Antibodies are very specific, that is, they will act against and neutralize only one particular protein. An antibody against a *Streptococcus* bacterium, for example, would be ineffective against a *Staphylococcus*. Measles antibodies are ineffective against chickenpox.

When the organism recovers from the disease, the antibodies remain for only a short time in the circulatory system, but the ability to produce them is greatly increased, so that a further invasion by bacteria or viruses is likely to be stopped at once and the person is said to be *immune* to the disease. People may acquire immunity after recovering from an attack, as in measles, or it may be induced in them by *vaccination* or *inoculation*. Naturally acquired immunity may occur because disease bacteria are present in the body without being sufficiently numerous or suitably placed to produce disease symptoms. A person might thus experience a mild form of disease without even noticing it, but his blood will have made antibodies which render him immune to any further attacks. A population that has never experienced a particular disease is likely to suffer acutely from it when it is first encountered. When the white man came first to the Fiji islands he also introduced the disease measles. This was a minor ailment for the European but a fatal and devastating disease to the native population who had no natural immunity.

A *vaccine* is a collection of disease bacteria or viruses, killed or inactivated by heat, chemicals or other methods to prevent their reproduction, or it may consist of relatively harmless strains of the disease organisms. When these are injected into the blood stream the organism undergoes a mild form of the disease and its cells manufacture antibodies. In this way immunity is artificially acquired. The period of immunity during which antibodies can be produced rapidly varies from a few months to many years, according to the nature of the infection. Artificial immunity induced by a vaccine is sometimes called *active immunity* because the person has to make the antibodies himself. *Passive immunity* can be acquired by the injection into the blood of antibodies already made by a donor organism, frequently the horse, in the form of a serum.

Serum. The blood of a person (or animal) who has recently recovered from a disease will contain antibodies. If the cells and fibrinogen are removed from a sample of this blood, a serum is obtained which, when injected into other people, may give them temporary (passive) immunity or cure them if they already have the disease. Sera for treating tetanus and

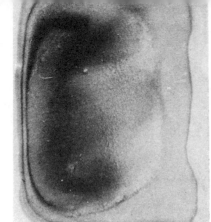

(a) The cells and serum are matched

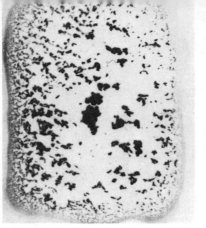

(b) Effect of a mis-match between cells and serum

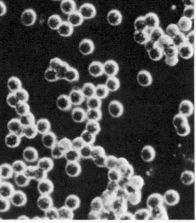

(c) The red cells are being agglutinated

(Philip Harris Biological Ltd)

Fig. 11.4   Agglutination; a and b show the appearance, to the naked eye, after compatible and incompatible cells and serum are mixed; c shows the red cells being agglutinated under the microscope.

snake bites are prepared from horses' blood. The horse is injected with diluted poison which stimulates the formation of antitoxins in its blood. Samples of the blood are then taken from the horse and serum prepared from the samples is used to treat cases. For further examples of active and passive immunity, vaccines and sera, see p. 38.

Blood groups and transfusion

Excessive loss of blood from the body may cause a condition known as 'shock' which often produces more serious effects on the patient than the direct effect of his injuries. This loss of blood can be made good by a transfusion in which blood from another person, the donor, is fed into the patient's veins.

Early experiments on transfusion often produced either spectacular successes or very distressing symptoms due to the coagulation of the donor's red cells in the blood vessels of the recipient. When this happens, the kidneys have difficulty in eliminating the products of the clumped and disintegrating red cells and in extreme cases they may cease to function normally.

In 1901, Dr Landsteiner mixed samples of blood serum with suspensions of red cells taken from different people. In some cases the serum and cells made satisfactory mixtures while in others the red cells were clumped together (Fig. 11.4). It was discovered that there were antagonistic substances on the surface of the red cells and in the serum. These behave in much the same way as antigens and antibodies in the blood. The substance on the cell is called the *agglutinogen* and that in the plasma is the *agglutinin*. Antagonistic agglutinogens and agglutinins do not occur in any one person's blood.

There are four main blood groups of this kind, called A, B, AB and O. In group A, the cells carry agglutinogen A on their surface while in the plasma is the agglutinin anti-B. In group B the cells carry the B agglutinogen and the plasma contains the anti-A agglutinin. The cells of group AB carry either agglutinogen A or B in about equal numbers and there is no agglutinin in the plasma. Group O cells have only a weak agglutinogen, not attacked by either anti-A or anti-B agglutinins but both of these antibodies are present in the plasma.

Group	Agglutinogen in cells	Agglutinin in plasma
A	A	anti-B
B	B	anti-A
AB	A and B	none
O	none	anti-A and anti-B

If group A blood is transfused into a group B person, the anti-A agglutinin in the recipient's plasma reacts with the agglutinogen A on the donor's cells and causes them to stick together. Similarly, group B cannot receive transfusions from group A. Group AB having no agglutinins in the plasma can receive blood from any group, while group O with both agglutinins in the plasma can receive blood only from group O donors whose cells have neither A or B agglutinogens. Conversely, group AB with both agglutinogens can donate blood only to their own group, whereas group O can donate to all groups since their cells cannot be agglutinated.

It is only the agglutination of the donor's cells that causes the pathological symptoms. Although the 'wrong' agglutinin in the donor's serum might be expected to react with the recipient's red cells, this does not appear to happen, or at least does not cause any ill effects. One possible reason is that the donor's serum with its antagonistic agglutinin is quickly diluted when it enters the recipient's blood stream, or that the foreign agglutinin does cause some cells to clump but in small, isolated and widely scattered groups.

To determine the blood group of a person, a little of his blood is mixed separately with sera from group A and group B. If the cells clump in A serum, he is group B; if they clump in group B serum he is group A. Agglutination in both indicates that he is group AB and if his cells react with neither, his group is O.

Group	Can donate blood to	Can receive blood from
A	A and AB	A and O
B	B and AB	B and O
AB	AB	all groups
O	all groups	O

A donor gives 420 cm³ of his blood from a vein in his arm. The blood is led into a sterilized bottle containing sodium citrate which prevents clotting. The blood is then stored at 5 °C for 10 days, or longer if glucose is added. Before blood is transfused, even though both groups are known, it is carefully tested against the recipient's blood to make sure that no unforeseen factors produce agglutination. Then it is fed into one of the patient's arm veins at the correct rate and temperature. In 50 days, the donor will have made up his blood to the normal volume and composition.

The ABO blood groups are subject to a fairly straightforward pattern of inheritance as described in Chapter 21. There are known to be subdivisions of the ABO blood groups as well as several other groups but these seem to be relatively unimportant in transfusions.

The Rhesus factor. In 1940 it was found that 85 per cent of white Americans carried an agglutinogen similar to one previously investigated in Rhesus monkeys. The remaining 15 per cent had no such factor and were called Rhesus negative (Rh−), while those possessing the factor were called Rhesus positive (Rh+). There is no natural Rh agglutinin in the plasma so that the first transfusion from Rh+ to Rh− is not likely to cause any harm. Exchange from Rh− to Rh+ is safe at all times. The Rh+ agglutinogen, however, stimulates the production of agglutinins in the plasma of a Rh− recipient so that a subsequent Rh+ transfusion could be as incompatible as a faulty ABO transfusion. The Rh− individual is said to have been *sensitized* by the first Rh+ transfusion.

If a Rh+ man marries a Rh− woman there is a chance that some of their children will be Rh+. In most cases this is of no consequence but sometimes the red cells of the Rh+ embryo get into the mother's circulation, possibly as a result of a fault in the placenta. The embryo's Rh+ cells in the mother's blood act as antigens and she makes antibodies (agglutinins) against them, i.e. she has been sensitized to the Rh+ factor. This will not affect the first embryo but if the mother conceives a second Rh+ child, whose cells enter her circulation, the antibody reaction is much more vigorous and if her antibodies reach the embryo they will destroy its red cells, causing it to be born jaundiced or even stillborn.

Usually, if expectant mothers are found to be Rh−, the husband's blood is tested so that if he proves to be Rh+ due precautions can be taken by suppressing the production of antibodies in the mother at the birth of the first child. About one in every ten marriages is between Rh+ men and Rh− women, but only about one in forty of these marriages is affected by the Rh incompatibility. It follows that Rh− women of child-bearing age should not be given Rh+ blood in a transfusion in case it sensitizes them.

The circulatory system

The blood is distributed round the body in vessels, mostly (but not all) tubular and varying in size from about 10 mm to 0.01 mm in diameter (Fig. 11.6). They form a continuous system, communicating with every living part of the body. Blood flows in them always in the same direction, passing repeatedly through the heart whose muscular contractions maintain the circulation (Fig. 11.9).

There are three types of blood vessel connected to form a continuous system, the arteries, veins and capillaries (Fig. 11.7), and also the lymphatic vessels which return lymph from the tissues to the heart.

Arteries (Figs. 11.5 and 11.7a). These are fairly wide vessels that carry blood from the heart to the limbs and organs of the body. They consist of a fibrous outer layer, a middle layer of elastic fibres and circular muscle, and an inner layer of smooth endothelium. In the big arteries there is more elastic tissue than circular muscle, a feature that enables them to absorb the energy of the pressure surges caused by the contractions of the ventricles of the heart. The stretched elastic tissue contracts in between heartbeats, and this squeezing further aids the flow of blood along the arteries. The arteries divide into smaller vessels called *arterioles*. In these there is more circular muscle than elastic tissue. The circular muscle is under the control of the nervous and endocrine systems, and when stimulated the muscle contracts, constricting the arterioles and reducing the flow of blood in them. The arterioles themselves divide repeatedly until they form a dense network of microscopic vessels permeating between the cells of every living tissue. These final branches are called capillaries.

Capillaries. Capillaries are tiny vessels with walls only one cell thick and not extensible (Figs. 11.7c and 11.8). Although the blood appears confined within the capillary walls, the latter are permeable, with the result that water and dissolved substances pass in and out, exchanging oxygen, carbon dioxide, dissolved food and excretory products with the tissues around the capillary (Fig. 11.10).

The capillary network is so dense that no living cell is far from a supply of oxygen and food. In the liver, every cell is in direct contact with a capillary. Some capillaries are so narrow that the flexible red cells are squashed and distorted in passing through them. The diameter of capillaries can be altered by both nervous stimulation which tends to close them, and by chemicals like histamine which dilate them. The change in diameter is brought about by a change in the shape of the cells constituting the walls.

Although the branching arterioles and capillaries are much smaller vessels than the arteries, their total volume is much greater. For example, the capillaries may be able to hold as much as 800 times the volume of blood in the aorta. One of the conditions of 'shock' resulting from serious injury, is that the capillaries and arterioles become so dilated that they can absorb all the blood delivered from the heart so that very little returns to the heart in the veins.

The friction between the blood and the capillary walls tends to reduce the intermittent surges of blood from the arteries to a steady flow. Eventually all the capillary branches join up again to form first *venules* and then veins.

Veins. Veins return blood from the tissues to the heart. The blood pressure in them is steady and less than that in the arteries. They are wider and have thinner walls than arteries.

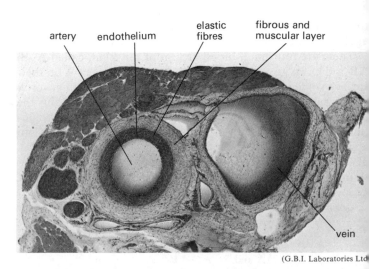

artery   endothelium   elastic fibres   fibrous and muscular layer

vein

(G.B.I. Laboratories Ltd)

Fig. 11.5   Transverse section through an artery and vein

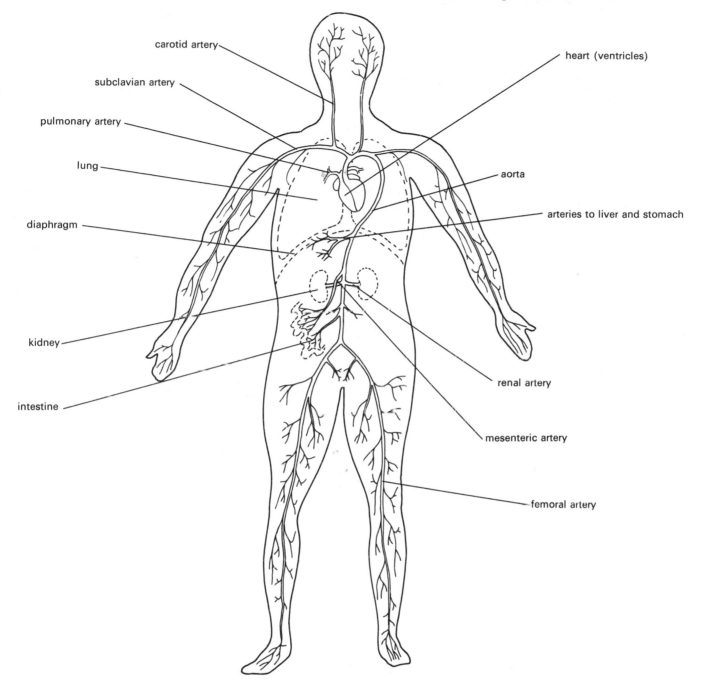

Fig. 11.6   Arterial system (in most cases the veins run parallel to the arteries)

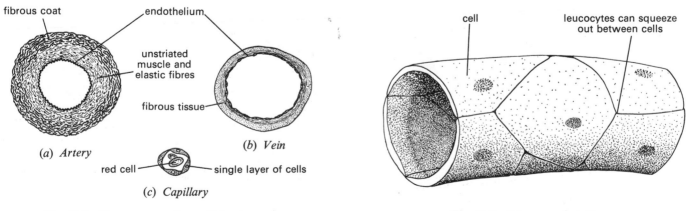

(a) *Artery*

(b) *Vein*

red cell — single layer of cells

(c) *Capillary*

Fig. 11.7   Transverse sections of blood vessels

Fig. 11.8   Diagram of capillary

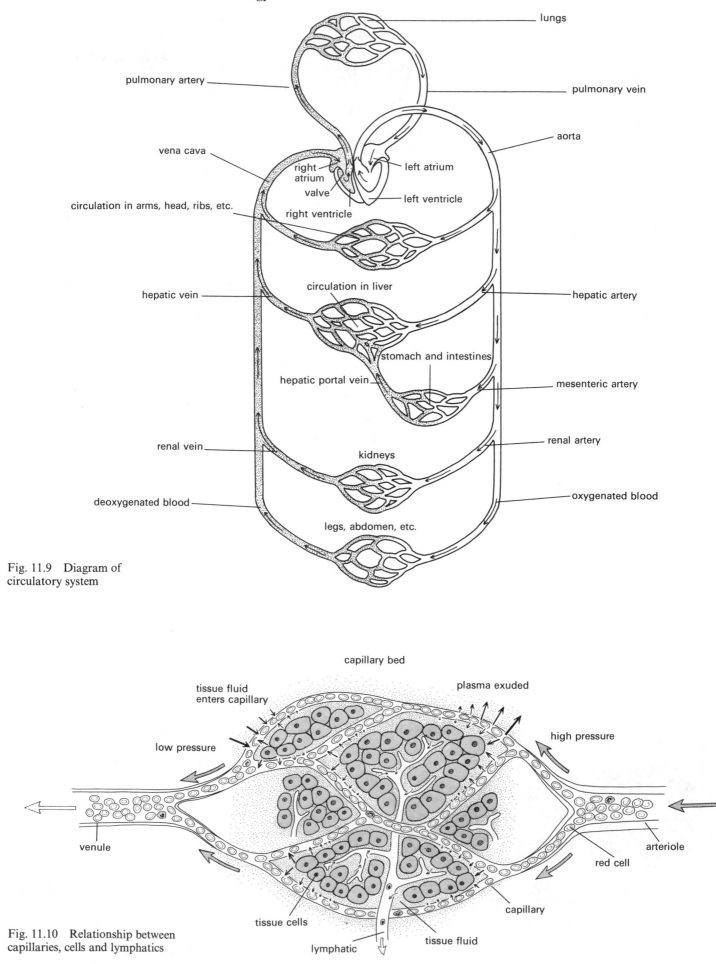

Fig. 11.9   Diagram of
circulatory system

Fig. 11.10   Relationship between
capillaries, cells and lymphatics

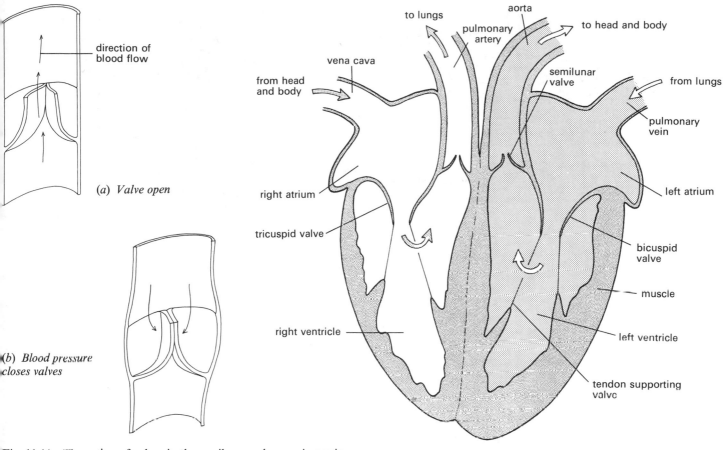

(a) *Valve open*

(b) *Blood pressure closes valves*

direction of blood flow

Fig. 11.11 The action of valves in the semilunar valves, or in a vein

to lungs

aorta

pulmonary artery

to head and body

vena cava

from head and body

semilunar valve

from lungs

pulmonary vein

right atrium

left atrium

tricuspid valve

bicuspid valve

muscle

right ventricle

left ventricle

tendon supporting valve

Fig. 11.12 Diagram of heart in longitudinal section

with an inextensible fibrous tissue replacing the elastic tissue of the latter (Fig. 11.7*b* and 11.5). Some veins also have valves in them (Fig. 11.11) which prevent blood flowing backwards, away from the heart, e.g. the veins of the limbs.

The pressure of surrounding muscles when they contract during activity tends to squash the veins and, since the valves prevent backward flow, assists the return of blood to the heart from the arms and legs. The positive pressure of the abdominal organs during inspiration of air also helps to keep the blood moving in the veins as does the simultaneous 'negative' (i.e. less than atmospheric) pressure in the thorax.

The blood in the veins usually contains less oxygen and food, and more nitrogenous waste and carbon dioxide, than arterial blood. The exceptions to this are (i) the pulmonary artery which carries deoxygenated blood to the lungs and (ii) the pulmonary vein which returns oxygenated blood from the lungs to the heart. Similarly, after a meal the hepatic portal vein from the intestines to the liver will have a higher concentration of glucose and amino acids than is present in any arteries. The renal vein leaving the kidney will have a reduced level of certain salts, nitrogenous waste and water.

The heart

The heart is a muscular pumping organ situated in the thorax. It develops in the embryo from a specialized region of an artery. The heart is enclosed in the *pericardium,* a tough membrane attached at its lower end to the diaphragm and at its upper region to the veins entering the heart. The fluid between the heart and the pericardium reduces friction with surrounding organs. The inextensible pericardium is also thought to prevent the heart becoming over-distended with blood in certain extreme conditions.

The heart itself consists of four chambers (Fig. 11.12); the left and right sides do not communicate. The upper chambers, the *atria,* are relatively thin-walled and receive blood from the veins. Oxygenated blood from the lungs enters the left atrium via the pulmonary vein, and deoxygenated blood from the body enters the right atrium from the vena cava. Each atrium opens into its corresponding *ventricle* through a large aperture guarded by a non-return valve (Fig. 11.11). Both ventricles are thick-walled and very muscular. They have the same capacity and expel the same volume of blood, i.e. about 70 cm^3 per stroke. The walls of the left ventricle, however, are three to four times thicker than those of the right, reflecting its function of pumping blood all round the body via the aorta. The right ventricle pumps blood to the lungs through the pulmonary artery. The muscle of the atria and ventricles is supplied with oxygenated blood from the *coronary artery* (Fig. 11.13) which branches from the aorta.

Coronary heart disease. If the coronary artery becomes obstructed by the formation of an internal blood clot, the blood flow is reduced and the heart muscle is deprived of oxygen.

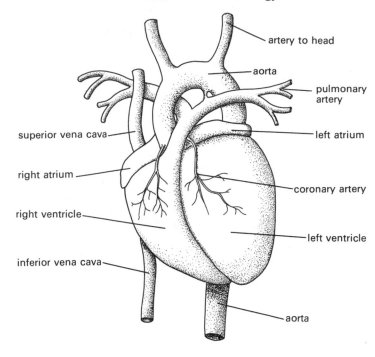

Fig. 11.13   External view of mammalian heart
(pulmonary veins not shown)

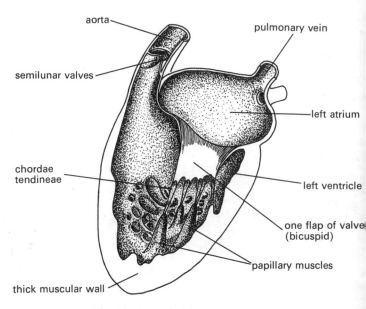

Fig. 11.14   Left side of heart cut open

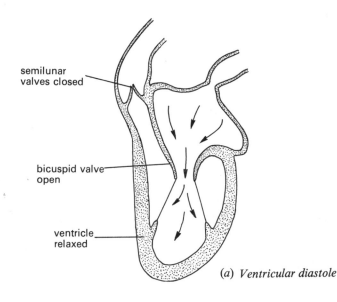

(a) *Ventricular diastole*

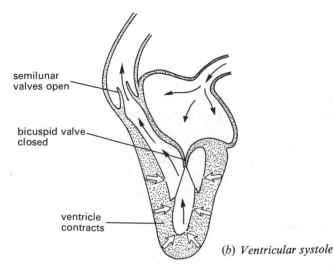

(b) *Ventricular systole*

Fig. 11.15   Heart action (left side only)

Ventricular contraction is so enfeebled that the person collapses and, unless he receives prompt medical attention, he may die. The condition is called *coronary thrombosis* and is one of the most familiar forms of 'heart attack' in industrialized societies.

Coronary heart disease is associated with a condition known as *atherosclerosis*. This is a deposition of fatty material on the internal lining of the arteries and it results in a decrease in their diameter. Consequently the blood flow through the affected arteries is diminished and if a blood clot forms it may block the artery completely. The direct causes of atherosclerosis are not certainly known but since it is a disease prevalent in industrialized communities, the causes are sought in the habits and diets of modern society.

Apart from any inherited predisposition to the disease, the main contributory factors are thought to be high blood pressure, lack of exercise, a high level of fats in the blood plasma and smoking. The fats are deposited on the arterial lining probably as a result of outward filtration of blood fluids through the arterial walls. High blood pressure increases this filtration rate and smoking makes the arteries more permeable so that the rate of deposition of fat is increased. Obesity and nervous tension both increase blood pressure.

Large amounts of fat in the diet, particularly fats from animal sources, produce a high level of fat in the plasma and so increase the chances of its being deposited on the arterial lining. Exercise probably reduces the level of fats in the blood as well as improving the blood supply to the heart muscle (p. 123).

Although none of these conditions is universally accepted as a proven cause of coronary heart disease there is enough circumstantial evidence to indicate that obesity, fatty diet, heavy smoking, lack of exercise and nervous stress predispose the subject to a heart attack.

Heartbeat. (a) *Diastole* (Fig. 11.15*a*). In this phase of the heartbeat, the atria and ventricles are relaxed. Each ventricle, as it relaxes, returns to a shape that increases its volume, allowing blood from the atria and main veins to flow into it. The valves between the atria and ventricles offer no resistance to flow in that direction.

(b) *Systole* (Fig. 11.15*b*). Contraction of the atria precedes, by a fraction of a second, that of the ventricles. This expels the blood from the atria into the ventricles and completes the filling of the latter. The flaps of the bicuspid and tricuspid valves are brought together by the back eddies from this flow of blood. The muscle of the ventricles now undergoes a powerful contraction and increases the blood pressure within them so that the tricuspid and bicuspid valve flaps are forced tightly together and prevent blood returning to the atria. The *chordae tendineae*, which are pulled taut by contraction of the *papillary muscles* (Fig. 11.14), prevent the valves being turned inside out by the pressure. When the ventricular blood pressure exceeds that in the aorta and pulmonary artery, the *semilunar* valves (Fig. 11.11) are forced open and blood enters these arteries, whose walls are consequently distended by the sudden rise in pressure. While the ventricles are contracting, the atria have relaxed and are once more filling with blood. When the ventricles relax and the pressure in them falls, return of blood from the arteries is prevented by the closure of the semilunar valves.

The closure of the bicuspid and tricuspid valves as the ventricles contract, followed by the shutting of the semilunar valves when the ventricles relax, gives rise to the heart sounds heard through the thorax either directly or by a stethoscope. They are usually described as 'lubb-dupp', the first sound (the bi- and tricuspid valves closing) being more prolonged and muffled than the second (the semilunar valves closing). Any deficiency in the closure of the valves, as in some forms of heart disease, is revealed by less clearly defined heart sounds as some of the blood leaks back.

During normal activity, the heart pumps about 5 litres of blood per minute while beating about 70 times. During exercise, the heartbeat may rise to more than 100 per minute and the output of blood to over 20 litres per minute.

The pulse. The sudden expansion of the main arteries as blood enters them from the contracting ventricles is transmitted as a pressure wave through all the principal arteries of the body. The wave can be felt as a pulse when an artery is near enough to the surface of the body and passing over a bone, as in the wrist. Such a region is known as a pressure point. Although the pulse rate corresponds to the heart beat it does not represent the arrival of blood just expelled from the heart. The pulse is a result of the elasticity of the arteries and is like a ripple on their surface travelling at about 7 metres per second from the heart. The blood in the arteries travels at only about 0.5 metres per second. A familiar pressure point is in the artery on the inside of the wrist just over the radius bone. Another is in the carotid artery on each side of the windpipe in the neck.

Control of the heartbeat. The heart's rhythmic muscular contraction is basically automatic and needs no nervous stimulation. If kept in the correct solution of salts, a frog's heart will continue to beat for some hours after removal from the body and the same is true of the mammalian heart at the correct temperature if an artificial circulation of nutrient and oxygenated liquid is maintained in the heart muscle. The natural rhythm of the atrium (75 per minute) is, however, faster than that of the ventricle (40 per minute) but the muscle fibres of the heart are able to conduct electrical impulses and the contraction of one region of muscle acts as a stimulus for the rest of the heart so that the atrial rhythm is imposed also on the ventricle.

The 'pace-maker' is a zone of tissue at the junction of the vena cava and the right atrium. It is called the *sinu-atrial node*, and it initiates contraction of the atria which in turn stimulates the ventricles. In the mammalian heart, the atria are separated from the ventricles by a ring of non-conducting fibrous tissue, and the only direct muscular connection between atrium and ventricle is a band of modified muscle fibres, the *atrio-ventricular bundle*, which conducts the impulse from atria to ventricles. These muscle fibres spread over the internal surface of the ventricles and cause them to contract as a whole rather than from top to bottom, since a stimulatory wave would pass only slowly through the ordinary heart muscle.

The normal sequence of events is thus as follows: the sinu-atrial node initiates contraction; the impulse from the SA node is conducted rapidly over both atria which contract together; the impulse is blocked by the fibrous ring between atria and ventricles except at one point, the *atrio-ventricular node*, where it is picked up by the atrio-ventricular bundle and distributed to the ventricles which contract shortly after the atria. The SA and AV nodes receive motor nerve fibres from the autonomic nervous system (p. 151). Sensory fibres carry impulses to the brain from pressure receptors in the aorta and carotid artery (Fig. 11.16). The motor fibres of the parasympathetic system (p. 151) carry impulses which originate in the cardiac centre in the medulla of the brain (p. 154); they run in the *vagus nerve*. The nerve fibres carry a constant stream of impulses which tends to slow down the natural rhythm of the heart. Any increase in the stimulation of the vagus nerve slows the heart rate even more. The sympathetic fibres come from the spinal cord. Stimulation of the sympathetic fibres or an increase in the adrenaline content of the blood promotes a more rapid rhythm.

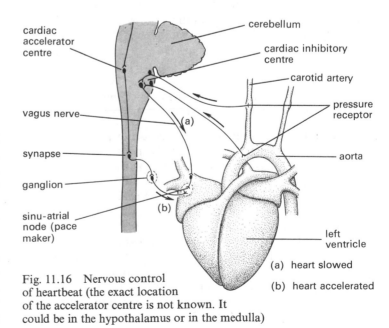

Fig. 11.16   Nervous control of heartbeat (the exact location of the accelerator centre is not known. It could be in the hypothalamus or in the medulla)

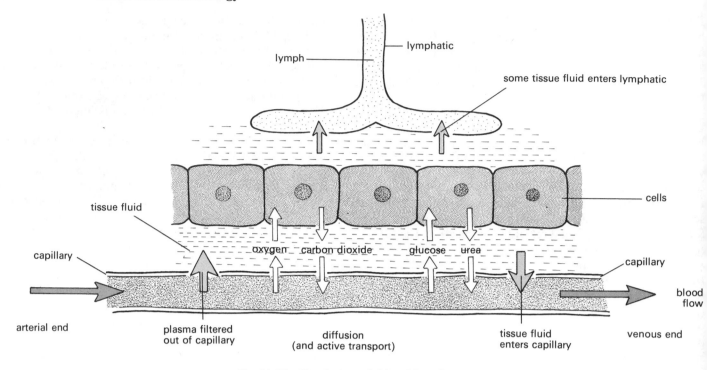

Fig. 11.17   Blood, tissue fluid and lymph

If the blood pressure in the aorta or carotid artery rises, impulses are sent from the pressure receptors through sensory fibres to the medulla. Here they make synaptic connections (p. 147) with other fibres and complete a reflex arc that causes impulses to be sent from the medulla to the heart, reducing the heart rate. By reducing the output of the heart, this reflex allows the blood pressure to fall to its normal level. Conversely, if the blood pressure in the arteries falls below a certain level, the pressure receptors send fewer impulses to the brain, stimulation of the heart by the parasympathetic motor fibres in the vagus nerve is diminished and the heart rate is permitted to increase. These reflexes tend to adjust the heart rate to meet the needs of the body and maintain the blood pressure.

At times of stress or excitement, the sympathetic nervous system sends motor impulses to the SA node and increases the heart rate. Adrenaline from the adrenal gland acts directly on the SA node and has the same effect. The output of the heart is thus increased and the muscles are supplied with additional oxygen and glucose which will be required during vigorous activity.

Thyroxine, the hormone from the thyroid gland, also has an excitatory effect on the SA node.

Blood pressure. In order to overcome atmospheric pressure, which compresses the tissues, and the resistance in the fine capillaries to the flow of blood, the heart has to maintain a relatively high blood pressure in the circulatory system. The pressure of the blood varies with (a) the region of the circulatory system under consideration, e.g. an artery or vein, (b) the phase of the heartbeat (diastole or systole), and (c) the physiological state of the body. The pressure in the arteries during systole, as measured by a doctor's sphygmomanometer (an inflatable cuff placed round the arm and connected to a pressure gauge), is usually in the region of 120 millimetres of mercury and the pressure during diastole is about 75 mmHg, but both vary considerably with age and from one individual to another. The blood pressure is regulated by, amongst other methods, the reflex nervous mechanism of the heart, described above.

Regulation of blood distribution. The total volume of blood in the body is less than the volume of the blood vessels that contain it. At any one time, the complete or partial constriction of arterioles and capillaries in a particular region will reduce the volume of blood reaching that region and help to maintain a steady circulation and return of blood to the heart. After a meal, for example, more blood will flow to the alimentary canal as a result of dilation of the arterioles and capillaries in that region. This facilitates the rate of digestion and absorption but tends to reduce the supply of blood to the muscles.

The arteries and arterioles receive motor fibres from the sympathetic nervous system under the control of the *vasomotor* centre in the medulla. Normally, the steady flow of impulses in these fibres keeps the vessels in a state of partial contraction. More intense stimulation may close the arterioles in a particular region (for example the fingers, making them white and numb). Nearly all the nervous stimuli that normally cause pain or emotion influence the vasomotor centre, and may cause constriction of the arterioles. Sensory impulses producing the sensations of fear act through the vasomotor centre and sympathetic system, causing the blood vessels of the skin and abdominal organs to constrict, leading to pallor and the 'hollow' feeling in the abdomen.

The blood supply to the brain and muscles, however, is not reduced and in fact is likely to be increased as a result of the rise in arterial pressure when such a large proportion of the system is shut down. This increased supply of blood to the brain and muscles enables a person to react quickly and vigorously in an emergency.

Adrenaline has an effect similar to the constrictor effect of the nervous system. The localized vasodilator effect of histamine has been mentioned on p. 74.

Fainting occurs when the return of blood to the heart and consequently to the brain is reduced, for example as a result of prolonged standing or loss of blood. Emotional shock (fright, horror) may also induce fainting as a result of reduced heart output because of the stimulation of the parasympathetic nervous system and the depressor action of the vagus nerve.

Exchange between capillaries, cells and lymphatics

At the arterial end of the capillary bed (Fig. 11.10) blood pressure is high and forces plasma out through the thin capillary walls. The fluid so expelled has a composition similar to plasma, containing dissolved glucose, amino acids and salts, but has a much lower concentration of plasma proteins. This exuded fluid permeates the spaces between the cells of all living tissues and is called *tissue fluid*. From it the cells extract the glucose, oxygen, amino acids, etc. which they need for their living processes, and into it they excrete their carbon dioxide and nitrogenous waste.

The narrow capillaries offer considerable resistance to the flow of blood. This slows down the movement of blood, so facilitating the exchange of substances by diffusion between the plasma and tissue fluid (Fig. 11.17). The capillary resistance also results in a drop of pressure so that at the venous end of a capillary bed the blood pressure is less than that of the tissue fluid and much of the latter passes back into the capillaries.

The fact that the plasma contains more proteins than the tissue fluid gives the blood a low osmotic potential (p. 23) which tends to cause water to pass from the tissue fluid into the capillary. At the arterial end of the capillary network the blood pressure is greater than this osmotic pressure, so forcing water out, but at the venous end water from the tissue fluid enters the capillary by osmosis.

Lymphatic system

The capillaries are not the only route by which the tissue fluid returns to the circulation. Some of it returns via the lymphatic system. The proteins in the tissue fluid are unable to re-enter the capillaries but can drain into thin-walled vessels with blind ends which are found between the cells. These *lymphatics* join up to form larger vessels which eventually unite into two main ducts and empty their contents into the large veins entering the right atrium.

The fluid in the lymphatic vessels is called *lymph*. Its composition is similar to plasma but it contains less proteins. It also contains a certain kind of white cell, the lymphocytes, which are made in the lymph nodes.

The larger of the two lymphatic ducts is the *thoracic duct* which collects lymph from the intestine and the lower half of the body (Fig. 11.19). The *lacteals* from the small intestine open into the lymphatic system. After a meal containing fats the lymph is a milky-white colour due to the emulsion of fat droplets absorbed in the lacteals.

On its way through the lymphatics to the ducts, the lymph passes through a number of *lymph nodes,* which appear as swellings on the lymphatics. The lymph nodes are particularly numerous in the armpit and groin. In each node there are spaces filled with a network of fibres, and attached to these fibres are white cells like macrophages which can trap and ingest foreign particles in the lymph. The lymph passing through a node is thus filtered of any invading bacteria before it is returned to the circulation. In addition the lymph node makes lymphocytes, some of which are added to the lymph while some enter the blood capillaries which permeate the node. As a result of a septic wound in a limb, the lymph node through which passes the lymph from the wound may become swollen and painful. A poisoned finger, for example, may give rise to a swollen lymph node in the armpit.

The tonsils and the spleen act in a similar way to lymph nodes.

The lymph flow takes place in one direction only, from the tissues to the heart, and there is no specialized pumping organ. The flow is caused partly by the pressure of the lymph which accumulates in the tissues, but one of the most important

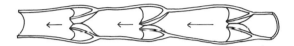

Fig. 11.18 Deep lymphatic vessel cut open to show valves

factors in the movement of lymph is muscular exercise. Some of the lymphatics have valves in them (Fig. 11.18) similar to those in veins and the pressure from contracting muscles around them compresses the lymphatic vessel and forces the lymph along in the direction determined by the valves.

If the accumulation of lymph exceeds the rate of removal in the lymphatics, a local swelling occurs. As a result of injury,

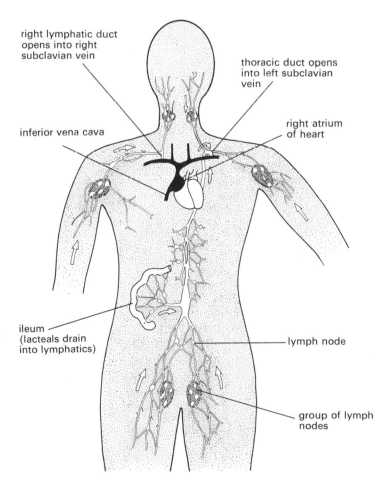

right lymphatic duct opens into right subclavian vein

thoracic duct opens into left subclavian vein

inferior vena cava

right atrium of heart

ileum (lacteals drain into lymphatics)

lymph node

group of lymph nodes

Fig. 11.19 Main drainage routes of lymphatic system

histamine is produced which makes the capillaries in the injured region more permeable, and the escape of fluid from them is too rapid for removal in the lymphatics.

Spleen. The spleen is a dark red, compact body about 12 cm long situated in the abdomen to the left of the stomach and protected by the lower ribs. It consists of spongy tissue enclosed in a fibrous capsule. The spleen produces lymphocytes and also contains other white cells, *macrophages*. The macrophages ingest and so remove from the blood worn-out red cells, cell fragments and any bacteria that may have entered the blood stream. The haemoglobin from the degenerating red cells is broken down and the iron-containing residue stored in the cells of the spleen and liver.

In diseases such as malaria (p. 213) in which many red cells are destroyed, the spleen in coping with the excess cell debris becomes considerably enlarged and projects beyond the rib cage and thus becomes more vulnerable to damage.

Practical Work

Experiment 1   Blood smear

To examine blood under the microscope a thin film must be spread on a slide. The finger is pricked with a sterile lancet which must be used by one person only. The method employed is one of personal preference. One technique is to squeeze the left little finger between fore-finger and thumb of the same hand and pierce the soft area at the tip. The capillaries are nearer the surface, however, on the back of the top joints of the fingers, just below the insertion of the fingernail.

The drop of blood is placed at one end of a clean, dry slide. A second slide is placed as shown in Fig. 11.20 so that the

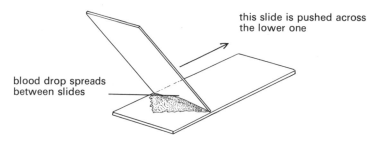

this slide is pushed across the lower one

blood drop spreads between slides

Fig. 11.20   Making a blood smear

blood drop spreads across the region of contact by capillary attraction. By pushing the top slide across the lower one, a thin film of blood is made which will show red cells quite clearly under the microscope.

To see white cells, it is best to study a prepared slide.

Experiment 2   Valves in the veins

If a light tourniquet is applied to the upper arm the veins in the forearm can be made to stand out. The lower end of one of these is blocked off near the wrist by pressing it with a finger. The blood can be expelled from the vein by running a finger with light pressure along its length towards the elbow. When

this has been done the vein will remain collapsed up to a certain point; above this the vein will fill up and swell once more. The boundary between the filled and collapsed regions indicates the position of a non-return valve.

Experiment 3   Effect of gravity on circulation

Allow the left arm to hang straight down at the side of the body. Open and clench the hand repeatedly between once and twice a second. It should be possible to continue these movements for 3 or 4 minutes or up to 500 times without feeling acute discomfort. After a period of rest, hold the arm straight up and repeat the exercises. After about one minute, or 100 closures, the movement becomes almost impossible. One reason for this is the reduced blood supply resulting from the retarding effect of gravity on the circulation. It is interesting to speculate on which particular aspect of circulation, i.e. oxygen transport, waste removal, etc., is responsible for the fatigue.

Experiment 4   Capillaries

These are best seen in the web of a frog's foot or a tadpole's tail where the red cells can be seen streaming through the narrow vessels.

Our own capillaries can be seen by soaking the back of the top joint of a finger in a clearing agent such as cedarwood oil and examining, by reflected light under a microscope, the area below the nail cuticle. Capillary loops can usually be seen even with a good hand lens.

Experiment 5   Pulse rate

The swelling of the arteries as a result of the surge of pressure from the heart can be felt in certain places and gives an indication of the rate of the heart's contractions. The pulse in the wrist is the most usual region for this. Count the number of pulsations over a period of 30 seconds and make a note of it. Then take some form of exercise, e.g. standing on and getting off a stool once in two seconds for about half a minute, and take the pulse rate again. Find out how long it takes to return to its original rate.

Questions

1 Although the walls of the left ventricle are thicker than those of the right ventricle, the volume of the ventricles is the same. Why is this necessary?
2 State in detail the course taken by (a) a glucose molecule and a fat molecule from the time they are ready for absorption in the ileum, and (b) a molecule of oxygen absorbed in the lungs, to the time when all three reach a muscle cell in the leg.
3 Why is a person whose heart valves are damaged by disease unable to participate in active sport?
4 A system for transporting substances in solution might as well be filled with water. What advantages has the blood circulatory system over a water circulatory system?
5 What is the advantage to an animal of having capillaries which are (i) very narrow, (ii) repeatedly branched and (iii) very thin-walled?
6 Study the paragraphs on homeostasis on pp. 72 and 92. Explain why transport by the blood of nitrogenous waste, carbon dioxide and heat can be considered to have a homeostatic function.
7 Explain what would happen in the following transfusions: (a) blood from an AB donor to an A recipient; (b) blood from an O donor to an AB recipient; (c) blood from a B donor to an AB recipient; and (d) blood from an O, Rh + donor to an A, Rh− recipient.

12
Breathing

The various processes carried out by the body, such as movement, growth and reproduction, all require the expenditure of energy. In animals this energy can be obtained only from the food they eat. Before the energy can be used by the cells of the body it must be transferred from the chemicals of the food. This process of energy transfer is called tissue respiration (p. 27) and involves the use of oxygen and the production of carbon dioxide.

Oxygen enters an animal's body from the air or water surrounding it. In the less complex animals the oxygen is absorbed over the entire exposed surface of the body, but in higher animals there are special respiratory areas such as lungs or gills. Excess carbon dioxide is usually eliminated from the same area.

In the respiratory organ, oxygen dissolves in the blood and is carried to all living parts of the body where it is used in tissue respiration. An efficient respiratory organ has a large surface area, a dense capillary network or similar blood supply, a very thin epithelium separating the air or water from the blood vessels and, in land-dwelling animals, a layer of moisture over the absorbing surface. All vertebrates and many invertebrates have some muscular mechanism whereby they can ventilate the breathing organs, i.e. exchange the water or air in contact with their lungs or gills. In man and other mammals, the respiratory organs are lungs.

Lungs

The lungs of man are two thin-walled elastic sacs lying in the thorax (Fig. 12.1). They can be expanded or compressed by changes of pressure in the thorax in such a way that air is repeatedly taken in and expelled. They communicate with the atmosphere through the windpipe or *trachea* which opens through the *glottis* to the *pharynx* (Fig. 10.3). In the lungs a gaseous exchange takes place; some of the atmospheric oxygen is absorbed and carbon dioxide from the blood is released into the lung cavities.

Lung structure. The trachea divides into two *bronchi* which enter the lungs and divide into smaller branches called *bronchioles* (Fig. 12.2). These divide further and terminate in a mass of little thin-walled, pouch-like air sacs or alveoli (Figs. 12.3 and 12.5).

(a) *Air passages.* Incomplete rings of cartilage keep the trachea and bronchi open and prevent their closing up when the pressure inside them falls during inspiration. The cartilaginous rings also stop the trachea from kinking when the

head is turned or inclined. The lining of the air passages is covered with numerous *cilia*. These are minute cytoplasmic filaments that constantly flick to and fro. Mucus is secreted by glandular cells also in the lining. Dust particles and bacteria which are carried in with the air during inspiration become trapped in the mucus film and are swept away in it at about 0.4 mm per second by the movements of the cilia up to the larynx and into the pharynx where they are swallowed. The ciliary beat is independent of the nervous system but can be arrested by tobacco smoke.

The epiglottis and other structures at the top of the trachea prevent large particles from entering the air passages, particularly during swallowing (p. 62). Choking and coughing are reflex actions that tend to remove any foreign particles which accidentally enter the trachea or bronchi.

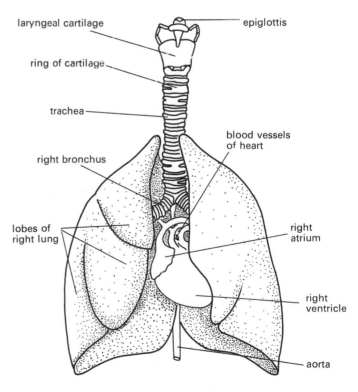

Fig. 12.1 Appearance of the lungs

(b) *Alveoli*. The alveoli have elastic walls consisting internally of a single layer of cells, or epithelium, 1 micron (1/1 000 mm) thick, and around each alveolus is a dense network of capillaries (Fig. 12.4) supplied with deoxygenated blood from the body pumped from the right ventricle through the pulmonary artery. There are about 700 million alveoli in a man's lungs with a total absorbing surface of about 50–80 square metres depending on the degree of expansion. There is evidence of minute cross-connections from one alveolus to another.

(c) *Pleural membranes* (Fig. 12.10). The pleural membrane is the lining that covers the outside of the lungs and the inside of the thorax. It produces pleural fluid which lubricates the surfaces in the regions of contact between lungs and thorax. As a result they can slide freely over one another with very little friction during the breathing movements.

Gaseous exchange

The lining of the alveoli is covered with a thin film of moisture (Fig. 12.6). The oxygen concentration of the blood in the lung capillaries is lower than in the alveolus, and oxygen in the air space dissolves in the film of moisture and diffuses through the epithelium, the capillary wall, the plasma and into a red cell, where it combines with the haemoglobin (p. 70). The capillaries reunite and eventually form the pulmonary vein which returns the oxygenated blood to the left atrium of the heart.

The carbon dioxide concentration in the alveoli is lower than in the lung capillaries. The enzyme *carbonic anhydrase* in the red cells breaks down the hydrogencarbonate (bicarbonate) salts and liberates carbon dioxide. This diffuses into the alveoli and is eventually expelled. About 250 cm³ oxygen is absorbed every minute and about the same volume of carbon dioxide expelled (Experiments 1 and 2).

Composition of inspired and expired air

	Percentage volume	
	Inspired	*Expired*
Oxygen	20.95	16.4
Carbon dioxide	0.04	4.1
Nitrogen	79.01	79.5
Water vapour	varies	saturated

There is no actual change in the volume of nitrogen in inspired and expired air but since the volume of carbon dioxide given out is slightly less than that of the oxygen absorbed, the percentage of nitrogen changes. The water vapour content of the air varies with the temperature and other atmospheric conditions but exhaled air is usually saturated with water vapour.

Diffusion gradient. A steep diffusion gradient (p. 22) of oxygen is maintained by (i) replenishment of air in the air passages by ventilation, (ii) the very short distance between the alveolar lining and the blood, (iii) the combination of oxygen with haemoglobin, so removing oxygen from solution, and (iv) the blood flow which constantly replaces oxygenated blood with deoxygenated blood. Similar factors work in the reverse direction for the diffusion of carbon dioxide. The conversion of hydrogencarbonate (bicarbonate) to carbon dioxide by carbonic anhydrase raises the concentration of carbon dioxide in the blood above that in the alveoli.

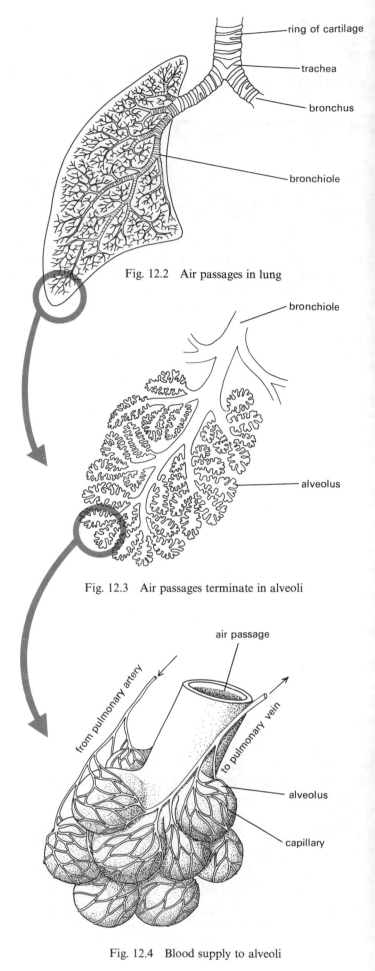

Fig. 12.2   Air passages in lung

Fig. 12.3   Air passages terminate in alveoli

Fig. 12.4   Blood supply to alveoli

Decompression. When the body is subjected to increased pressure as in deep sea diving or working under water in pressurized compartments, a greater proportion of the atmospheric gases oxygen and nitrogen dissolve in the blood and tissues. When the pressure returns quickly to normal, the extra oxygen can be taken up by the red cells and escapes in the usual way through the lungs. There is no special transport mechanism for nitrogen, however, and it tends to come out of solution as small bubbles of gas in any part of the body, rupturing tissues, blocking blood vessels and giving rise to acute pain at the joints. This decompression sickness or 'bends' is relieved by returning the victim to high pressure and reducing it very slowly, thus allowing the excess dissolved nitrogen to escape naturally from the lungs.

Smoking and health

There is little doubt today that smoking is injurious to health. There is overwhelming statistical and experimental evidence to associate smoking with the incidence of lung cancer and coronary heart attacks (p. 79). Quite apart from early death from these two diseases, heavy smokers suffer from persistent coughs which damage the lungs, and an increased susceptibility to bronchitis and pneumonia. The absorptive surface is so much decreased by the damage done to the lungs that the individual becomes 'short of breath', i.e. the least exertion causes excessive panting and discomfort. The immediate effect of tobacco smoke on the lungs and respiratory passages is to inhibit the ciliary action that removes mucus and dust particles. Consequently, the fluid remains and accumulates in the lungs making them liable to infection. In the long term, certain of the chemicals in tobacco smoke induce a cancer in the lung tissue which destroys the lung.

Carbon monoxide in tobacco smoke combines with the haemoglobin in the blood to form a compound called *carboxy-haemoglobin*. The raised level of carboxy-haemoglobin in the blood of smokers increases the permeability of their blood vessels and this in turn leads to a higher rate of deposition of fats in the artery walls and an increased risk of coronary heart attack (p. 79).

Giving up smoking progressively reduces the health hazards described above so that ten years after giving up, the death rates for ex-smokers are the same as for non-smokers.

The nose

The ciliated epithelium and film of mucus that line the nasal passages help to trap dust and bacteria. The air is also warmed to about 30 °C, depending on the external temperature, and moistened before it enters the lungs. In addition there are in the upper part of the nasal cavity sensory organs which respond to chemicals in the air and confer a sense of smell.

Inflammation of the mucous membrane lining the nasal cavity results in its swelling and blocking the free flow of air. This nasal congestion, characteristic of the common cold, can also give rise to discomfort in a warm but badly ventilated room.

Voice

The vocal cords are two folds protruding from the lining of the larynx. They contain ligaments which are controlled by muscles. When air is passed over them in a certain way, they vibrate and produce sounds. The controlling muscles alter the tension in the cords and the distance between them, and in this way they vary the pitch and quality of the sounds produced. Precise co-ordination of the breathing movements, vocal cords, lips, tongue and jaws is required to produce articulate speech. The ability to make sounds is inborn, but speech has to be learned.

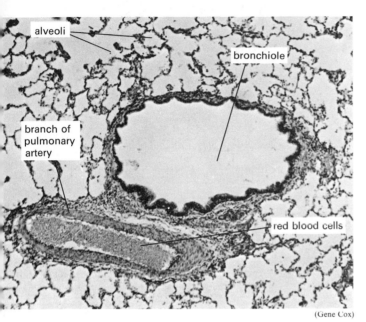

(Gene Cox)

Fig. 12.5 Appearance of lung tissue under the microscope (section)

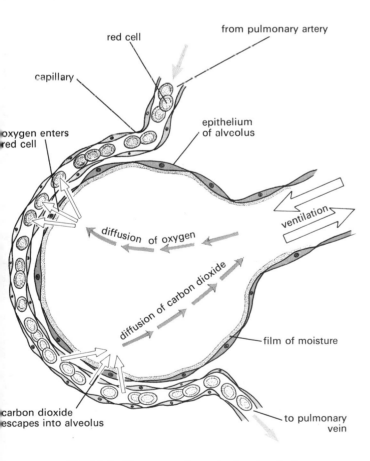

Fig. 12.6 Gaseous exchange in the alveolus

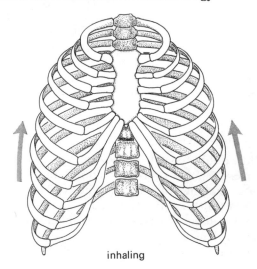

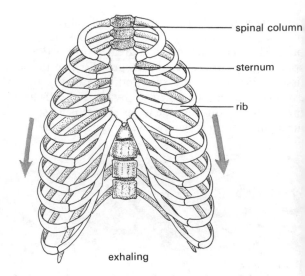

(a) Inspiration. Ribs swing up and increase volume of thorax

(b) Expiration. Ribs swing down and reduce volume of thorax

Fig. 12.7   Movement of rib cage during breathing

Fig. 12.8   Side view
of rib cage to show
intercostal muscles

Fig. 12.9   Model to show action of
intercostal muscles

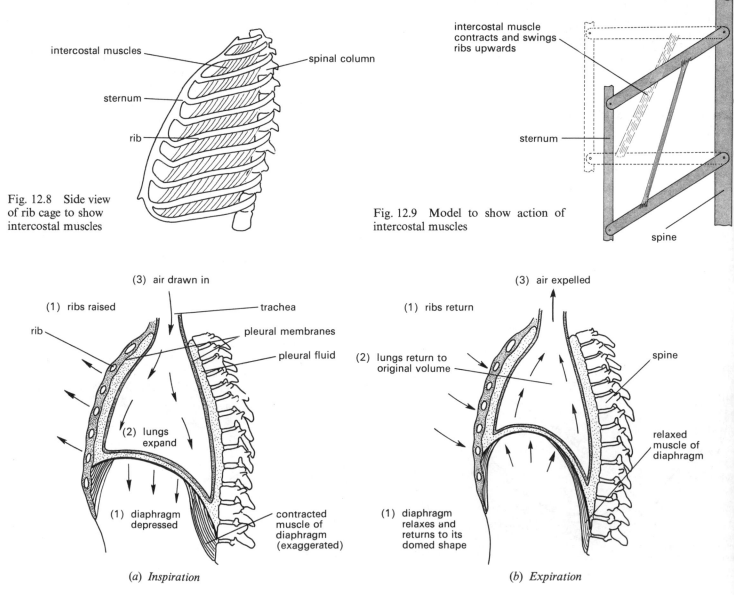

(a) Inspiration

(b) Expiration

Fig. 12.10   Sections through thorax to show mechanism of breathing

Ventilation of the lungs

The exchange of air in the lungs is brought about by movements of the thorax that alter its volume. The thorax is an airtight cavity enclosed by the ribs at the sides and the diaphragm below. The *diaphragm* is a muscular sheet of tissue extending across the body cavity between the thorax and abdomen. When relaxed it is a flattened dome shape extending upwards into the thoracic cavity with the liver and stomach immediately below it. The muscle fibres of the diaphragm radiate from a central sheet of fibrous tissue to the margins of the lower thorax, where they are attached to the ribs and body wall. Any change in the volume of the thorax is followed by the lungs which are too thin and elastic to oppose the movements.

Inspiration. During inspiration, the volume of the thorax is increased by two movements:

(a) the muscles round the edge of the diaphragm contract and pull it downwards rather like a piston (Fig. 12.10a). This movement incidentally has the effect of pushing the abdominal organs down so making the abdomen swell slightly.

(b) The lower ribs are raised upwards and outwards (Fig. 12.7) by contraction of the *intercostal muscles* which run obliquely from one rib to the next (Figs. 12.8 and 12.9).

Both these movements increase the volume of the thorax and also the volume of the lungs which follow the movements. The increase in volume lowers the air pressure in the lungs so that atmospheric pressure forces air into them through the nose and trachea. The cartilaginous rings of the trachea keep it open despite the fall of pressure inside it.

Expiration. Expiration, or breathing out, results mainly from a relaxation of the muscles of the ribs and diaphragm. Released from these constraints the elasticity of the lungs makes them contract and so expel air. The ribs move down under their own weight and the organs below the diaphragm, under pressure from the muscular walls of the abdomen, push the diaphragm, which has now relaxed, back into its original position (Fig. 12.10b).

More controlled and forcible expiration is achieved by contraction of the abdominal muscles, as in coughing, blowing up a balloon or playing a wind instrument. Expiration, either active or passive, expels from the lungs air containing less oxygen and more carbon dioxide and water vapour than when it entered. Usually, in quiet breathing, the movements of the diaphragm alone are mainly responsible for the ventilation of the lungs. X-ray studies show that the centre of the diaphragm moves down by only 12 mm during quiet breathing.

Lung capacity (Fig. 12.11). The total capacity of the lungs when fully inflated is about 5.5 litres in an adult man, but during quiet breathing only 0.5 litres of air is exchanged. This is called *tidal air*. During activity, the thoracic movements are more extensive, and deep inspiration can take in another 2 litres while vigorous expiration can expel an additional 1.3 litres. The thorax cannot collapse completely so that one litre of air can never be expelled. This *residual air* remaining in the alveoli exchanges carbon dioxide and oxygen by diffusion with the tidal air that sweeps into the bronchioles and air passages.

The 140 cm³ air which enters the trachea and bronchi at the end of each inspiration is expelled without having exchanged any oxygen or carbon dioxide with the lungs. This region is called the *dead space. Vital capacity* is the maximum volume of air which can be exchanged, i.e. the volume of air which can be expelled by forcible expiration after deep inspiration (Experiment 3).

Control of breathing rate

The rhythmical breathing movements are usually carried out quite unconsciously from 12 to 20 times a minute in an adult. A respiratory centre in the medulla of the brain is thought to control these reflex breathing movements, and experiments with the detached brains of animals have shown a pattern of nervous activity which corresponds to the breathing rhythm. These results suggest that the respiratory rhythm is initiated by the brain, but it is known also that the rate can be influenced by reflex action, the chemical composition of the blood and conscious control.

(a) **Nervous reflex.** There is some evidence of the presence in the lungs of nerve endings which, when stretched, fire off sensory impulses to the medulla via the vagus nerve. These impulses appear to bring inspiration to a halt and allow the lungs to return to their relaxed volume. The motor nerves for breathing pass from the respiratory centre to the diaphragm and intercostal muscles via the spinal cord in the neck and thoracic region.

(b) **Chemical effect.** (i) *Carbon dioxide.* Relatively small increases in the carbon dioxide content of the blood stimulate the respiratory centre and produce at first deeper breathing and then more rapid breathing. If the breath is held, the carbon dioxide concentration builds up in the blood and stimulates the respiratory centre until one is compelled to start breathing again. Forced breathing, i.e. deep inspiration and expiration for a minute, enables the breath to be held for much longer, probably as a result of the 'flushing out' of carbon dioxide from the blood so that a longer time is needed for the carbon dioxide concentration to build up to 'bursting point' in the medulla. Since the blood is normally 95 per cent saturated with oxygen it seems unlikely that forced breathing achieves its effects by increasing the oxygen content of the blood, and experiments show that breath-holding is very little improved by breathing oxygen beforehand.

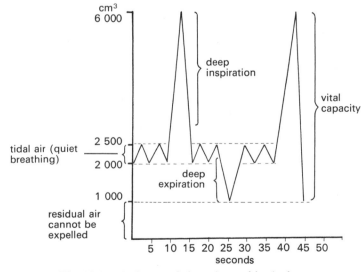

Fig. 12.11   Volumes of air exchanged in the lungs

The carbon dioxide concentration of the blood is most likely to rise during vigorous activity because of the rapid breakdown of carbohydrates in the muscles to provide energy. The accelerated breathing rate which results from the rise in carbon dioxide concentration helps to expel this gas as fast as it accumulates and also to maintain the amount of oxygen in the blood, so meeting the demands of increased tissue respiration. The increased rate of breathing which prevents the carbon dioxide rising above a certain level is an example of homeostasis (p. 92).

(ii) *Oxygen*. The oxygen concentration in the air can fall from 21 to 13 per cent with very little effect on the rate of breathing. In the carotid arteries are bodies containing chemical receptors which are stimulated by gross oxygen shortage and send sensory impulses to the medulla resulting in an increased breathing rate.

Flying at high altitudes may lead to oxygen shortage and is dangerous because the pilot is usually unaware of the deficiency since the carotid sensory receptors respond only to a severe fall in oxygen tension.The oxygen deficiency in the blood leads to errors of judgement, hilarity or aggressiveness similar to drunkenness. Pressurized cabins or supplementary oxygen prevent this condition.

(c) **Conscious control.** 'Higher', conscious, parts of the brain can influence the respiratory centre and bring the breathing rhythm under conscious control, as in speaking and singing or simply holding the breath.

Acclimatization. Mountain sickness results from oxygen deficiency at high altitudes. The body becomes acclimatized by the kidneys' adjusting the acidity of the blood and, over a longer period, by the production of more red cells by the bone marrow.

Other factors affecting breathing. Swallowing momentarily interrupts breathing. Stimulation of the lining of the larynx produces a reflex contraction of the abdominal muscles leading to coughing. Air is expelled violently from the lungs so dislodging and removing the foreign body. Sneezing is a comparable reflex action induced by the stimulation of the mucous membrane in the nasal cavity.

Breathing of the embryo. Although the mammalian embryo derives its oxygen and eliminates its carbon dioxide via the placenta (p. 105) by exchanges between the maternal and embryonic blood circulatory systems, the human foetus has been demonstrated to make irregular and intermittent breathing movements during which amniotic fluid is breathed in and out.

At birth, the change from floating in warm amniotic fluid (p. 106) to being exposed to the air and to touch stimuli, sends sensory impulses to the respiratory centre of the brain which then relays motor impulses to the rib muscles and diaphragm so that breathing begins.

Artificial 'respiration'

The effect of severe electric shock or partial drowning can result in the arrest of the breathing movements. If the brain cells are deprived of oxygen for more than a few minutes they are permanently damaged and full recovery of the victim becomes unlikely. Breathing can be restarted by a method of artificial 'respiration' or resuscitation which should be applied without delay. The most effective method is for the rescuer to apply his mouth to the victim's mouth and blow air into the lungs. The victim's head must be tilted well back to open the air passages and the nostrils pinched shut with the fingers. In this way the victim's lungs are inflated about 20 times per minute until his breathing begins once more. Although the air breathed into the unconscious person's lungs is 'used' air, it will contain about 16 per cent oxygen which is sufficient to nearly saturate the blood in the alveoli.

When the breathing muscles are paralysed as a result of some disease such as poliomyelitis which affects the nervous system, the patient's breathing is maintained by an 'iron lung' in which the breathing movements are induced by intermittent decompression on the outside of his thorax.

Practical Work

Experiment 1   **Composition of exhaled air (1)**

Two large test-tubes (boiling tubes) are prepared as shown in Fig. 12.12 and 10 cm³ lime water placed in each. Check that the rubber tubing is connected to the long glass tube in one case and to the short glass tube in the other. Place both pieces of rubber tubing in the mouth and breathe in and out through the tubing for about 30 seconds. Air breathed out will bubble through the lime water in tube B, whereas air breathed in will pass through tube A.

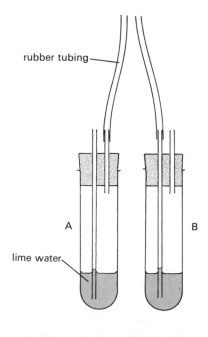

rubber tubing

A   B

lime water

Fig. 12.12   Testing exhaled air for carbon dioxide

Result. The lime water in tube B will go milky while that in A will remain clear.

Interpretation. Since it is carbon dioxide that turns lime water milky, the results suggest that exhaled air contains more carbon dioxide than inhaled air.

Experiment 2 Composition of exhaled air (2)

Prepare a large glass jar with two lids, one holding a bent wire with a candle stub as shown in Fig. 12.13*b* (a gas jar and deflagrating spoon will do if these are available). Light the candle, lower it into the jar and count the number of seconds it stays alight. Collect exhaled air in the jar as follows:

(a) lie the jar on its side in a basin of water and place a rubber tube inside it (Fig. 12.13*a*);

(b) stand the jar upside down in the basin so that it remains full of water;

(c) blow down the tube to fill the jar with exhaled air;

(d) remove the rubber tube and put the lid on the jar still upside down and under water.

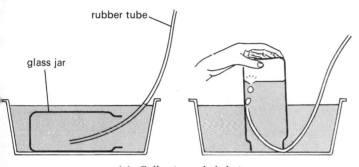

(a) Collecting exhaled air

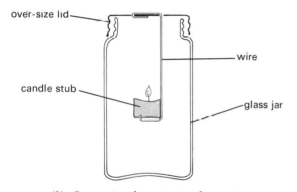

(b) Comparing the amounts of oxygen

Fig. 12.13 Testing air for its oxygen content

Remove the jar from the basin and test the air in it with a lighted candle as before.

Collect and test a further sample of exhaled air, but this time expel nearly all the air from the lungs before blowing down the rubber tube into the jar.

Result. The candle will burn for a shorter time in exhaled air than in atmospheric air, and for a shorter time still in the air from the deeper regions of the lungs.

Interpretation. The candle needs oxygen in order to burn. The less oxygen is present the sooner will the flame go out. Exhaled air therefore contains less oxygen than inhaled air.

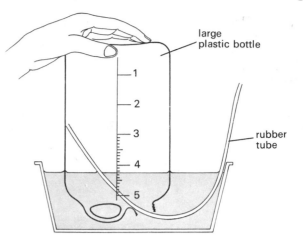

Fig. 12.14 Measuring lung capacity

Experiment 3 Lung capacity

Calibrate a large (plastic) bottle up to five litres by filling it with water one litre at a time and marking the levels. Invert the bottle full of water in a basin of water, remove the stopper under water and insert a rubber tube through the neck. Take a deep breath and exhale through the tube so that the exhaled air collects in the bottle, displacing the water. The level of water left in the bottle will give a measure of the lung capacity (*vital capacity*) (Fig. 12.14).

Push the rubber tube half-way up inside the bottle so that its end is clear of the water and blow out any water remaining in the tube. Support the bottle with your hand and breathe in and out through the tube as normally as possible. The bottle will rise and fall in the basin with each breath giving some idea of the volume of air exchanged during quiet breathing (*tidal air*).

Questions

1 Outline the events that take place in the course of vigorous exercise leading to a change in the rate and depth of breathing both during and after the activity. (*See also* Chapter 5, pp. 27 and 28.)

2 The lungs and ileum are adapted for absorption. Point out the features they have in common which facilitate absorption.

3

	inhaled air	*exhaled air*	*alveolar air*
oxygen (%)	21	16	14
carbon dioxide (%)	0.03	4	5.5

The table above gives the approximate percentage volume composition of air inhaled, exhaled or retained in the lungs. Explain how these differences in composition are brought about by events in the lungs.

4 An artificial pneumothorax is a method of resting an infected lung. Air is injected into the pleural cavity and the lung collapses. After a few months, the air is absorbed and the lung works normally again. Try to explain why the introduction of air into the pleural cavity should cause the lung to stop working and say why it is possible for a person with a collapsed lung to lead a normal life.

13

Excretion and the Kidneys

The processes which constitute 'life' can generally be described as chemical reactions that perpetuate themselves. Many of these reactions, respiration for example, result in energy transfer to activate other processes. All these chemical changes give rise to end products, some of which are poisonous or could affect the normal body chemistry if allowed to accumulate.

The chemical units of living protoplasm are constantly being renewed. Even the apparently permanent structures of the body, like muscles, blood, skin and internal organs, are in fact changing from day to day. New molecules are being added, old molecules and entire cells are being broken down. For example, an amino acid in some protein eaten on one day may be built into the living protoplasm of a muscle fibre the next day. Later the same amino acid may be broken down and the products carried off in the blood stream. The products of this kind of protein decomposition contain nitrogen, urea being one of the most common nitrogenous compounds in the mammalian body. Accumulation of these compounds could upset the delicate balance of the tissue fluids and they are removed by the kidneys as soon as their concentration reaches a certain level. Excess protein taken in during a meal and absorbed as amino acids is deaminated in the liver (p. 69), producing urea and other nitrogenous compounds.

Excretion is the process by which such excess or harmful substances are removed from the body as fast as they exceed a certain concentration.

Excretory products. The main excretory products in animals are carbon dioxide and water from respiration and nitrogenous compounds from the breakdown of proteins or excess amino acids. Ammonia is a nitrogenous compound formed in the kidneys and intestine but it is converted in the liver into urea which is less poisonous to the body.

Excretory organs. In man, the excretory organs are the kidneys and the lungs. The lungs eliminate excess carbon dioxide from the body and in this sense may be considered excretory. Water also is lost from the lungs, and water, sodium chloride, a little urea and lactic acid are lost from the skin in the sweat. It can hardly be claimed that these losses are excretory since they do not take place in response to changes in the chemical composition of the body fluids. Loss of water vapour from the lungs is inevitable with every breath expired and sweat production is a response to increase in temperature. It could be maintained that the green bile pigments derived from the breakdown products of haemoglobin are excretory products,

since these pigments are released into the intestine with the bile from the liver and contribute to the colour of the faeces. This could be described as an excretory function of the liver.

Homeostasis

Although most cells of the body are adaptable to changes in their environment, their delicately balanced chemical reactions work best within narrow limits of temperature, acidity etc. A fall in temperature will slow down all the chemical reactions in the cell; a drop in pH may inhibit some enzyme systems; a rise in the concentration of solutes may withdraw water from the cells by osmosis. Homeostasis is the name given to the processes whereby such changes of the internal medium are kept within narrow limits, and many organ systems of the body contribute to this control.

The internal medium of most animals is the tissue fluid (p. 83) which is in contact with all the living cells of the body. The composition of the tissue fluid depends on the composition of the blood from which it is derived and, therefore, the homeostatic mechanisms of many animals act by adjusting the composition of the blood.

The skin helps to regulate blood temperature (p. 98), the liver adjusts its glucose concentration (p. 69), the lungs keep the carbon dioxide concentration down to a certain level (p. 90), and the kidneys control its composition in three principal ways: they (a) eliminate all soluble nitrogenous waste compounds above a certain concentration, (b) remove excess water, (c) expel salts above a certain concentration, and (d) excrete excess hydrogen ions to maintain its pH. These activities are both excretory, in that they remove the unwanted waste products of metabolism, and osmoregulatory (p. 23), in that they keep the osmotic potential of the blood more or less constant.

Kidney structure and function

The two kidneys are compact, oval structures with an indentation on the side nearest the mid-line of the body. They are red-brown, enclosed in a transparent membrane and attached to the back of the abdominal cavity (Fig. 13.1). The *renal artery* branching from the aorta brings oxygenated blood to them, and the *renal vein* takes deoxygenated blood away to the vena cava. A tube, the *ureter,* runs from each kidney to the base of the bladder in the lower part of the abdomen.

The kidney tissue consists of many capillaries and tiny tubes

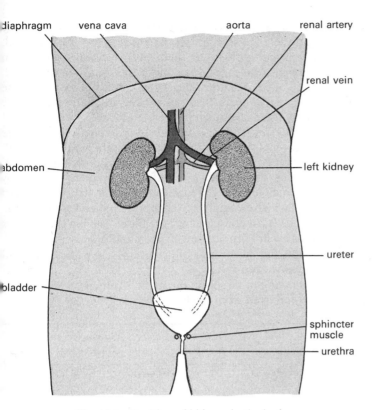

Fig. 13.1   Position of kidneys in the body

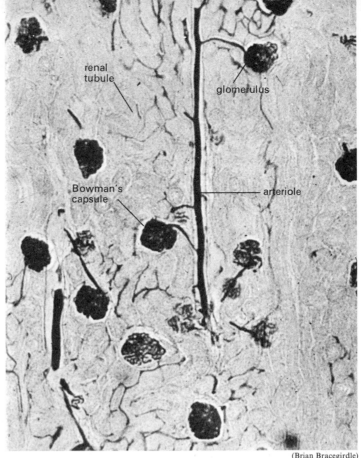

(Brian Bracegirdle)

Fig. 13.3   Section through kidney cortex

called renal tubules, held together with connective tissue. A section through the kidney shows an outer darker region and a lighter inner zone, the medulla. Where the ureter leaves the kidney is a space called the *pelvis*, and projecting into this are cones or pyramids of kidney tissue.

Detailed structure. The renal artery divides up into a great many arterioles and capillaries, mostly in the cortex (Fig. 13.2). Each arteriole leads to a *glomerulus* which is a capillary repeatedly branching and coiled into a small knot of vessels

(Fig. 13.3). The glomerulus is almost completely surrounded by a cup-shaped structure called a *Bowman's capsule* which leads to a coiled renal tubule. This tubule, after a series of coils and loops, joins other tubules and passes through the medulla to open into the pelvis at the apex of a pyramid (Fig. 13.4). The glomerulus, Bowman's capsule and associated renal tubule are called a *nephron*.

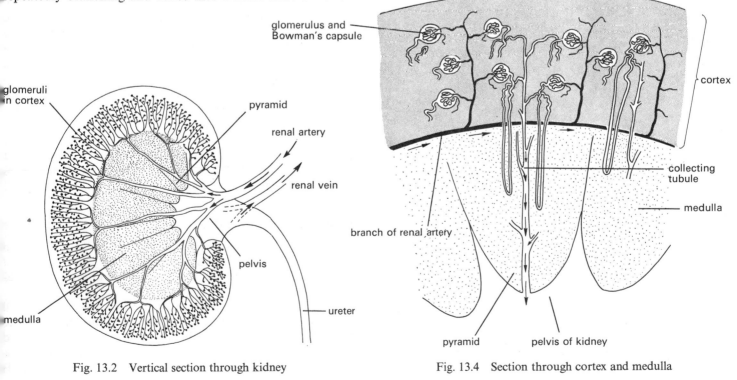

Fig. 13.2   Vertical section through kidney

Fig. 13.4   Section through cortex and medulla

93

Mechanism of excretion in the kidney. The pressure of blood in the capillaries of the glomerulus is high because (a) the renal artery is short and the blood pressure from the heart is little diminished, and (b) the tortuous path through the glomerular capillaries offers a resistance to the flow of blood. This pressure causes fluid to filter out through the capillary walls and to collect in the Bowman's capsule. The filtered fluid contains glucose, amino acids, salts and nitrogenous waste dissolved in water, but the blood cells and large molecules such as fibrinogen and other proteins remain in the blood in the capillaries. Experiments show that the composition of this filtrate is more or less the same as blood plasma minus its proteins, and that the fluid is forced by blood pressure through the capillaries and porous walls of the Bowman's capsule which do not usually permit large molecules to pass. In man, 180 litres per day of this filtrate, carrying 145 g glucose and 1 100 g sodium chloride, pass into the Bowman's capsules.

As the filtered serum passes down the renal tubule, all amino acids and glucose with much of the water and some of the salts are absorbed into a network of capillaries surrounding the tubule (Fig. 13.5). This selective reabsorption prevents the

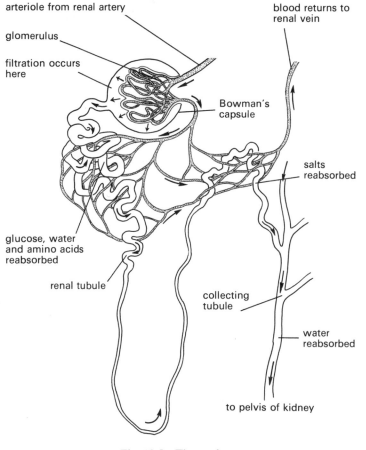

Fig. 13.5   The nephron

loss of useful substances from the blood serum and regulates its composition. The remaining liquid, now called *urine,* contains only the waste products such as urea, uric acid, excess salts and water, and traces of substances such as hormones. It passes down the collecting tubule where more water is reabsorbed and, consequently, the concentration of the blood plasma is regulated. If the blood is too dilute, e.g.

after drinking a great deal, less water is absorbed back into the blood and the urine is dilute. If the blood is too concentrated, e.g. after sweating profusely, more water is reabsorbed from the collecting tubules, making the urine more concentrated. From the collecting tubes, the urine enters the pelvis of the kidney where it collects. Peristaltic waves of contraction in the ureter carry the urine down to the bladder.

The capillaries from the glomeruli and renal tubules unite to form the renal vein. It is the cells of the kidney tubules which selectively reabsorb substances from the glomerular filtrate. They do this often against a diffusion gradient (p. 22) by methods which are not fully understood, e.g. active transport (p. 29), but which certainly need energy supplied by respiration within the cells. In consequence, the blood leaving the kidneys in the renal vein contains less oxygen and glucose, more carbon dioxide and, as a result of excretion, less water, salts and nitrogenous waste.

The following table shows the main nitrogenous substances which are removed from the blood by the kidneys.

	Nitrogenous compounds in blood (%)	Nitrogenous compounds in urine (%)
Proteins	7–9	0
Urea	0.03	2
Uric acid	0.005	0.05
Ammonia	0.0001	0.05
(Water	90–93	95)

The bladder

The bladder is an extensible sac with elastic tissues and muscle in its walls. The accumulation of urine entering the bladder from the ureters extends its elastic walls to a volume of 400 cm³ or more but without increasing the pressure very much. When the volume of urine reaches 400–600 cm³, waves of contraction pass down the bladder resulting in an urge to urinate. Nerve impulses are sent to the sphincter muscle (Fig. 19.13) at the mouth of the bladder, causing it to relax and allow the urine to escape through the urethra. Voluntary control over the sphincter can be maintained until the fluid volume in the bladder (of an adult) reaches about 600 cm³. Attempts to retain urine in the bladder beyond this stage result in a back pressure being developed through the ureters to the kidneys where damage to the tubules may occur.

In babies, the contraction of the bladder and the relaxation of the sphincter are under reflex control only, being triggered off by the stretched walls of the full bladder. After about 2 years or less, the reaction can be brought under voluntary control.

Water balance and osmoregulation

Water is lost from the body in urine, faeces, sweat and exhaled breath. It is gained by eating, drinking and as a product of tissue respiration. These losses and gains will produce corresponding changes in the blood.

An increase in the salts in the blood or a loss of water will cause its osmotic potential to rise. When this blood passes through the hypothalamus in the brain, the rise is detected by osmoreceptors and the posterior pituitary gland is stimulated to release a hormone called *antidiuretic hormone* (ADH) into the circulation. When the ADH reaches the kidney it increases the amount of water reabsorbed into the blood from the filtrate in the renal tubules. Thus, more water is retained in the blood helping to reduce its osmotic potential, and less water is excreted in the urine which thus becomes more concentrated. If the osmotic potential of the blood falls, e.g. as a result of drinking a large quantity of water, the osmo-receptors in the hypothalamus detect the change and cause the posterior pituitary to release less ADH. Consequently less water is reabsorbed into the blood from the kidney tubules and more is excreted in the urine.

The mechanism that produces the sensation of thirst is not well understood but it undoubtedly serves to regulate the intake of water and so maintain the concentration of the blood.

The artificial kidney

Although a person can survive and lead a more or less normal life with only one functional kidney, failure of both kidneys leads to death in about ten days, largely due to accumulation in the blood of excess potassium which adversely affects the heart function. A temporary failure of the kidneys sometimes results from an accident which leads to such a fall in blood pressure that filtration in the glomeruli is greatly reduced. Permanent failure results from kidney disease. In both cases the condition can be alleviated by the use of an 'artificial kidney' which eliminates the excess salts and nitrogenous waste from the patient's blood.

In one form of artificial kidney, perhaps better called a dialysis machine, the patient's blood is led from the radial artery in his arm through a coiled cellophane tube and then returned to a vein in the same arm. The cellophane tube is immersed in a solution warmed to body temperature and containing a very carefully regulated amount of dissolved salts and sugars. The cellophane tubing is differentially permeable so that salts, sugars, urea, hydrogen ions, etc. can diffuse out from the patient's blood into the solution. The diffusion gradient for any particular substance can be controlled by dissolving more or less of the substance in the external solution. For example, the glucose concentration outside the tubing is the same as in the blood so that there is no loss of sugar from the blood. The sodium and potassium salts in the external solution are at a level characteristic of a healthy person so that any excess of these salts in the patient's blood will diffuse out and restore his blood to a normal composition. The pH of the external solution is adjusted so that excess hydrogen ions are lost from the patient's blood preventing its becoming too acid. The external solution is changed regularly so that substances that diffuse out of the blood are removed. Excess water is removed by artificially raising the blood pressure in the cellophane tubing.

The dialysis machine enables the victim of a temporary kidney failure to recover before the imbalance of salts in his blood leads to heart failure. People with permanent kidney damage can survive and, with strict dieting, lead a relatively normal life if they circulate their blood through a dialysis machine for about twelve hours twice a week.

Questions

1 In an experiment, a man drank a litre of water. His urine output increased so that after 2 hours he had eliminated the extra water. When he drank a litre of 0.9 per cent sodium chloride solution, there was little or no increase in urine production. Explain the difference in these results.
2 In cold weather one may need to urinate frequently, producing a fairly colourless urine. In hot weather, urination is infrequent and the urine is often coloured. Explain these observations.
3 Consult pp. 69, 94 and 157 and then explain briefly why glucose does not normally appear in the urine.
4 Explain why the elimination of water by the kidneys may be considered to be both excretion and osmoregulation.

14
Skin and Temperature Control

The skin is a continuous layer of tissue over the surface of the body. It has many functions:

(a) it protects the tissues beneath from mechanical injury and abrasion; from toxic chemicals and bacterial invasion; from desiccation as a result of evaporation; and from the destructive effects of ultraviolet radiation in sunlight;

(b) it contains numerous sense organs which are sensitive to temperature, touch and pain, so making man aware of changes in his surroundings. This sensitivity has a generally protective aspect in that it initiates voluntary or involuntary withdrawal actions, e.g. voluntarily moving away from a hot fire or reflex withdrawal of the fingers from a hot object thus preventing further damage;

(c) it helps to keep the body temperature constant by sweat production and changes in its blood flow.

In addition, in man, vitamin D can be synthesized in the skin. Teeth, hair, nails and mammary glands all develop from modifications of the skin.

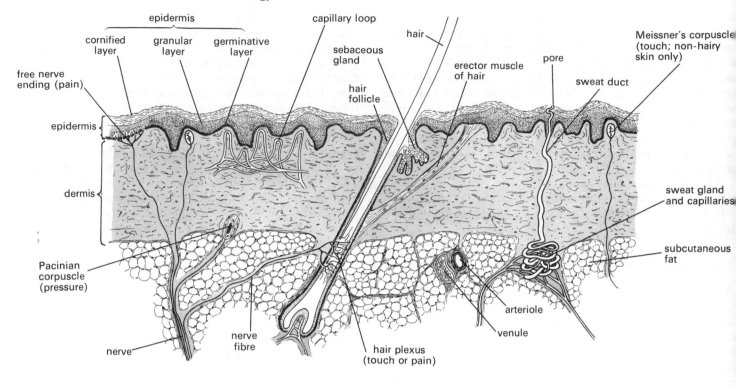

Fig. 14.1   Generalized section through skin

Skin structure

The skin consists of two main layers, an outer *epidermis* and an inner *dermis*. The details of skin structure vary, however, with the region of the body under consideration but the following description applies to most regions (*see* Fig. 14.1).

Epidermis

(a) **Germinative layer.** This is a continuous layer of cells which can divide actively and so produce new epidermis. In this layer also occurs the pigment *melanin* which determines the skin colour and absorbs the ultraviolet radiation. Infoldings of the germinative layer produce the sweat glands, the sebaceous glands, hair follicles and fingernails. Since the epidermis contains no blood vessels, the germinative cells must derive their food and oxygen by diffusion or active transport from the capillary networks in the dermis.

(b) **Granular layer.** This layer consists of living cells recently produced from the germinative layer. As these cells are gradually pushed to the outside by the accumulation of new cells beneath them, deposits of a substance called *keratin* are formed in them and they lose their nuclei, become flat and finally wear away or fall off.

(c) **Cornified layer.** These flat, dead cells full of keratin granules constitute the cornified layer which makes a tough, bacteria-resisting, waterproof coat, so forming a barrier between man and his environment. The cells of this region are continually worn away and replaced from beneath. In non-hairy skin, i.e. the palms of the hands and soles of the feet, the cornified layer may be very thick (Fig. 14.2). Non-hairy skin also has a thick epidermis with a regular pattern of ridges (fingerprints), and a relatively thin dermis with numerous

sweat glands but few or no hair follicles. Hairy skin has a thick dermis and a thin epidermis with numerous hair follicles (Fig. 14.3) and covers the whole body except the palms and soles.

Dermis

The dermis is a layer of connective tissue with relatively few cells but many collagen fibres and a small number of elastic fibres in it. The collagen fibres give the skin its tensile strength and its tough, slightly elastic properties. These fibres are probably made by cells called *fibroblasts* whose appearance varies according to age but are usually apparent only as nuclei. Fibroblasts are important in wound healing. Apart from fibroblasts, the only other cells generally distributed in the dermis appear to be *macrophages,* cells similar to white blood cells which can destroy foreign particles and bacteria by engulfing them and can move about to some extent.

In the dermis are also blood capillaries, nerve endings and lymphatic vessels, Sweat glands, hair follicles and sebaceous glands, although they appear in the dermis, are in fact produced by the epidermis.

Capillaries. The capillaries supply the skin with the necessary food and oxygen and remove its waste products. The sweat glands and hair follicles have a network of capillaries supplying them. The capillaries beneath the epidermis not only nourish it but play an important part in temperature control (p. 98).

Sweat glands. The sweat gland is a coiled tube consisting of secretory cells which absorb fluid from the surrounding cells and capillaries and pass it into the tube, through which it reaches the skin surface. The composition of sweat varies but it consists mainly of water with some salts dissolved in it, notably sodium chloride (0.3 per cent), and small quantities of urea (0.03 per cent) and lactic acid (0.07 per cent).

In hot conditions accompanied by hard work, a man may lose up to 10 litres of sweat, containing 30 g sodium chloride per day. Both the liquid and the salt must be replaced or the circulatory system may fail. If water alone is taken to replace the lost sweat, the salt and water balance of the blood and tissues is upset leading to heat cramp, sometimes called 'miner's cramp', i.e. cramping pains in the muscles most frequently used.

Hair follicle. This is a deep pit of granular and germinative layers whose cells multiply and build up a cylindrical hair inside the follicle. The cells of the hair become impregnated with keratin and they die. The constant adding of new cells to the base of the hair causes it to grow. The hairs on the head continue to grow for up to four years after which the hair falls out and a new period of growth begins. The growth of a body hair may be for only a few months. The colour of the hair depends on the amount, if any, of the melanin incorporated in the cells. The curliness of hair depends on the shape of its cross-section; a circular cross-section is characteristic of straight hair, an elliptical section produces wavy hair and a flattened or kidney-shaped section produces woolly hair. Contraction of the hair muscle pulls the hair more upright and at the same time compresses the sebaceous gland forcing a little of its secretion, sebum, on to the skin.

Sebaceous glands. The sebaceous glands open into the hair follicles and produce an oily secretion, *sebum*, which gives the hairs water-repelling properties, keeps the epidermis supple and reduces the tendency for it to become dry through evaporation. The fatty acids in sebum are thought to be effective in preventing the multiplication of harmful bacteria and fungi.

Fingernails. These consist of a modified granular layer produced by a groove lined with germinative cells. They grow at the rate of about 0.5 mm per week.

Subcutaneous fat. The layers beneath the dermis contain numerous fat cells in which fat is stored. Apart from being a reserve of food, this layer, by virtue of its insulating properties, has the effect of reducing heat losses.

Damage and repair

Burns. Superficial burns which affect only cornified or granular layers are soon repaired by the normal division of the germinative cells. Deeper burns which destroy the germinative layer heal more slowly as the new germinative layer has to grow out from the undamaged hair follicles to cover the exposed area.

If the burns are so deep that the hair follicles are destroyed, new epidermis cannot grow although scar tissue will be formed by the dermis. In this case skin grafting is used. Even superficial burns, if they occur over a wide area, can be dangerous if not given expert attention. This is partly due to the increased chances of bacterial invasion through the unprotected dermis, and partly a result of the leakage of blood plasma which may affect the concentration and volume of the blood causing impairment of the circulation.

Repair. (a) *Natural.* When the skin is damaged, as in a cut, the formation of a blood clot (p. 73) reduces both the escape of blood and the entry of germs. The capillaries of the damaged region dilate and become more permeable allowing plasma, its proteins and its white cells to escape into the tissues giving rise to the familiar reddening and swelling. The white cells of the blood and the macrophages of the dermis combat any bacteria which have gained access, aided by antibodies which may be present in the blood plasma (*see* p. 74). Bacteria which escape these defences may enter the lymphatics and on passing through a lymph node may be ingested by the phagocytic cells contained there. Beneath the scab, macrophages and fibroblasts move in, the former digesting the blood clot and cell debris, the latter laying down new collagen fibres. Nerve endings and capillaries invade the new dermis so formed. The epidermis is restored by multiplication and migration of cells from the margins of the undamaged germinative layer at the rate of about 0.5 mm per day until the wound is closed and the scab is ready to fall off. With deep wounds, healing takes place more or less as described, with the difference that far more collagen fibres are laid down making a tough, rather inflexible and insensitive scar.

Fig. 14.2   Section through non-hairy skin (the sweat ducts are contorted in passing through the cornified layer)

(Brian Bracegirdle)

Fig. 14.3   Section through hairy skin

(Brian Bracegirdle)

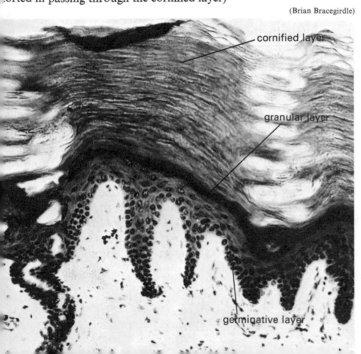

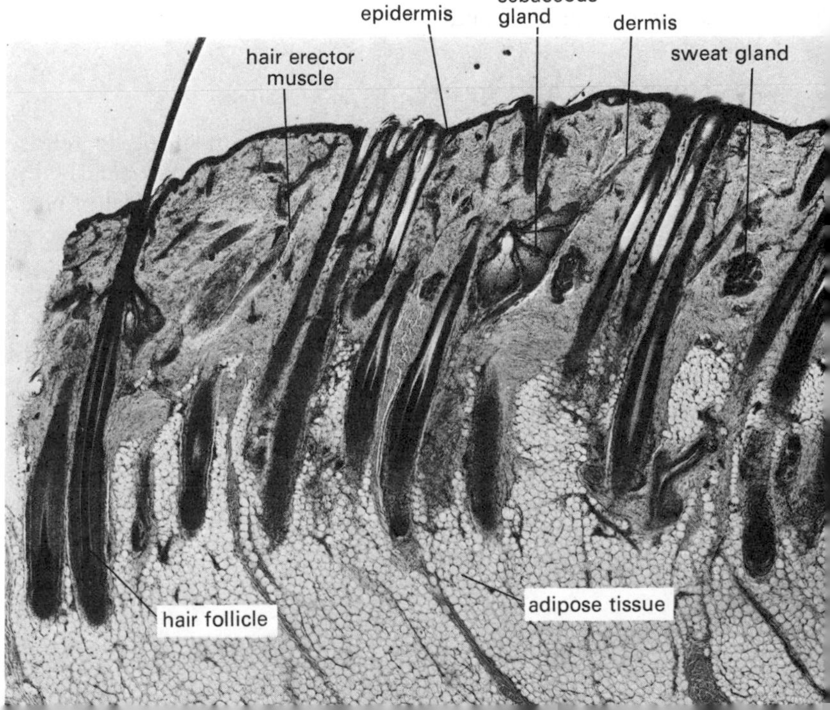

cornified layer

granular layer

germinative layer

hair erector muscle

epidermis

sebaceous gland

dermis

sweat gland

hair follicle

adipose tissue

(b) *Skin grafting*. Extensive wounds and burns in which the hair follicles are destroyed can be repaired by skin grafts. Small slices of skin, deep enough to include the germinative layer and some dermis, are taken from a donor area such as the abdomen, arm or thigh and placed over the region to be covered. After a few days, the capillaries of the receiving area have invaded and made connections with the capillaries in the donated skin and in a few weeks the graft has become a part of the damaged area. The donor area heals normally by overgrowth of the germinative layer from the hair follicles or, if a deeper layer of skin has been removed, healing is promoted by sewing the edges of the wound together. Grafted skin cannot be transferred from one person to another with success; the graft must come from the injured person's own body.

A transplant of skin from anyone other than an identical twin is rejected. Blood vessels fail to grow into it, it dies and falls away. The body reacts to transplants of skin and most other organs or tissues as it would to bacteria, incorrect red cells and foreign proteins. The transplant is attacked by phagocytes and antibodies and eventually destroyed.

The transplanting of kidneys, hearts, livers, etc. depends on using drugs to suppress this immune reaction of the body and this, in turn, leaves the patient very susceptible to attack by disease organisms.

Temperature control

Fish, amphibia, reptiles and all the invertebrate animals are *poikilothermic*. That is to say their body temperature is the same as or only a few degrees above that of their surroundings and varies accordingly. This makes them very dependent on external temperature changes. For example, in cold conditions their low body temperature slows down most chemical changes and reduces the organism to a state of inactivity. Insects can be quite immobilized by a sudden fall in temperature.

Homoiothermic or constant-temperature animals are more independent of their surroundings as their body temperature is higher and does not alter with fluctuations in external temperature. Man by both voluntary and involuntary means is able to maintain his internal temperature even in extremes of heat or cold and it may be for this reason that humans have a wider distribution over the Earth's surface than any other vertebrate, being able to maintain a stable temperature in arctic or tropical conditions.

Heat loss and gain

Many of the chemical changes in living protoplasm release heat energy. Chemical changes in glands, particularly the liver, and in contracting muscle produce a great deal of heat; in fact, over a period of 24 hours, 95 per cent of the energy transferred in chemical reactions in the body appears as heat. The circulatory system distributes this heat round the body. If no heat were lost from the body, the temperature of even a totally inactive person would rise by about 1°C per hour. In fact, the body loses heat from its surface to the atmosphere mainly by convection and radiation, though in tropical conditions heat may be gained by these means. Fluid is constantly diffusing through the skin and evaporating into the air so removing heat from the body. This is not the same as sweating,

as the sweat glands are not in constant activity. An outer layer of fur, feathers or clothing reduces these heat losses.

With an inactive subject in an environmental temperature of about 29–30 °C, the rates of heat loss and gain are about the same and the body temperature remains between 35.8 °C and 37.3 °C. The temperature of the body is not the same in all regions but is usually measured in the mouth, armpit or rectum and taken as an indication of the blood temperature. The mouth temperature is the most reliable indicator of changes in the temperature of the blood. Body temperature also varies during the day with activity and from one person to the next. The specific marking of 98.4 °F (36.9 °C) on a clinical thermometer represents an average temperature of healthy individuals but since their temperatures may range from 96.6 to 100 °F (35.9–37.8 °C), readings of 2 °F (1 °C) above or below this average do not indicate ill-health. When heat loss and gain do not balance, regulatory mechanisms in the body under the control of the brain come into action and compensate for overheating or overcooling.

Overheating

This may be brought about by a high environmental temperature, vigorous activity, disease, by absorbing radiation from the sun, or by many other external causes. If the temperature of the blood reaching the hypothalamus of the brain (p. 155) is a fraction of a degree higher than 'normal', nerve impulses are sent to the skin producing two marked effects.

1 **Vasodilation.** Certain of the arterioles beneath the epidermis dilate (get wider). Consequently more blood flows near the surface, losing heat through the epidermis into the air by convection and radiation (Fig. 14.4a). In white-skinned

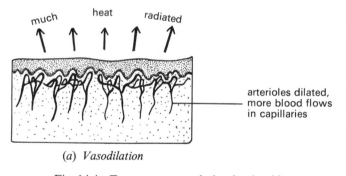

(a) *Vasodilation*

Fig. 14.4 Temperature regulation by the skin

people, vasodilation may cause obvious flushing (reddening) of the skin on account of the increased volume of blood just beneath the epidermis. With an environmental temperature of 34 °C about 12 per cent of the blood pumped out by the heart may pass to the skin.

2 **Sweating.** Vasodilation and vasoconstriction are effective in controlling the body temperature when external conditions vary between 25 °C and 29 °C. Above this range sweating begins, and below 25 °C shivering sets in, depending on other factors such as clothing and activity. Sweating begins when the external temperature rises above 29–31 °C, depending on the weight of clothing, or when for any reason the blood reaching the hypothalamus is 0.5–1.0 °C above 'normal'. Nerve impulses starting mainly in the hypothalamus and conveyed by the autonomic nervous system (p. 151) stimulate the sweat

glands into activity. Fluid from the blood is filtered into the glands and passes through their ducts so that a layer of moisture is produced on the skin surface. As the sweat evaporates it takes its latent heat from the body and so reduces the body temperature. Evaporation from the forehead, upper lip, neck, chest and trunk is responsible for temperature regulation. Sweating from the palms, soles and armpits seems more dependent on emotional stress than on body temperature.

In humid conditions, the air contains so much water vapour that the sweat may not evaporate rapidly enough to produce an adequate cooling effect, and may lead to *heat stagnation* in which the body temperature rises to over 41 °C, causing collapse and sometimes death. *Heatstroke* is a similar result of extreme overheating when, after prolonged sweating due to vigorous activity at high temperatures, sweat production ceases and the body temperature rises to a lethal level. Both conditions may be called 'sunstroke' but it is not the effect of direct sunlight on the body so much as the high temperatures produced.

Overcooling

If the body begins to lose more heat than it is generating, the following compensatory changes may take place:

1 **Decrease in sweat production,** thus minimizing heat lost by evaporation.

2 **Vasoconstriction.** Constriction, or closing, of the arterioles that supply the surface capillaries in the skin reduces the volume of blood flowing near the surface and hence diminishes heat losses (Fig. 14.4*b*). Vasoconstriction makes a white-skinned person look pale or blue.

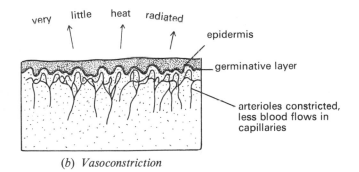

(*b*) *Vasoconstriction*

3 **Increased metabolism.** An increase in the rate of chemical changes in the body, particularly in the liver, releases more heat.

4 **Shivering.** This reflex action operates when the body temperature begins to drop. It is a spasmodic contraction of the muscles. These contractions produce heat which helps to raise the body temperature.

Furry mammals and birds can fluff out their fur or feathers by contraction of the erector muscles which are attached to them in the skin. This increases the layer of trapped air round the skin and so improves insulation by reducing convection and conduction. In man, a similar contraction of the muscles of the hairs produces only 'goose-pimples' but adding layers of clothing increases the thickness of the insulating air layer round the skin.

Voluntary temperature control

By constructing houses with efficient heating and ventilation, by adding or removing clothing, by taking exercise or cold showers, man exerts conscious, voluntary control over his rate of heat loss or gain. Vigorous exercise can produce a rise of from 1 to 4 °C.

Comfort. The sensations of feeling hot or cold result from the stimulation of receptors in the skin. The body temperature remains virtually constant even though the brain is registering heat loss or gain through the skin. A person *feels* cold when the skin temperature receptors respond to a loss of heat to the atmosphere and the skin may become cold as a result of vasoconstriction, but the temperature of the blood does not alter.

A comfortable environment is one which results in a skin temperature of about 33 °C. The humidity of the environment is an important factor in temperature regulation and comfort. If the air is saturated with water vapour little or no sweat will evaporate from the body and this important means of temperature control is ineffective. A hot, humid environment may lead to overheating of the body and sensations of discomfort.

Hypothermia

In some conditions where heat loss exceeds heat production, the body is unable to compensate rapidly enough and the deep body temperature begins to fall. This is a dangerous condition known as *hypothermia*. It may occur in elderly people spending long hours inactive in cold buildings. It is also the main cause of death due to 'exposure' in cold, wet conditions. The affected person becomes tired and weak and loses consciousness. Unless the victim's temperature is raised carefully, hypothermia leads in a few hours to heart failure.

In certain heart operations the patient's body is deliberately cooled to 27 °C. At this temperature the rate of metabolism is slowed by 30 to 40 per cent and the oxidation of glucose ceases. In these conditions the demand of the tissues for oxygen is much reduced and the circulation can be interrupted for 10 to 15 minutes without damaging the nerve cells of the brain which are particularly affected by lack of oxygen. The patient is given a light anaesthetic and an injection to suppress the shivering reflex; the body is cooled by ice packs or by rubber tubing carrying chilled brine. The low temperature is sufficient to ensure the maintenance of unconsciousness.

Questions

1 Why is it more accurate to describe fish as 'variable-temperatured' animals rather than 'cold-blooded'?
2 When a dog is hot, it hangs its tongue out and pants. Why should this have a cooling effect?
3 Why do you think we experience more discomfort in hot humid weather than we do in hot dry weather?
4 You may 'feel hot' after exercise or 'feel cold' without your overcoat and yet your body temperature is not likely to differ by more than 0.5 °C on the two occasions. Explain this apparent contradiction. (*See also* p. 130.)
5 Draw up a balance sheet showing all the possible ways in which the human body can gain and lose heat.
6 In what ways does the skin contribute to the homeostasis of the body? (*See* p. 92.)

15
Reproduction

Sexual reproduction involves the fusing together of two cells called *gametes*. One of these reproductive cells comes from a male and the other from a female. The fusion of two gametes is called *fertilization* and the resulting composite cell is called a *zygote*. The most important aspect of fertilization is the fusion of the nuclei of these male and female gametes, since in these nuclei is the genetic information that determines the inherited characteristics of the individual that develops from the zygote.

Fertilization then is the fusion of the nuclei of male and female gametes to form a zygote from which a new individual can develop. In animals the male gametes are *sperms* which are produced in the reproductive organs called *testes*. The female gamete is an *ovum* which is produced in reproductive organs called *ovaries*. (Some animals such as earthworms and snails are *hermaphrodite*, that is they have both testes and ovaries, but in the majority of animals the sexes are separate.)

Internal and external fertilization. In most fish and amphibia fertilization is external. The female lays the eggs first and the male fertilizes them by shedding sperms over them afterwards. A behaviour pattern that brings the sexes close together usually ensures that sperms are shed near the eggs and so increases the chances of fertilization.

In birds and reptiles, the eggs are fertilized inside the body of the female by the male passing sperms into the egg ducts. The sperm meets the ovum and fertilizes it before it is laid. However, very little development of the egg takes place before laying and the embryo grows in the egg after it has left the mother's body.

In mammals, sperms are placed in the vagina of the female and the eggs are subsequently fertilized internally. They are not laid after fertilization but are retained in the female's body while they develop to quite an advanced stage. They are born more or less fully formed and are protected by their parents and fed on a secretion of milk from the mammary glands until they can feed independently.

Sexual reproduction in man

Female reproductive organs (Figs. 15.1–15.3). The *ovaries* are two oval bodies each about 35–40 mm long, lying in the lower part of the abdomen. They are attached by a membrane to the uterus and supplied with blood vessels. Close to each ovary is the expanded funnel-shaped opening of an oviduct, also known as the *Fallopian tube*. This is the tube down which the ova pass after they are released from the ovary.

Both oviducts open into a wider tube, the *uterus* or *womb*,

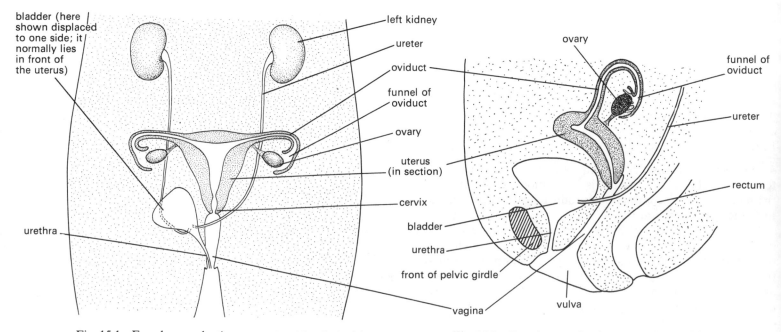

Fig. 15.1   Female reproductive organs (position in body)

Fig. 15.2   Female reproductive organs (vertical section)

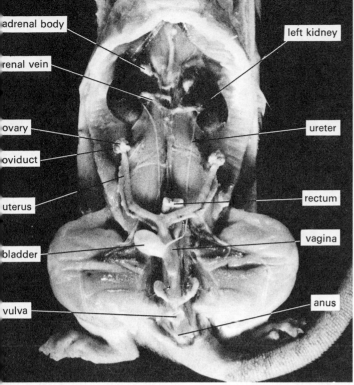

adrenal body
renal vein
ovary
oviduct
uterus
bladder
vulva
left kidney
ureter
rectum
vagina
anus

(Dissection by Gerrard and Haig Ltd)

Fig. 15.3   Dissection of female reproductive organs of a rat (note that there are two uteri in the rat)

lower down in the abdomen. When there is no embryo developing in it, the uterus is only about 80 mm long with walls 10 mm thick consisting of unstriated (involuntary) muscle and a glandular lining. The uterus communicates with the outside through a muscular tube, the *vagina*. The *cervix* is a ring of muscle closing the lower end of the uterus where it joins the vagina. There is normally only a very small aperture

joining these two organs at this point. Two folds of skin, the *labia majora* and the *labia minora*, enclose the *vulva* at the entrance to the vagina. The urethra from the bladder opens into the vulva just in front of the vagina.

Male reproductive organs (Figs. 15.4 and 15.5). The two testes lie outside the abdominal cavity in man, in a special sac called the *scrotum*. This enables the testes to remain at a temperature about 2 °C lower than the rest of the body, a condition which favours sperm production. Each testis consists of a large number of sperm-producing tubules. Between these tubules are interstitial cells which produce a male hormone, *testosterone*, and possibly other substances. The sperm-producing or *seminiferous* tubules join to form sperm ducts leading to the *epididymis*, a coiled tube about 6 metres long on the outside of the testis. The epididymis in turn leads into a muscular *sperm duct* (Fig. 15.6). The two sperm ducts, one from each testis, open into the top of the urethra just after it leaves the bladder. Surrounding the urethra at this point are the *prostate gland* and, further down, *Cowper's gland*. The urethra at different times conducts both urine and sperms, and is prolonged through the penis which consists of connective tissue with numerous small blood spaces in it.

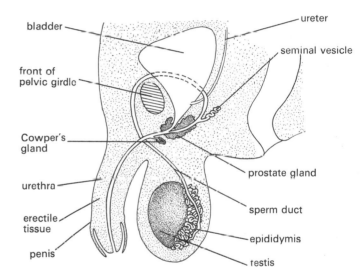

bladder
front of pelvic girdle
Cowper's gland
urethra
erectile tissue
penis
ureter
seminal vesicle
prostate gland
sperm duct
epididymis
testis

Fig. 15.5   Male reproductive organs (vertical section)

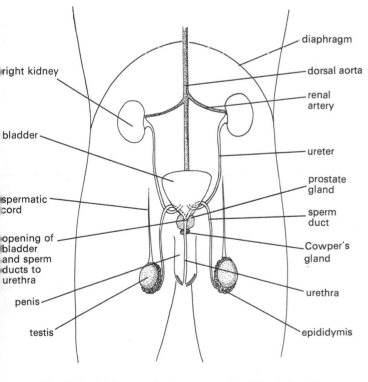

right kidney
bladder
spermatic cord
opening of bladder and sperm ducts to urethra
penis
testis
diaphragm
dorsal aorta
renal artery
ureter
prostate gland
sperm duct
Cowper's gland
urethra
epididymis

Fig. 15.4   Male reproductive organs (position in body)

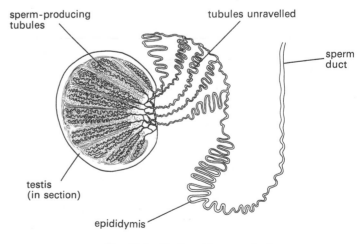

sperm-producing tubules
testis (in section)
epididymis
tubules unravelled
sperm duct

Fig. 15.6   Testis and sperm duct

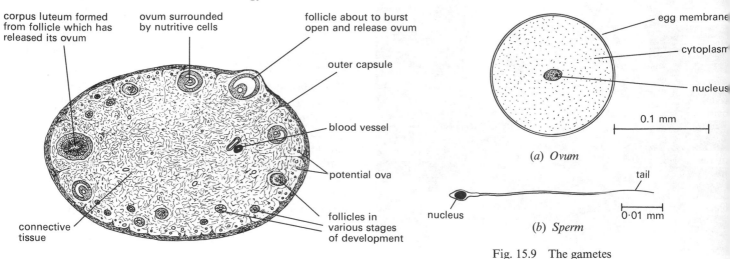

corpus luteum formed
from follicle which has
released its ovum

ovum surrounded
by nutritive cells

follicle about to burst
open and release ovum

outer capsule

blood vessel

potential ova

follicles in
various stages
of development

connective
tissue

Fig. 15.7   Section through ovary

egg membrane

cytoplasm

nucleus

0.1 mm

(a) Ovum

tail

nucleus

0·01 mm

(b) Sperm

Fig. 15.9   The gametes

Ovulation. The ovary consists of connective tissues, blood vessels and potential egg cells (Fig. 15.7). It is thought that 70 000 potential egg cells are already present at birth and are not, like sperms, formed continuously during adult life. Of these potential egg cells only about 500 will ever become mature ova. The ovaries also secrete hormones called *oestrogens* which control the secondary sexual characters (p. 108) and initiate the thickening of the lining of the uterus which occurs each month.

Between the ages of about eleven and fourteen years, the ovaries become active and begin to produce mature eggs. The beginning of this period of life is called *puberty* and is characterized by a series of physiological and psychological changes (*see* p. 108). In the ovary, some of the ova start to mature and the cells around them divide rapidly. A fluid-filled cavity is eventually produced, which partly encircles the ovum and its coating of follicle cells. This structure is now called a *Graafian follicle*. When the Graafian follicle is ripe it is about 10–20 mm in diameter and projects as a clear vesicle from the surface of the ovary (Fig. 15.8). Finally it bursts and releases the ovum into the funnel of the oviduct whose ciliated cells waft it into

the tube. At this stage the ovum (Fig. 15.9a) is a spherical mass of protoplasm about 0.13 mm in diameter, with a central nucleus and with some of the cells from the follicle still adhering to the outside (Fig. 15.12a). An ovum is produced from one or other of the ovaries every four weeks and it may spend several hours travelling down the oviduct to the uterus. The oviduct is lined with ciliated cells whose cilia help to propel the ovum towards the uterus.

Sperm production (Fig. 15.10). The lining of the seminiferous tubules making up the testis consists of actively dividing cells which give rise ultimately to sperms (Fig. 15.9b). A sperm is a nucleus surrounded by a little cytoplasm which extends into a long tail (Fig. 15.11). The sperms are quite immobile when first produced and pass into the epididymis where they are stored. During copulation, muscular contractions of the epididymis, sperm duct and accessory muscles force the accumulated sperms through the urethra. Here, the secretion of fluids from the prostate gland and seminal vesicles adds nutrients and enzymes to the sperms, so diluting them and possibly stimulating them into their swimming action in which lashing movements of their tails propel them along. Sperms not ejaculated in this way are broken down and their products reabsorbed in the sperm ducts at the same rate as they are produced in the testis.

Fig. 15.8   Mature Graafian follicle

(Brian Bracegirdle)

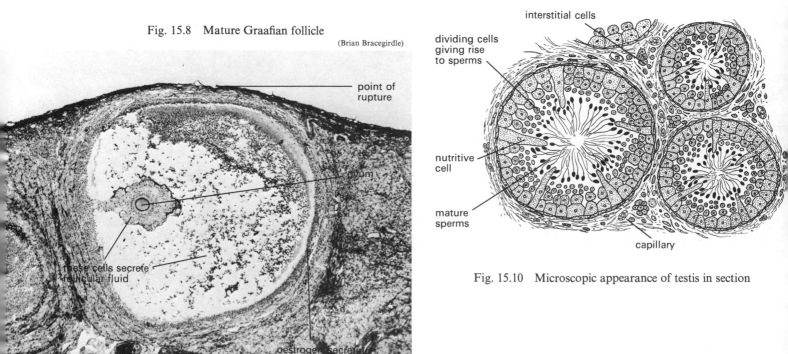

point of
rupture

ovum

these cells secrete
follicular fluid

oestrogen secreting
layer

interstitial cells

dividing cells
giving rise
to sperms

nutritive
cell

mature
sperms

capillary

Fig. 15.10   Microscopic appearance of testis in section

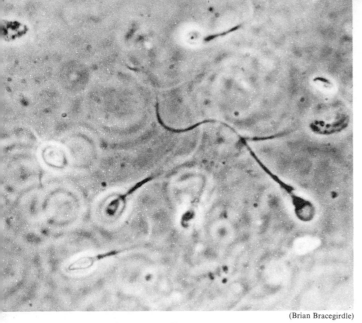

(Brian Bracegirdle)

Fig. 15.11   Human sperms

being ejaculated into the vagina. This event is the climax of copulation. The sperms deposited in the vagina swim through the cervix into the uterus and up the oviduct, assisted probably by contractions of the uterus. If an ovum is present in the oviduct, many of the sperms swim towards it. Eventually, the head of one sperm sticks to the ovum. The sperm's head passes into the cytoplasm of the ovum and fuses with the female nucleus there (Fig. 15.12).

Although a single ejaculation may release more than a hundred million sperms, only one will actually fertilize the ovum. Experiments with animals suggest that each sperm produces a minute quantity of enzyme, which disperses the remaining follicle cells adhering to the ovum, so facilitating fertilization. Whether this is an important process in man is not clear. In other mammals, such as the rabbit, several ova are released from the ovary at the same time and may be fertilized by the corresponding number of sperms.

In the ovary, the cells of the follicle from which the ovum was released continue to divide and grow for a while, filling the follicle with a solid mass of tissue called the *corpus luteum*. The corpus luteum produces a hormone, *progesterone,* which acts on the uterus causing its lining to thicken and its vascular supplies to increase in preparation for the implantation and nourishment of the embryo. If fertilization does not occur, the corpus luteum degenerates and gives way to ordinary ovary tissue. If, on the other hand, fertilization occurs, the corpus luteum persists and produces progesterone for another three months.

The period during which a released ovum can be fertilized is thought, by some authorities, to be as little as eight hours and by others to be up to forty-eight hours. Results of artificial insemination suggest that sperms can fertilize an ovum only up

Fertilization. Fertilization occurs internally when the sperms meet the ovum as it passes down the oviduct. They are introduced into the female by the penis which is placed in the vagina. To facilitate this action the penis becomes erect and firm, largely as a result of the arterioles dilating and so allowing blood to enter the blood spaces more rapidly than it escapes, which increases the turgidity of the tissues round the urethra. Similarly, the lining of the vulva and vagina secrete mucus which makes entry of the penis easier. Contact with the walls of the vagina stimulates the sensory endings in the penis and sets off a reflex action that results in the *semen* (consisting of 60 per cent fluid from the seminal vesicles, 20 per cent prostatic secretion, and the accumulated sperms)

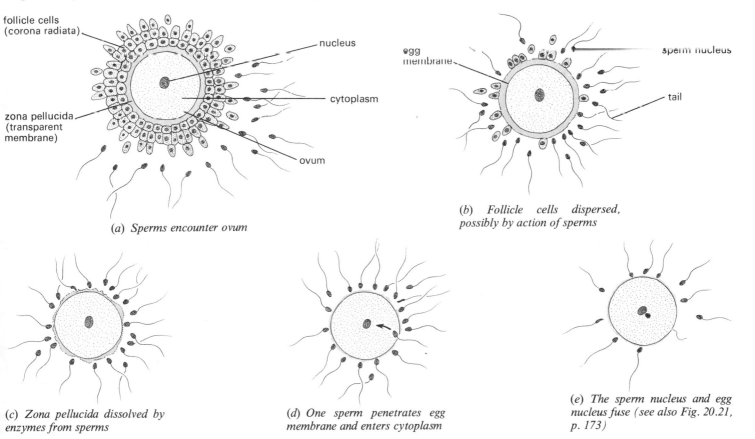

(a) *Sperms encounter ovum*

(b) *Follicle cells dispersed, possibly by action of sperms*

(c) *Zona pellucida dissolved by enzymes from sperms*

(d) *One sperm penetrates egg membrane and enters cytoplasm*

(e) *The sperm nucleus and egg nucleus fuse (see also Fig. 20.21, p. 173)*

Fig. 15.12   Fertilization of human ovum (the diagrams show what is thought to happen but the events are not known for certain)

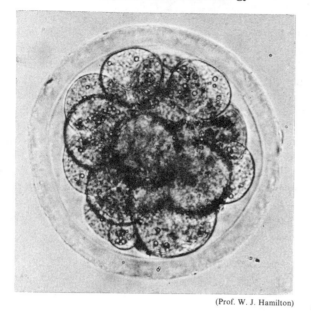

(Prof. W. J. Hamilton)

Fig. 15.13 Early stages of cell division in zygote of sheep

to twenty-four hours after arriving in the female tracts even though they may live for about three days. Thus there is a relatively short period in which fertilization can occur. Since the times of ovulation cannot be determined exactly, it is not easy to ensure that copulation takes place within a period of twenty-four hours before or thirty-two hours after ovulation, if children are wanted, or outside this period if they are not.

Pregnancy and development. The zygote undergoes rapid cell division (Fig. 15.13) as it passes down the oviduct and into the uterus. At first it floats freely, absorbing nutriment from the uterine secretions and then, four to seven days after its release from the ovary, it adheres to and sinks into the uterine lining. This is called *implantation* and may take place at various points in the uterus, but frequently it is high up on the posterior surface. As the embryo begins to form, finger-like processes grow from it into the uterine lining, digesting the epithelium and then absorbing nourishment. These villi do not form part of the embryo but, later, contribute to a special organ called the *placenta* which supplies the embryo with both food and oxygen (Fig. 15.14).

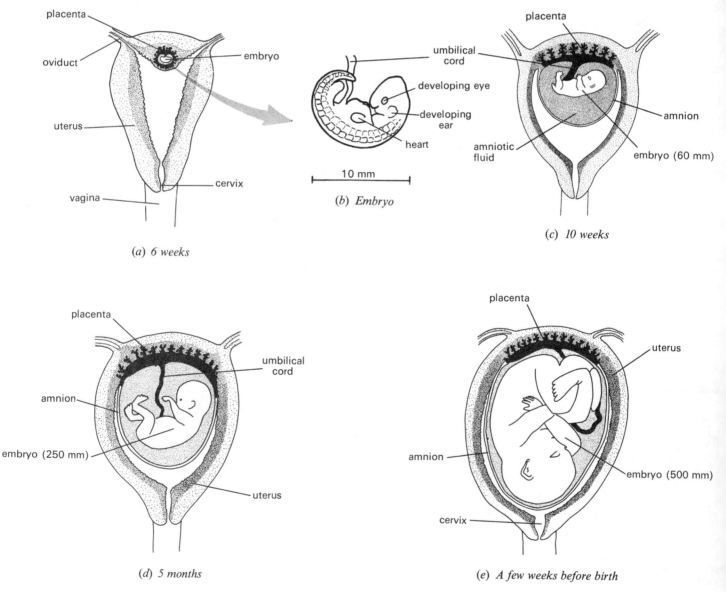

Fig. 15.14 Growth and development in uterus (not to scale)

The uterus, which at first has a volume of only 2 to 5 cm³, extends with the growth of the embryo to 5 000–7 000 cm³, enlarging the abdomen and displacing the organs in it to some extent. The uterus lining at the same time develops a rich supply of blood vessels and becomes increasingly muscular.

The embryo's cells divide to form tissues; the tissues swell, roll, extend and so form organs of the body. By the end of five weeks the heart and a circulatory system have formed, the heart is beating and circulating the blood but the embryo is still only about 10 mm long. After two months, the limbs and the main organ systems have been laid down and the embryo is now referred to as a foetus.

Although the foetus depends for its food and oxygen on the mother's blood, its circulatory system is never directly connected with the maternal blood vessels. If it were, the adult blood pressure would burst the delicate capillaries forming in the foetus and many substances in the mother's circulation would poison it.

The placenta. The placenta becomes a large disc of tissue, adhering closely to the uterine lining (Fig. 15.15). From the foetal part of the placenta, villi protrude into the uterine lining which has thickened and in which capillaries have broken down to form more extensive blood spaces. The membranes separating the foetal capillaries from the maternal blood spaces are very thin so that dissolved substances can pass across in both directions (Fig. 15.16). In the placenta, oxygen, glucose, amino acids and salts in the mother's blood pass from the uterine blood spaces into the capillaries of the foetus, while carbon dioxide and urea from the foetus pass across in the opposite direction (Fig. 15.17). The differences in concentration on either side of the placenta are sufficient to account for the diffusion of oxygen and carbon dioxide, but do not entirely explain the quantities of glucose transferred, and the method by which fats cross the placenta is not yet known. Amino acids are passed from uterine to foetal blood against a diffusion gradient presumably by some form of active transport.

In addition, the membrane in the placenta which separates foetal and maternal blood seems to exert a selective influence over the substances that pass into the foetal circulation, and so prevents harmful material from reaching the embryo. Vitamins have been shown to pass from mother to child, and also some antigens and antibodies such as the diphtheria toxin and the Rhesus positive antibody (p. 76).

A pregnant woman will absorb more iron than usual from her diet and pass it to the foetus. The demands of the latter for calcium and phosphorus may be so great that if the mother's diet is deficient in available forms of these elements they will be taken from her own bones and teeth.

The placenta, as well as exchanging food, waste products

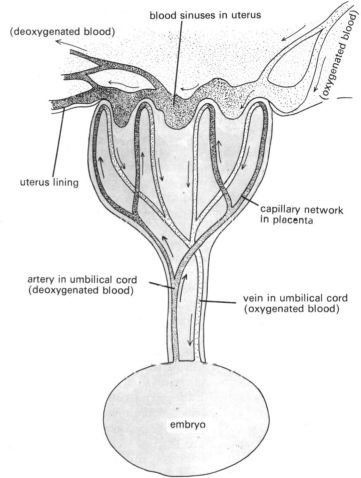

Fig. 15.16 Diagram of relationship between blood supply of embryo, placenta and uterus

Fig. 15.15 Human foetus, 7 weeks

(Prof. W. J. Hamilton)

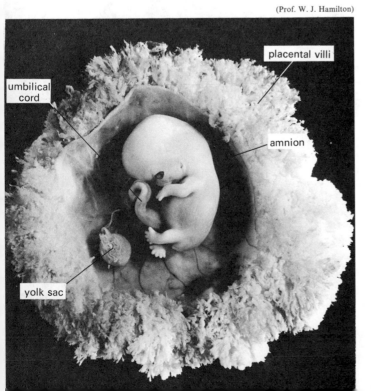

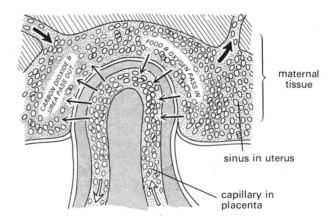

Fig. 15.17 Diagram to show exchange of oxygen and food from uterus to placenta

and respiratory gases, also produces hormones similar to oestrogen and progesterone that prevent menstruation and ensure continued pregnancy. The capillaries in the placenta are connected to an artery and vein which run in the *umbilical cord* from the placenta to the abdomen of the foetus. The foetus is surrounded by a 'water sac', the *amnion,* whose fluid buoys it up while the delicate organs and tissues are growing. It also evens out the pressure changes resulting from the contractions of the uterus which go on all the time and it protects the foetus from mechanical damage, while enabling it to move about fairly freely. The foetus swallows this fluid and also takes it in and out of its lungs with shallow, irregular 'breathing' movements. It also excretes foetal urine into the amniotic fluid but does not defaecate. After about five months' growth, the foetus moves its limbs quite vigorously inside the amniotic cavity and uterus.

The time from fertilization to birth, the *gestation period,* lasts about nine months in humans, but over half the weight of the foetus is gained in the last six to eight weeks. In fifty per cent of pregnancies, birth occurs within seven days either side of the 280 days from the last menstrual period. The mechanism which starts *labour* is not yet known. It seems, however, that the distension of the uterus in the latter months of gestation restricts the blood supply in it, and the output of hormones which retain the foetus is reduced. The corpus luteum has degenerated and the concentration of progesterone falls to a level at which the uterus is more readily stimulated to contract. It is also suspected that a hormone produced by the pituitary body has some influence on the beginning of labour.

A baby born after only seven months of gestation has a good chance of survival if given special care and extra oxygen. If born earlier than this, the baby's chances of survival are slight. The average birth weight of a baby is about 3 kg.

Birth. A few weeks before birth, the foetus has come to lie head downwards in the uterus with its head just above the cervix (Fig. 15.18). The uterus makes rhythmic contractions even when empty but before birth these contractions become more frequent and more regular. This is the onset of labour, and the interval between the contractions becomes shorter and the contractions themselves more forcible. The opening of the cervix gradually dilates enough to let the child's head pass through and the uterine contractions are then reinforced by voluntary contractions of the abdominal muscles. The amnion breaks at some stage during labour and the fluid escapes through the vagina. Finally, the muscular contractions of the uterus and vagina expel the child, head first, through the dilated cervix and vagina.

In a few minutes, the arteries in the umbilical cord constrict and the latter can be tied and cut. About 10 to 20 minutes later the placenta breaks away from the uterus and is expelled separately as the 'afterbirth'. The uterus contracts to its normal size soon after the birth, but bleeding from the placental area continues for some days and the raw area is very liable to infection, so commonsense precautions must be taken such as refraining from sexual intercourse for about six weeks. Before the nature of infection was properly understood, many mothers died of 'childbirth' fever as a result of infections of the uterus.

The sudden fall in temperature and other new sensations from the skin and muscles experienced by the newly born baby stimulate it to take its first breath, usually accompanied by crying, when amniotic fluid is expelled from its lungs. In a few days, the remains of the umbilical cord attached to the baby's abdomen shrivel and fall away, leaving in the abdominal wall a scar called the *navel.*

For the first three to four days there is a loss in weight but once feeding is properly established the weight increases rapidly. The child does not grow uniformly, however, since the proportions at birth are quite different from those at maturity. For example, the relative increase in the legs is × 5, arms × 4, trunk × 3, but the head only × 2.

Foetal circulation (Fig. 15.19). The circulatory system of a foetus shows marked differences from that of an adult as a result of the connection to the placenta and the non-functioning of the lungs. Much of the blood flowing down the foetal aorta passes via two *umbilical arteries* to the placenta, where its composition changes as indicated on p. 105. The oxygenated blood returns from the placenta to the foetus through the *umbilical vein,* passing through the liver or bypassing the latter in the *ductus venosus,* to reach the vena cava. Only a small fraction of the blood from the inferior vena cava reaches the right ventricle; most of it passes through the *foramen ovale* between the two atria to enter the left atrium (Fig. 15.20). The deoxygenated blood from the head enters the right atrium through the superior vena cava and passes into the right ventricle in the usual way. From the right ventricle the blood is pumped into the pulmonary artery, but the *ductus arteriosus* which in the foetus connects the pulmonary artery to the aorta, allows blood to bypass the lungs and enter the aorta. At birth, the blood supply to the placenta is cut off by the constriction of the umbilical arteries and the blood pressure rising in the left side of the heart closes the valve in the foramen ovale which seals up within a week. The ductus arteriosus begins to close within a few hours so that all the blood from the right ventricle passes through the lungs.

Fig. 15.18   Model of human foetus just before birth

(Reproduced with permission from the Birth Atlas published by Maternity Centre Association, New York)

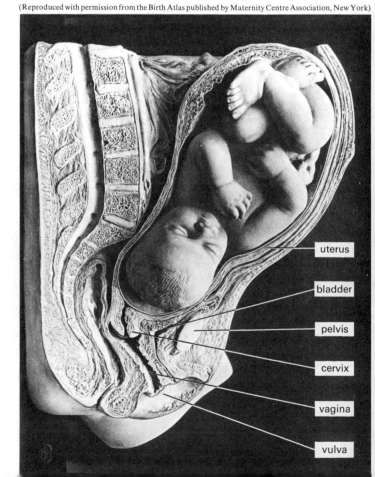

uterus

bladder

pelvis

cervix

vagina

vulva

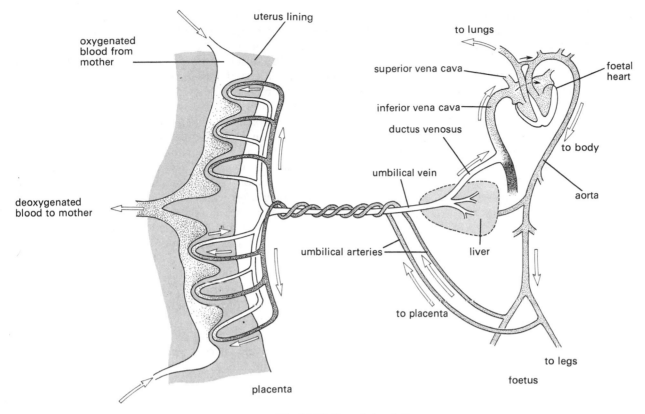

Fig. 15.19 Foetal circulation

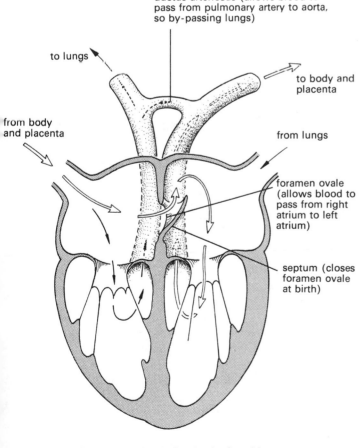

Fig. 15.20   Circulation in the foetal heart

Feeding and parental care. About twenty-four hours after birth, the baby starts to suckle at the breast. During pregnancy the mammary glands of the breast have developed and are stimulated to secrete milk by the first sucklings. In fact, the production of milk is under hormonal control but the volume produced is related to the quantity removed by the child during suckling.

All mammals suckle their young and protect them in various ways until they are old enough to move about efficiently and obtain their own food. Most mammals prepare a nest in which to bear their young, and in this way the babies are protected from animals of prey and from temperature changes. It reduces the chances of their wandering away and prevents them injuring themselves. Young mammals are often born without fur but the presence of the mother's body prevents them losing too much heat. The food at first is entirely milk, suckled from the mother. Milk contains nearly all the food, vitamins and salts that the young need for their energy requirements and tissue building but there is no iron present for the manufacture of haemoglobin. All the iron needed for the first weeks or months is stored in the body of the foetus during gestation. The parent's milk supply increases as the demands of the young increase (in the case of man it reaches up to one litre per day) and is gradually supplemented and eventually entirely replaced by solid food.

In man, parental care follows the basic pattern common to all mammals but is conscious and planned. The period of dependence of the young on the parents is very prolonged compared with other mammals and involves not only food, warmth and shelter but also education, training and concern for the psychological and moral welfare of the offspring.

Puberty and secondary sexual characters. In addition to producing gametes, the ovaries and testes make hormones. At puberty these hormones are released into the blood stream, and as they circulate round the body they give rise to the physical and mental changes which we associate with masculinity or femininity. Although the sex chromosomes X and Y (*see* p. 172) are known to determine sex, the means by which they do so has not been discovered. For the first seven weeks after implantation the embryo has reproductive bodies which are neither testes nor ovaries, but after seven weeks they continue development in one direction or the other. A working hypothesis is that the XY constitution determines whether testes or ovaries develop from embryonic tissue and that the remaining organs depend on the production of specific hormones from the testis or ovary. It is known that a hormonal imbalance can upset the genetically pre-determined sex, but it is unlikely that the explanation is as simple as this. Until the foetus is three months old, the sex cannot be determined by examination of the external genitalia.

Puberty in girls is marked by the onset of menstruation and this is an indication of the beginning of ovulation and sexual maturity. In most cases, menstruation starts between twelve and fourteen years but it may begin at any time between nine and eighteen years. The breasts may have started to enlarge prior to puberty, largely due to deposition of fat. Other changes are the increase in the size of the uterus and vulva, the growth of hair in the pubic region and the armpits (axillae) and the widening of the pelvic girdle.

Comparable changes take place at about the same time in boys. There is an increase in growth rate, hair grows in the pubic region, in the axillae and on the face. Enlargement of the larynx causes the voice to 'break', i.e. become deeper. The penis, scrotum and prostate gland enlarge and sperms are produced by the seminiferous tubules in the testes.

The external genitalia and the perceptible changes which take place at puberty are called the *secondary sexual characters.*

The psychological changes associated with adolescence are probably the results, in the first instance, of the physiological change from sexual immaturity to maturity, with an increase in sexual desire and a revised attitude to the opposite sex. In civilized society, the frustration resulting from the very long interval between attainment of sexual maturity at the age of about thirteen and its fulfilment at the time of marriage is likely to be responsible for some of the other manifestations of adolescent behaviour in a society that places an economic and moral taboo on premarital sexual relations. A study of the adolescents growing up in Samoa leads one anthropologist to conclude that most of the so-called difficulties of adolescence are a product of modern society and are not a natural result of the beginnings of sexual maturity.

Menstruation. Of the five hundred or so ova produced in the life of a woman, not more than about twelve are likely, even in theory, to be fertilized and form embryos; in practice the number is far less than this. Nevertheless, at the time of release of each ovum, the lining of the uterus becomes thicker with additional layers of cells, into which the ovum will sink if fertilized. The blood supply is increased at the same time. If the ovum is not fertilized, however, production of progesterone by the corpus luteum decreases and the new uterine lining disintegrates (Fig. 15.21).

The unwanted cells and 50 to 250 cm³ blood (which does not clot) are lost through the cervix and vagina. This *menstruation,* as it is called, occurs twelve to fourteen days after the ovum is released, about once in four weeks. The periodicity varies with individuals and from one period to the next. After fertilization, menstruation ceases and this is one of the first indications of pregnancy.

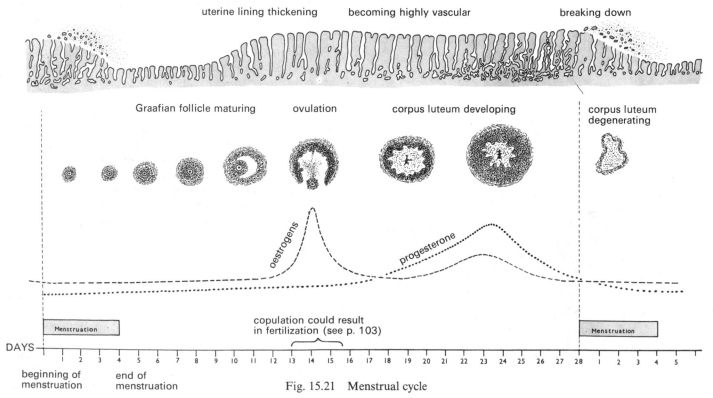

Fig. 15.21 Menstrual cycle

(After G. W. Corner, *The Hormones in Human Reproduction,* Princeton)

Menopause. Between the ages of about forty-two and fifty-two a woman loses her ability to reproduce. Ovulation ceases and so does menstruation. The uterus, breasts and genitalia decrease in size and sexual desire declines.

Twins. (a) *Identical twins.* Sometimes a developing embryo divides into two groups of cells at an early stage in cell division and the two parts each develop into a normal embryo, though often they share the same placenta. Such 'one-egg' twins are the same sex and are identical in nearly every physical respect, although differences in position and blood supply in the uterus may cause them to be different initially in weight and vigour.

(b) *Fraternal twins.* If two ova are released from the ovary and fertilized simultaneously, twins will result. These twins may be of different sexes and are not necessarily any more alike than other brothers and sisters of the same family.

About one in every eighty-eight births results in twins of which one-third are identical twins. Triplets and other multiple births may result from simultaneous fertilization of several ova or the separation of a single zygote into four or more cell masses, one of which subsequently fails to develop.

Contraception. Copulation in humans is accompanied by pleasure. Man has therefore sought to enjoy sexual intercourse while avoiding the birth of unwanted children. Many parents also wish to limit the size of their families to their economic means. Most people would probably agree that the creation of human beings is a sufficiently important matter not to be left to chance and the growth of populations today seems to necessitate a widespread acceptance of some means of contraception.

If copulation is restricted to times when an ovum is unlikely to be present in the oviduct, e.g. just after menstruation, then conception (i.e. fertilization and implantation) is unlikely. Since, however, it is not possible to determine accurately the extent of this period, called the 'safe period', it cannot be regarded as a reliable means of birth control. Another method of preventing conception, called *coitus interruptus,* involves withdrawal of the penis from the vagina before ejaculation so that sperms cannot reach the ovum. This practice is both unreliable and psychologically unsatisfactory.

The principal effective methods of contraception are as follows:

(a) *The sheath or diaphragm.* A thin rubber sheath worn on the penis, or a small rubber diaphragm inserted in the vagina prevents the sperms from reaching the cervix.

(b) *Intra-uterine loop.* A small plastic strip bent into a loop or coil is inserted and retained in the uterus. Whether it interferes with fertilization or implantation is not certain but it is very effective.

(c) *The contraceptive pill.* The pill contains chemicals which have the same effect on the body as the hormones oestrogen and progesterone. When mixed in suitable proportions, these hormones suppress ovulation and so prevent conception. The pills need to be taken each day for the twenty-one days between menstrual periods and are almost one hundred per cent effective.

Conception can also be prevented by simple surgical means. In the male, the sperm ducts are tied or cut *(vasectomy)*; in the female, the oviducts are tied. Vasectomy is the more common operation, but either method prevents ova and sperms from meeting, and apart from this, sex life is unaffected. The operation in most cases is irreversible.

World population. With the increasing application of medical knowledge, fewer people are dying from infectious diseases. The birth rate, however, has not fallen off in proportion, with the result that the world population is doubling every fifty years or less. In the developing countries with limited natural resources, this leads to shortages of food and living space. In the industrialized countries, the population increase has contributed to the pollution of the environment as a result of waste disposal and intensive methods of food production.

There is clearly a physical limit to the number of people who can live on the Earth, though authorities may differ in their estimates of this number. Therefore it seems essential, at the very least, to educate people (a) into accepting the need to limit their families and (b) in methods of achieving this. The alternative to voluntary population control is control by famine and disaster.

Infertility. This condition may result from various causes, from blockage of the oviduct to failure to produce adequate amounts of living sperms. Many of these causes may be corrected by simple surgery or drugs.

Miscarriage and abortion. Miscarriage, or spontaneous abortion, are terms applied to the birth of a foetus at a stage too early to survive, e.g. after only three or four months' gestation. Treatment with the appropriate hormones may prevent this in women with whom miscarriages are prevalent. The term abortion is usually applied to the deliberate killing of a foetus in the uterus by drugs or surgery or to the induction of its birth at a stage when it could not possibly survive. Abortion is a common practice as a measure of family limitation in some countries and it is also carried out when a continued pregnancy could endanger the mother's health or life.

Caesarian section. In some women, the gap between the spinal column and the front of the pelvic girdle is too small to permit the passage of the foetus. In such cases, at the normal time for birth, the abdomen and uterus are opened surgically and the baby removed. Two or three children in succession may be born in this way.

Questions

1 In what ways does a zygote differ from any other cell in the body?

2 What is the advantage to the embryo of the early development of its heart and circulatory system?

3 What differences are there in the numbers, structure and activity of the male and female gametes in man?

4 What do you consider are the advantages of (a) internal fertilization over external fertilization, and (b) development of the embryo in the uterus rather than in the egg?

5 In what ways is parental care in man similar to and different from parental care in other mammals?

6 List the changes in the composition of the maternal blood that are likely to occur when it passes through the placenta.

7 Explain why there are only a few days in each menstrual cycle when fertilization is likely to occur.

8 What changes in diet should be made by a woman once she becomes pregnant? Suggest reasons for these changes.

16
The Skeleton, Muscles and Movement

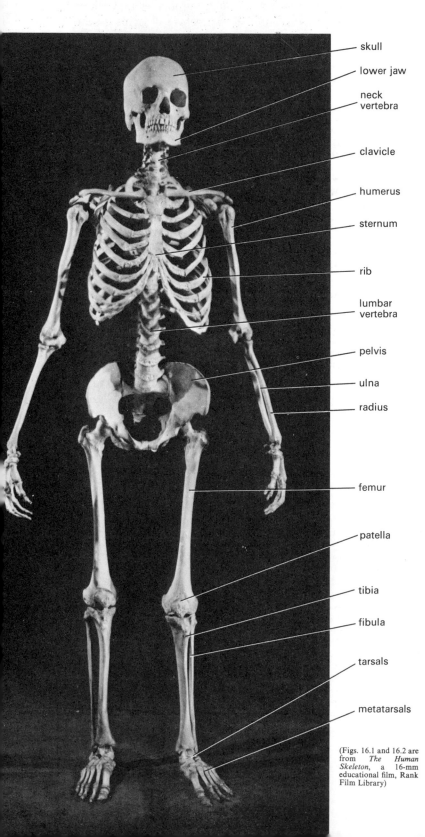

skull
lower jaw
neck vertebra
clavicle
humerus
sternum
rib
lumbar vertebra
pelvis
ulna
radius
femur
patella
tibia
fibula
tarsals
metatarsals

(Figs. 16.1 and 16.2 are from *The Human Skeleton*, a 16-mm educational film, Rank Film Library)

Skeletal tissues are hard substances formed by living cells. Frequently they contain non-living mineral matter such as calcium salts. The structures made of such non-living material can nevertheless grow and change as a result of the activities of living cells which dissolve away and replace the hard materials.

Exoskeletons. Where the hard material is formed mainly on the outside of the body it is often called an exoskeleton. Insects and crustaceans such as crabs have exoskeletons or cuticles, though there are projections from the exoskeleton into the body cavity for muscle attachment. Animals with exoskeletons increase their size periodically by dissolving and absorbing most of the cuticle, splitting and shedding the outermost layers, and forming a new cuticle on the exposed surface.

Endoskeletons. Vertebrate animals have skeletons within their bodies. These animals can grow by a continuous increase in size. The skeleton is made of bone and cartilage; it is covered and manipulated by muscles.

Functions of the skeleton

The functions can be grouped conveniently under the headings of support, protection, movement and locomotion, and muscle attachment.

Support. There are many invertebrate animals that have no skeleton. Those living in water may become fairly large because the water supports them and buoys them up to a certain extent. In others, e.g. the earthworm, they are supported by the pressure of fluid in their body cavities acting outwards against a muscular body wall. In larger land-dwelling animals a rigid skeletal support raises the body from the ground and allows rapid movement; it suspends some of the vital organs, prevents them from crushing each other, and maintains the shape of the body despite vigorous muscular activity (Fig. 16.1).

Protection. Certain delicate and important organs of the body are protected by a casing of bone. The brain is enclosed in the skull, the spinal cord in the vertebral column, while the heart and lungs are surrounded by a cage of ribs between the ster-

Fig. 16.1   Skeleton of man

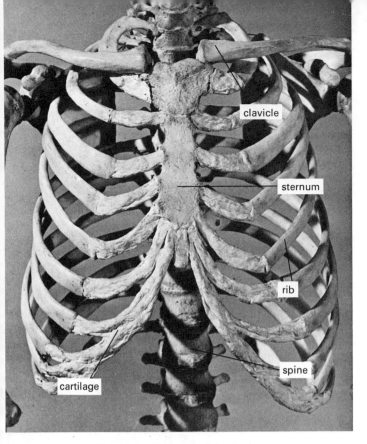

Fig. 16.2 Skeleton of the thorax

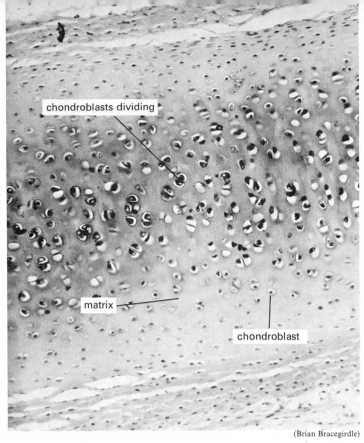

(Brian Bracegirdle)

Fig. 16.3 Photomicrograph of section through cartilage

num and spine (Fig. 16.2). The organs are thus protected from distortion resulting from pressure and injury resulting from impact. The rib cage plays a positive part in the breathing mechanism (p. 89) in addition to protecting the organs of the thorax.

Movement. Many bones of the skeleton act as levers. When muscles pull on these levers they produce movements, such as the chewing action of the jaws, the breathing movements of the ribs and the flexing of the arms. Locomotion is the result of the co-ordinated action of muscles on the limb bones and is discussed more fully on p. 120. Movements of the skeleton require a system of joints and muscle attachments.

Muscle attachment. To produce effective movement of any part of the skeleton, the muscles must be attached securely to it at each end. One end of the muscle must be attached to the part of the skeleton to be moved while the other end is anchored to a part of the skeleton to be held stationary with respect to the moving part. This is discussed more fully on p. 118.

Cartilage, bone and muscle

Cartilage, typically, is a semitransparent, firm, elastic but somewhat gelatinous material found in the ear pinna, the epiglottis, the trachea and on the surface of bones where they form a joint. In fish of the shark family the entire skeleton is composed of cartilage, but in mammals, although the skeleton of the embryo is first laid down as cartilage, it is replaced by bone long before birth.

The gelatinous material or *matrix* of cartilage is secreted by cells called *chondroblasts,* which come eventually to lie in cavities within the matrix (Figs. 16.3 and 16.5a). The chondroblasts can divide and produce new cells which secrete more matrix and so bring about the growth of cartilage. Such growth, in humans, takes place in the embryo when the skele-

ton is first formed in cartilage, and later, only at the junctions between the head and shaft of bones that are still growing in length. Capillaries do not penetrate the matrix and in consequence the chondroblasts must receive their food and oxygen by diffusion through the matrix.

Fibres of two kinds, tough, inextensible *collagen* fibres and stretchy, elastic fibres, are dispersed to varying degrees in the cartilaginous matrix. Since, for the most part, they run in different directions to each other, they prevent the cartilage splitting under pressure.

Elastic fibres are abundant in the ear pinna, while collagen fibres are predominant in the fibro-cartilage of a tendon insertion (p. 118); here, the fibres are lined up in the direction of the pull, thus transmitting the full force of muscular contraction to the bone.

Bone formation and structure. Most of the bones of the human embryo are formed in cartilage which is then replaced by bone, leaving cartilage only on the joint surface. The early cartilaginous model first of all undergoes calcification by precipitation of calcium phosphate in the matrix. Next, since the calcified matrix is impermeable to dissolved food and oxygen, the chondroblasts die and the calcified cartilage starts to disintegrate. Finally, cells called *osteoblasts* invade the space so formed (Fig. 16.4) and lay down bone on what is left of the calcified cartilage, using calcium and phosphate ions supplied by the blood. This is called *ossification.* At the same time, capillaries penetrate the cavities of the ossifying cartilage bringing food, oxygen and the necessary calcium and phosphate compounds with which the osteoblasts make bone. Eventually each osteoblast surrounds itself with bone and at this stage is called an *osteocyte.*

The process of ossification is more complicated than suggested above and the final product is by no means simply a homogeneous mineral deposit of calcium phosphate. The bone is penetrated by collagen fibres which give far more tensile strength to bone than a simple mineral could possess.

111

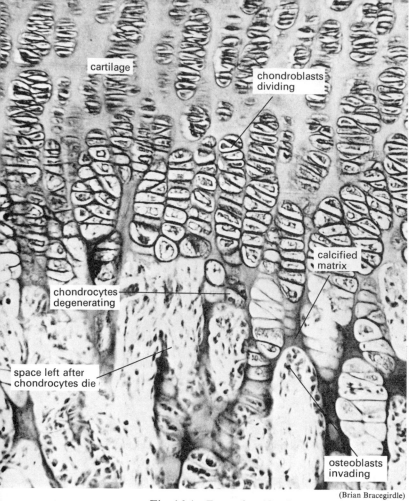

cartilage

chondroblasts dividing

calcified matrix

chondrocytes degenerating

space left after chondrocytes die

osteoblasts invading

(Brian Bracegirdle)

Fig. 16.4 Zone of ossification

If a bone is placed in dilute acid the calcium salts are dissolved out, leaving the collagen fibres and other connective tissues intact. The bone retains its shape but (while it is moist) it is quite flexible. Ossification is depicted diagrammatically in Fig. 16.5.

Certain bones, such as those roofing the skull, are not modelled first in cartilage but produced by ossification directly in the dermis of the skin. In the skull this gives rise to a series of plates which grow at the margins until they meet and join at the sutures to form a continuous skeletal system.

Periosteum. Surrounding each bone is a tough, fibrous sheath. Its outer regions consist principally of collagen fibres, while its inner surface contains osteoblasts whose activities can produce growth in thickness of the bone. The periosteum is continuous across joints where it forms a capsule whose inner surface secretes synovial fluid which lubricates the surfaces of the joint (*see* p. 115).

Centres of ossification and growth of bone. The conversion of cartilage to bone in a limb begins first in the centre of the shaft and, shortly after, at the two ends which will form the heads or *epiphyses* of the bone. As ossification proceeds from these three centres (Fig. 16.6) the newly formed bone of the shaft approaches that of the epiphyses until only a narrow band of cartilage, the *metaphysis,* is left. This cartilaginous disc persists, however, and is the means by which a bone grows in length. In the metaphysis, the chondroblasts divide and make the cartilaginous disc thicker. This new cartilage in its turn is ossified from the side nearest the shaft and so extends the shaft (Figs. 16.6*d* and 16.7). Only when the skeleton has attained its full proportions do the shaft and epiphyses fuse together (Fig. 16.8).

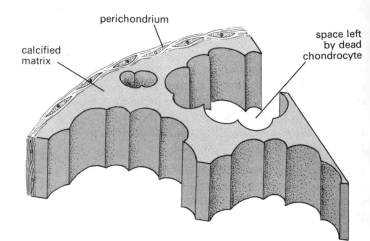

perichondrium (cells and fibrous tissue surrounding cartilage)

gelatinous matrix

chondrocyte (mature chondroblast)

(a) *Cartilage*

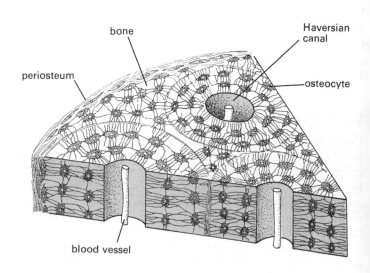

perichondrium

calcified matrix

space left by dead chondrocyte

(b) *The chondrocytes die and the matrix is eroded*

bone

Haversian canal

periosteum

osteocyte

blood vessel

(c) *The spaces are invaded by osteoblasts which lay down bone in concentric cylinders*

Fig. 16.5 Conversion of cartilage to bone (ossification)

cartilage

(a) A 'model' of the bone is first laid down in cartilage

centres of ossification

(b) The cartilage is invaded and replaced by bone at three centres of ossification, in the shaft and two heads of the bone

this cartilage continues growing

the newly produced cartilage is ossified (see Fig. 16.7)

bone in centre of shaft breaks down and is replaced by fatty marrow

(c) Ossification proceeds but cartilage remains covering the heads of the bone where they make joints and between the heads and the shaft to allow for growth

(d) Growth takes place by the internal cartilage extending and becoming ossified

Fig. 16.6   The growth of a long bone

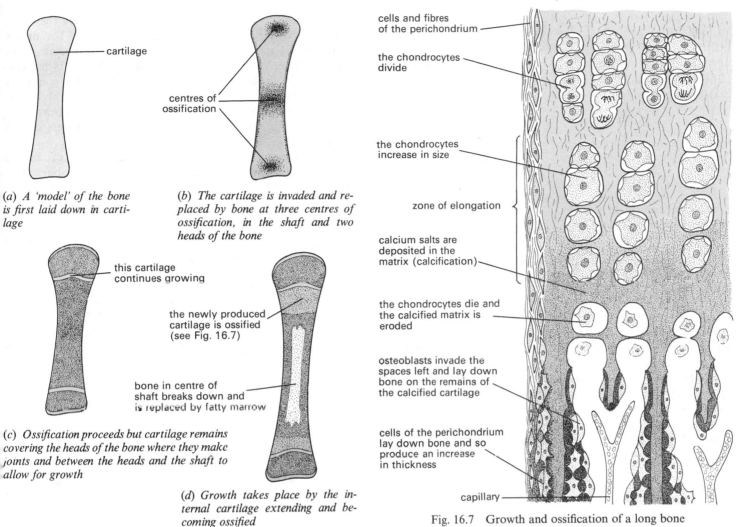

cells and fibres of the perichondrium

the chondrocytes divide

the chondrocytes increase in size

zone of elongation

calcium salts are deposited in the matrix (calcification)

the chondrocytes die and the calcified matrix is eroded

osteoblasts invade the spaces left and lay down bone on the remains of the calcified cartilage

cells of the perichondrium lay down bone and so produce an increase in thickness

capillary

Fig. 16.7   Growth and ossification of a long bone

(b) Adult (epiphyses fused)

(a) Six years old (epiphyses unfused)

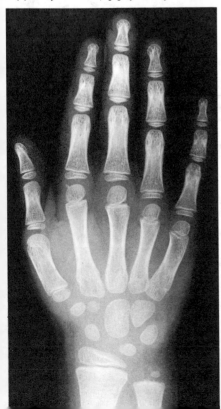

Fig. 16.8   X-ray photograph of the hand

(St Bartholomew's Hospital, Department of Medical Illustration)

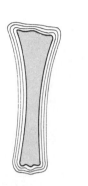

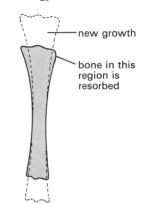

new growth

bone in this region is resorbed

(a) *Uniform increase in thickness would produce a distorted shape*

(b) *Growth in length exceeds growth in width*

Fig. 16.9   Pattern of growth in long bones

It is clear from Fig. 16.9 that increase in length from the metaphysis and increase in thickness from the periosteum do not account for the necessary change in the shape of the bone as it grows, particularly the change in the expanded ends of the shaft. During growth, parts of the bone are added to as described above, and parts are dissolved and resorbed. There is no universal agreement on the precise mechanism by which resorption takes place. It may be that parts of the bone are dissolved away by tissue fluid or that special cells, the *osteoclasts,* erode away the areas of bone.

Bone resorption also takes place in the centre of the shaft, leaving a cylindrical space occupied by marrow. The finally formed bone may be of two kinds, *compact* or *cancellous.* Compact bone is formed on the outside of the shafts and epiphyses, while cancellous bone is in the centre of the epiphyses and the centre of most bones other than the long limb bones, e.g. in the ribs and vertebrae. Cancellous bone appears as a network of thin, bony columns, *trabeculae,* interspersed with the tissues that form the blood cells (Fig. 16.10).

In its final form, bone consists of living osteocytes occupying spaces, *lacunae,* in the ossified matrix which they have produced (Fig. 16.11). Withdrawal of fine cytoplasmic processes

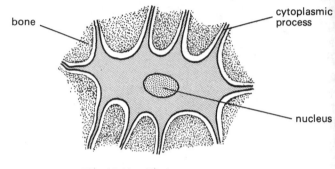

bone

cytoplasmic process

nucleus

Fig. 16.11   Single osteocyte

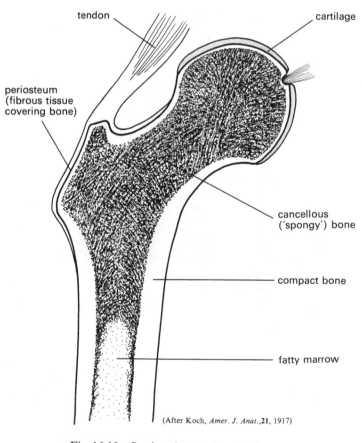

tendon

cartilage

periosteum (fibrous tissue covering bone)

cancellous ('spongy') bone

compact bone

fatty marrow

(After Koch, *Amer. J. Anat.,***21**, 1917)

Fig. 16.10   Section through head of femur

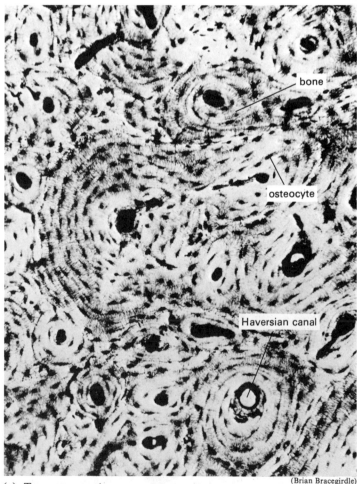

bone

osteocyte

Haversian canal

(a) *Transverse section*

(Brian Bracegirdle)

Fig. 16.12   Photomicrographs of sections through bone tissue (the

which once united the osteocytes leaves a delicate network of channels through which tissue fluid can penetrate, bringing nutrients, salts and oxygen to the osteocytes and removing their excretory products. The osteocytes are so arranged that they form cylinders of bone, not more than six cells thick (Figs. 16.12 and 16.5c); through these cylinders run capillaries which extend into the bone from the periosteum, having been incorporated into the bone tissue as it was laid down by the periosteum. The presence of this capillary network allows the bone to continue growth, repair fractures and effect a continual turnover of bone substance. Injection of radioactive phosphorus into experimental animals shows that phosphate in the blood is incorporated into existing bones within a few hours even though they have ceased growing. After about three weeks, the radioactive phosphorus has almost entirely disappeared from the bone. These results indicate that bone tissue is not an inert solid but in a state of constant change, its minerals being continually removed and replaced.

Rickets. If either calcium, vitamin D, or both are deficient in the diet, bone growth continues but ossification is inadequate. That is, the osteoblasts lay down a fibrous matrix that is not hardened by deposition of calcium salts. Such bones, if subjected to normal stresses of muscular action or body weight, distort easily leading eventually to crippling deformities (p. 36). Absence of vitamin C also prevents normal bone formation in the shafts of bones, which are subsequently more liable to fracture.

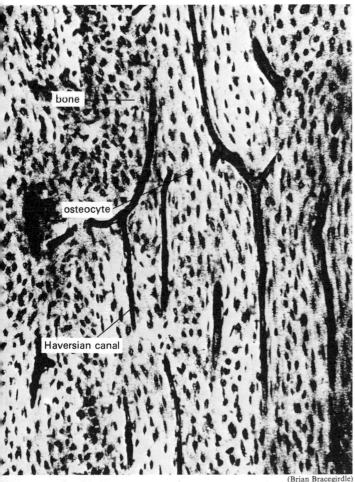

(Brian Bracegirdle)

(b) Longitudinal section

canals are blocked with dust produced while cutting the section)

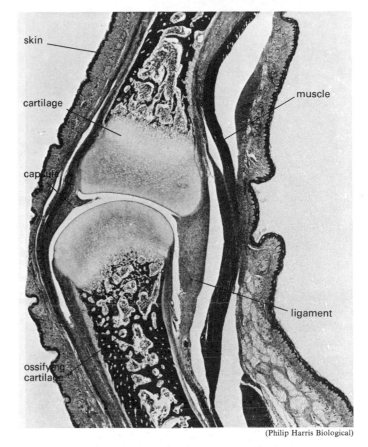

(Philip Harris Biological)

Fig. 16.13   Finger joint of human foetus

Fractures. That bone can so readily repair fractures is evidence of its living properties and adaptability to new situations and stresses. When a limb bone is fractured, blood leaking from the torn ends of capillaries forms a clot which occupies the damaged area. Macrophages invade the clot and ingest red cells and cell debris. Shortly after, capillaries penetrate the clot. Osteoblasts in the periosteum round the margins of the fracture begin to reproduce rapidly both outside the shaft and in the marrow cavity. These osteoblasts start to lay down bone on the shaft and also migrate towards the blood clot where they lay down cartilage, forming a thickened layer or *callus* over the break and so uniting the bones. After this, ossification takes place in the normal way, with calcification, resorption and deposition of bone. The bone at the broken ends has died, probably as a result of the cessation of the normal blood supply. This dead bone is resorbed and replaced as the callus forms and, finally, the callus itself is resculptured by resorption to conform to the normal shape of the limb.

The time taken for healing depends on the diameter of the bone, its blood supply and the age of the individual. A rib heals quickly, a femur slowly, particularly the neck of the femur with its restricted blood supply.

Joints. Where two bones meet a joint is formed. Sometimes, as in the sutures between the bones of the skull, no movement is permitted (Fig. 16.27); in others, e.g. the vertebrae of the spine, only a very limited movement can occur; while the most familiar joints, called *synovial joints* (Fig. 16.13), allow a considerable degree of movement. The ball and socket joints

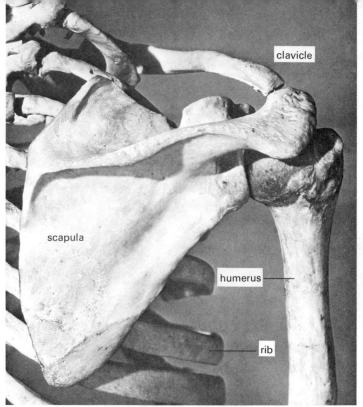

Fig. 16.14   The shoulder joint

also surrounds the joint, secreting and retaining the synovial fluid.

The vertebrae of the spine can also move slightly so that the spinal column as a whole is flexible (Fig. 16.19). The vertebrae are separated by discs of cartilage.

Girdles. To produce movement of the body as a whole, the upwards or backwards thrust of the limbs against the ground must be imparted to the body. The force is transmitted through a skeletal structure called a girdle which is attached to the spinal column. The *pelvic* girdle (Fig. 16.20) is rigidly fused to the base of the spine so that in walking or jumping the force of the leg thrust is transmitted to the spine, which is the central support of the whole body. By this means also the weight of the body is supported when at rest. The shoulder blades which form part of the *pectoral* girdle (Fig. 16.14) are not fused to the spine but bound by muscles to the back of the thorax. This is not so effective a means of imparting a force to the body, but this function is not so important with the arms as it is with the legs and the free movement of the shoulders allows greater mobility of the arms. The shoulder in man is more mobile than in most mammals and the clavicle serves to limit these movements.

of the humerus and scapula at the shoulder (Fig. 16.14) and the femur and pelvis at the hip (Figs. 16.15 and 16.16) allow movement in two planes. The hinge joints of the ulna and humerus at the elbow (Fig. 16.17), and the femur and tibia at the knee (Fig. 16.18) allow movement in only one plane.

The surfaces of the heads of bones, which move over each other, are covered with cartilage which is slippery and smooth. This, together with the liquid in the joint, called synovial fluid, allows friction-free movement. The relevant bones of the joint are held together by strong *ligaments* (Figs. 16.16*b* and 16.18*b*) which prevent dislocation during normal movement. A *capsule* of fibrous tissue, continuous with the periosteum,

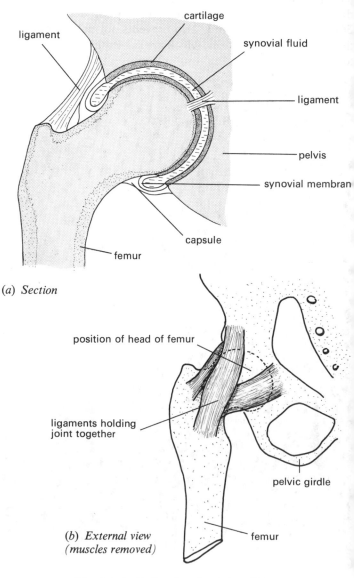

(a) *Section*

position of head of femur

ligaments holding joint together

pelvic girdle

(b) *External view (muscles removed)*

femur

Fig. 16.16   Ball and socket joint of hip

Fig. 16.15   The hip joint

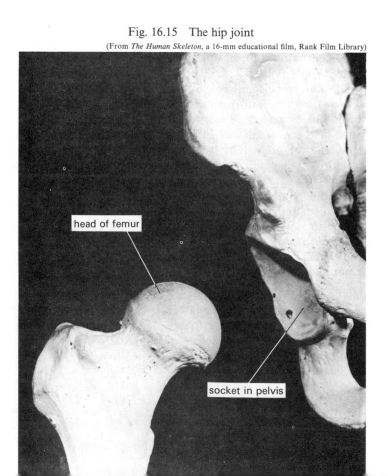

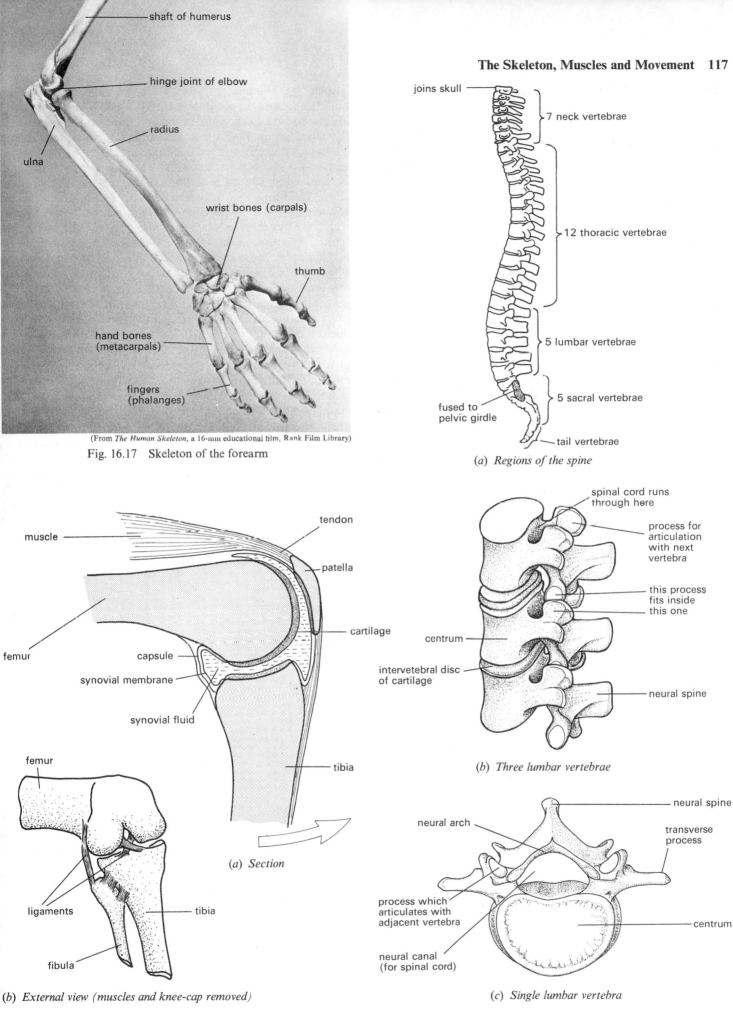

shaft of humerus

hinge joint of elbow

radius

ulna

wrist bones (carpals)

thumb

hand bones (metacarpals)

fingers (phalanges)

(From *The Human Skeleton*, a 16-mm educational film, Rank Film Library)

Fig. 16.17   Skeleton of the forearm

joins skull

7 neck vertebrae

12 thoracic vertebrae

5 lumbar vertebrae

5 sacral vertebrae

fused to pelvic girdle

tail vertebrae

(a) *Regions of the spine*

muscle

tendon

patella

cartilage

femur

capsule

synovial membrane

synovial fluid

tibia

(a) *Section*

femur

ligaments

tibia

fibula

(b) *External view (muscles and knee-cap removed)*

Fig. 16.18   Hinge joint of the knee

spinal cord runs through here

process for articulation with next vertebra

this process fits inside this one

centrum

intervetebral disc of cartilage

neural spine

(b) *Three lumbar vertebrae*

neural spine

neural arch

transverse process

process which articulates with adjacent vertebra

centrum

neural canal (for spinal cord)

(c) *Single lumbar vertebra*

Fig. 16.19   The spinal column

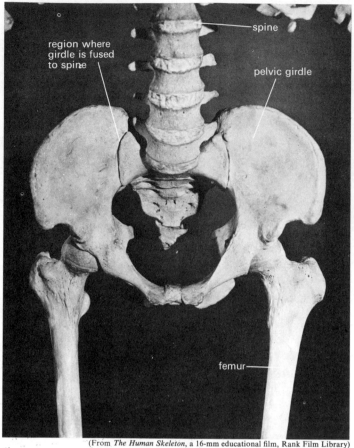

region where
girdle is fused
to spine

spine

pelvic girdle

femur

(From *The Human Skeleton*, a 16-mm educational film, Rank Film Library)

Fig. 16.20   The pelvic girdle

Muscle. (a) *Voluntary muscle*. Contractions of voluntary muscle are brought about as a result of nerve impulses reaching the muscle (although the contraction itself may often be described as involuntary if it results from a simple reflex). Voluntary muscle consists of elongated cells up to 40 mm long and 10–40 microns in diameter. The cells are grouped into bundles and enclosed in sheaths of fibrous connective tissue (Figs. 16.21 and 16.22). At the ends of the limb muscles, the connective tissue sheaths are drawn out to form *tendons* which are attached to the periosteum covering the bone. At a tendon insertion collagen fibres of the periosteum are embedded in the bone substance giving a very firm anchorage. Muscle cells if stimulated by a nervous impulse will contract to about two thirds or one half of their resting length. This makes the muscle as a whole shorter and thicker and, according to its attachments at each end, it pulls on a bone and so produces movement.

Muscles that produce movement usually act across joints in such a way that the bones are worked as levers with a low mechanical advantage. Fig. 16.23 makes this clear. The muscles can only contract a short distance, but since they are attached near a joint the movement at the end of a limb is greatly magnified. The biceps muscle of the arm may contract only 80 or 90 mm but the hand will move about 60 cm (Fig. 16.24).

Muscles can only contract and relax, they cannot elongate. A muscle that has contracted has to be pulled back to its resting length when it relaxes. Consequently, most muscles are in pairs, one of them producing movement in one direction

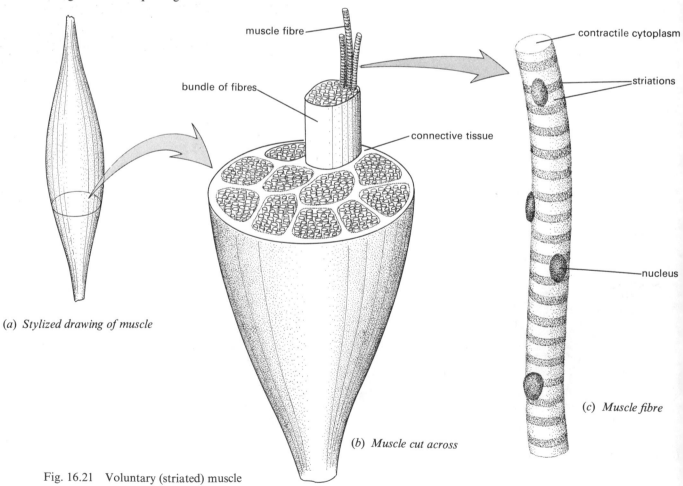

muscle fibre

bundle of fibres

connective tissue

contractile cytoplasm

striations

nucleus

(a) *Stylized drawing of muscle*

(b) *Muscle cut across*

(c) *Muscle fibre*

Fig. 16.21   Voluntary (striated) muscle

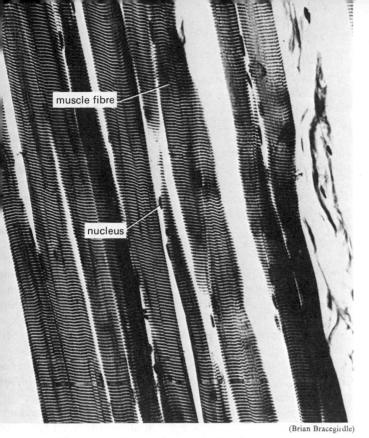

muscle fibre

nucleus

Fig. 16.22   Photomicrograph of striated muscle

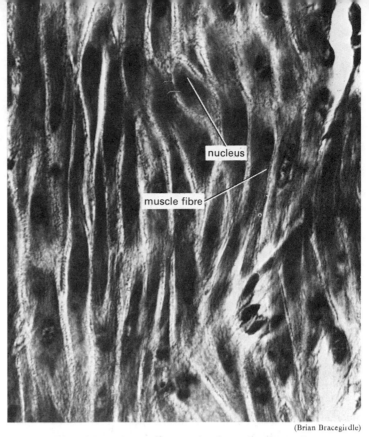

nucleus

muscle fibre

Fig. 16.25   Photomicrograph of unstriated muscle

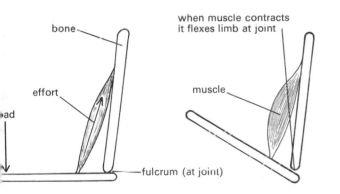

bone

when muscle contracts
it flexes limb at joint

effort

muscle

load

fulcrum (at joint)

Fig. 16.23   Lever action of limb

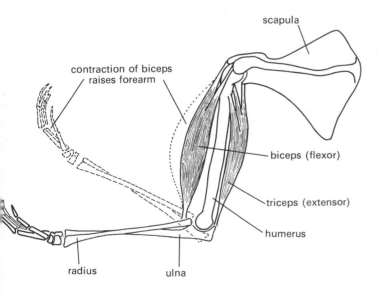

scapula

contraction of biceps
raises forearm

biceps (flexor)

triceps (extensor)

humerus

radius   ulna

Fig. 16.24   Antagonistic muscles of the forearm

and the other producing the opposite movement. When one partner contracts, it will extend the other if it is in a relaxed state. Such pairs of muscles are called *antagonistic*: in the case of a limb they may be called *flexor* and *extensor* muscles, according to whether they bend (flex) or straighten (extend) the limb; they may be called *adductors* and *abductors* if they pull a limb towards or away from the body respectively. Often, the antagonistic muscles are in groups; e.g. both the *brachialis* and the *biceps* muscles flex the arm at the elbow and antagonize the *triceps,* but the biceps does so only when the palm is facing upwards. The biceps serves, therefore, both to rotate the lower arm and to flex the elbow. Combinations of other pairs of muscles acting at the joints may produce rotary or circular movements.

Of such pairs or groups of antagonistic muscles, one is usually much stronger than the other. The biceps which flexes the arm is larger and more powerful than the triceps which extends it; the *gastrocnemius* and *soleus* of the calf muscles which extend the foot at the ankle are stronger than the *peroneus* muscles which flex it.

Locomotion is brought about by the co-ordinated movement of limbs, by sets of antagonistic muscles contracting and relaxing alternately. When the body is at rest, a proportion of the fibres in the antagonistic muscles remain in a state of contraction producing a *muscular tone* which holds the body in position.

(b) *Involuntary muscle.* The muscle in the walls of the arteries, arterioles and the alimentary canal has a structure different from that of voluntary muscle, being made up of shorter cells (Figs. 16.25 and 2.8c, p. 11) and arranged with connective tissue in continuous sheets rather than in discrete muscles. Their distribution in circular and longitudinal muscle sheets, however, allows an antagonistic action. Contraction of fibres running in a circular manner round a cylindrical organ causes a reduction in diameter, while shortening of the longitudinal fibres brings about a reduction in length and, in some cases, an increase in diameter.

Involuntary muscle produces rather slow contractions which may be under the control of the autonomic nervous system (p. 151) as in vasoconstriction (p. 99), or stimulated in other ways to produce rhythmic contractions, as in peristalsis (p. 62). The bladder, ureters, arteries, arterioles, alimentary canal and iris diaphragm of the eye all contain involuntary muscle. Contraction of this muscle cannot be brought about by the conscious will.

(c) *Heart muscle.* This tissue is different from both voluntary and involuntary muscle. Its rhythmic contraction can take place without nervous stimulation although the heartbeat is under the control of the central nervous system. All muscle fibres can conduct electrical impulses to some extent, but in the heart muscle this property is of particular importance since the majority of cells have no direct contact with nerves. The impulse that causes the muscle cells to contract in unison is conducted by the cells themselves.

Muscle attachment. The skeletal muscles must be attached to the limb bones at one end in order to produce movement but, in addition, they must have a rigid attachment at the other end so that only one part of the limb moves when the muscle contracts. Sometimes the 'stationary' end is attached to the upper part of the limb; e.g. the extensor muscles which extend the foot are attached to the top of the tibia or lower end of the femur. The muscles that move the femur, however, are attached to the pelvic girdle. Bones frequently have projections or ridges where muscles are attached (Figs. 16.26 and 16.27).

Locomotion

When a quadruped walks, its four limbs move in a co-ordinated sequence, each one in turn thrusting backwards on the ground, so propelling the animal forwards. Usually, one fore-limb and the opposite hind-limb are moved forwards while the body is supported on its other two limbs. Man has to maintain his upright posture on one leg while the other leg is swinging forwards during walking. Consequently, the action of the leg muscles during walking is rather complicated to describe and it will be clearer to consider how muscles and bones effect locomotion in a simpler situation, in this case, a runner at the start of a sprint race. While waiting for the starting gun, the legs are flexed and, on the starting signal, one of them is violently extended, thrusting against the ground to push the runner upwards and forwards. In Fig. 16.28 a simplified diagram of the leg and some of its muscles is shown. When muscle A contracts it pulls the femur backwards. Contraction of muscle B straightens the leg at the knee and contraction of C extends the foot at the ankle. Friction between the ground and the foot prevents the foot slipping backwards so that contraction of these three muscles produces a thrust which is transmitted through the pelvic girdle to the spine and thence to the whole body, propelling it forwards.

At the end of this thrusting leap, muscles A, B and C relax and allow the knee and ankle to be flexed and the femur to swing forwards by contraction of antagonistic muscles to A, B and C, of which only b and c are shown in the diagram. There are, of course, many more muscles involved than are shown in Fig. 16.28 and their co-ordinated action is more subtle and complex than can be described here.

To produce effective movement, it is essential that the contraction of the many sets of muscles is co-ordinated so that, for example, antagonistic muscles do not contract simultaneously. Contributing to this co-ordination there is a system of stretch receptors (p. 131) in the muscles; these fire nervous impulses to the spinal cord when the muscle is being stretched. Such internal sensory organs or *proprioceptors,* linked to the nervous system, feed back information to the brain about the position of the limbs and enable a pattern of muscular activity to be computed by the brain, so producing effective movement.

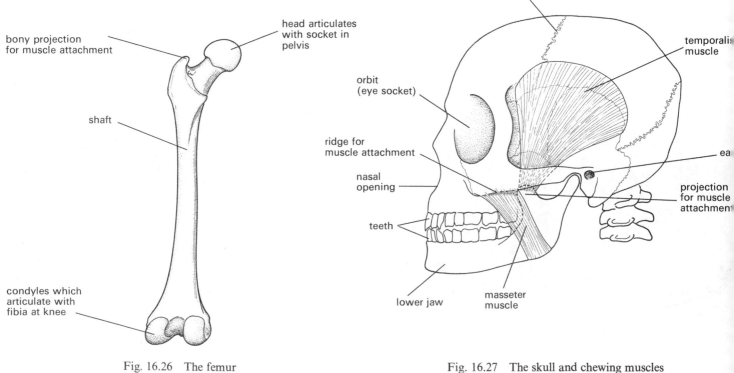

Fig. 16.26   The femur

Fig. 16.27   The skull and chewing muscles

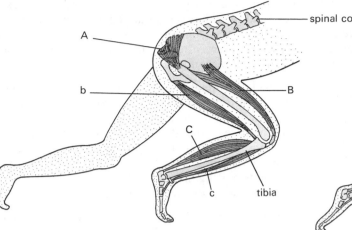

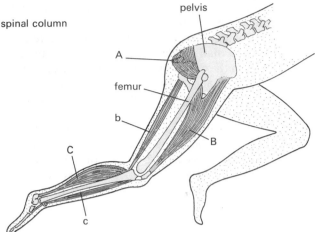

Fig. 16.28   Action of leg muscles in producing movement (the action could be the start of a sprint; only a few of the muscle systems have been drawn)

Posture

It is generally accepted that during the course of evolution, man or his immediate predecessor took to walking on his hind legs instead of all fours. This had the great advantage of leaving his hands free for collecting and manipulating materials essential to life. The adoption of a two-footed stance was accompanied by many changes in skeletal structure which made it possible to maintain the upright posture. However, a jointed skeleton alone cannot maintain posture, upright or otherwise, and if a man were to relax all his muscles, he would buckle at the knees and ankles, his spine would sag and he would fall to the ground. The upright posture is maintained mainly by the simultaneous contraction of appropriate sets of antagonistic muscles.

Fig. 16.29 shows some of the antagonistic muscles of the leg which contribute to walking and standing. It can be seen that contraction of the *tibialis anterior* would flex the ankle (i.e. tend to raise the foot) whereas contraction of the *soleus* and *gastrocnemius* (not shown) would extend it. When both sets of muscles contract or, rather, maintain themselves in a state of tension (*isometric contraction*), the tibia is held at about 90° to the foot. Similarly the controlled tension in the *rectus femoris* and the *biceps femoris* keeps the leg straight at the knee, while the *gluteus maximus* and the rectus femoris, acting together, prevent the pelvic girdle from rotating forward or backward. Thus, since the spine is fused to the pelvis, the trunk is kept upright.

If this were the whole story, a great deal of muscular energy would have to be expended just to keep the body stationary and upright but in fact the energy expenditure in maintaining posture is greatly reduced by (a) using only part of each muscle, (b) exploiting the ligaments and (c) balance.

(a) The postural tension of a muscle is maintained by only a small number of its fibres and this fraction is constantly changing with the result that fatigue is minimal.

(b) Certain of the ligaments in the knee joint allow the knee to flex (bend) and extend (straighten), but because the ligaments are inextensible they prevent the knee from bending the 'wrong way'. At rest, the centre of gravity of the body falls just in front of the knee joint (Fig. 16.30) and so keeps the joint fully extended and held in this position by the ligaments. Muscles such as the rectus femoris are then almost completely relaxed. Ligaments in the hip joint, similarly, tend to stop the pelvis rotating backwards and thus help to maintain upright posture when the centre of gravity falls behind the joint.

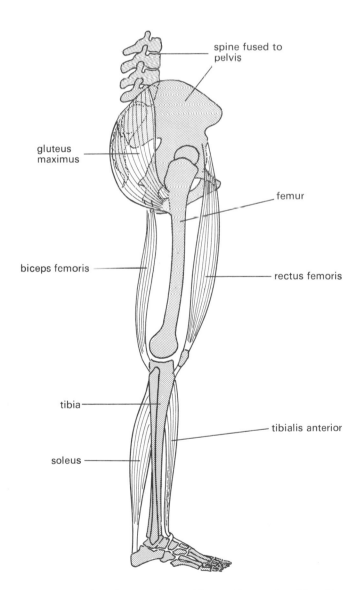

Fig. 16.29   Some of the leg muscles used in standing and walking (the many other muscle systems of the leg have been omitted for clarity)

(c) The weight of the body is considered, for theoretical purposes, to act through the *centre of gravity* (the point at which an object can be balanced). Fig. 16.30 shows where the centre of gravity is for a man. When the posture is adjusted so that a vertical line from the centre of gravity passes just behind the hip joint and just in front of both knee and ankle, the joints are in their most stable position and minimal muscular energy is needed to maintain the posture.

The centre of gravity will only be in the position shown if the upper half of the body is held correctly, with the head of the humerus and a point on the skull just behind the ear directly above the indicated centre of gravity. Since the lower part of the spine is fused rigidly to the pelvic girdle, the position of the head and shoulders is maintained by the curvature of the spine. An excessively curved or straight spine will necessitate muscular intervention to maintain balance and so result in fatigue and discomfort.

The feet. The weight of the body is ultimately supported by the feet. Each foot is a kind of three-dimensional arch, with the three main points of support at the heel, the base of the big toe and the base of the little toe. When the posture is correct the weight is distributed appropriately between these three points (Fig. 16.31) but incorrect posture leads to unequal stresses on the joints and ligaments of the foot, causing discomfort and in some cases distortion and flattening of the arches.

Dynamic posture. Even when the skeleton is well balanced and the muscles are as relaxed as possible, there are bound to be small involuntary movements since the body is flexible and

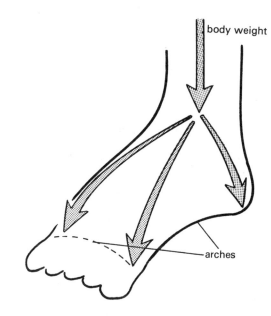

Fig. 16.31　Distribution of weight on the foot

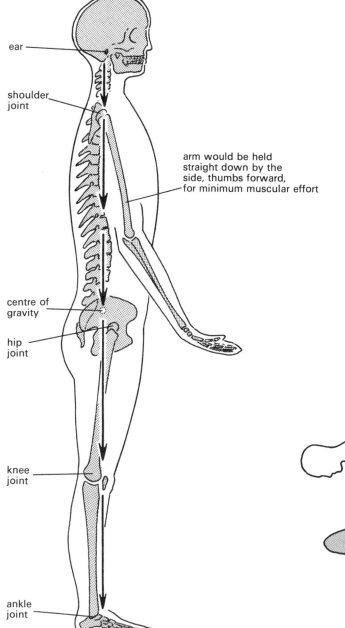

Fig. 16.30　Standing posture involving minimal muscular energy

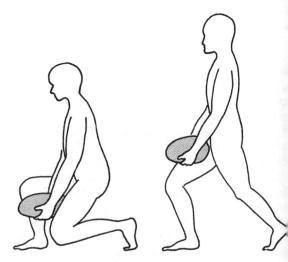

(a) *Incorrect*

(b) *Correct; the weight is close to the body and the back is nearly upright*

Fig. 16.32　Lifting heavy objects

not a rigid structure. The movements are detected by the organs of balance (p. 142) and the stretch receptors (p. 131) of the muscles. These sensory organs send nerve impulses to the brain and spinal cord and automatic adjustments are made by the muscles, returning the body to a stable position. For example, if the body were to sway forward, the soleus would be stretched and cause a reflex action (p. 148) to make the same muscle contract slightly and bring the centre of gravity once again to a stable position.

Postural defects. Any deviation from the balanced posture described above will necessitate expenditure of muscular energy to maintain an upright stance and so lead to fatigue and perhaps discomfort and muscular pain. Small, temporary deviations are of little importance. In pregnancy, for example, the centre of gravity moves forward and the muscles of the back have to work harder to maintain an increased curvature of the lower spine. In very fat people, however, similar adaptations lead eventually to permanent postural defects such as the flattening of the arches of the foot with the difficulty and discomfort in walking that this entails. Any position, standing or sitting, in which the head is not balanced easily on the spine leads to strain of the neck muscles. Poor lighting, short sight or low working surfaces may necessitate prolonged leaning forwards and so cause fatigue and pain of the neck muscles, sometimes registered as a headache, and in the long term may induce permanent distortion in the alignment of the upper vertebrae in the neck and thorax.

The treatment of established postural defects is difficult and time-consuming, particularly as the defect may have been present for several years before the symptoms become severe enough for the patient to seek medical advice. Prevention is therefore all-important. The maintenance of mobility and muscle strength by exercise and the awareness of what constitutes a good posture are the key factors.

Lifting and carrying. It seems likely that through thousands of years of evolution, the human skeleton and musculature are well adapted to an upright posture both at rest and during locomotion. Disorders of the back and feet can generally be attributed to a misuse of the body rather than to natural defects. The daily work of civilized man often involves sitting for long hours at a desk or production line, and if good posture is not practised, this may lead to disorders as described above.

Other work and leisure activities often involve lifting heavy objects, carrying and digging for which the body seems ill-adapted. Consequently, the common ailments of the back such as distorted intervertebral discs can usually be attributed to long-term static or active bad posture. Fig. 16.32a shows a method of lifting heavy objects that subjects the spinal column to stresses which it is ill-adapted to withstand. Fig. 16.32b shows a far better method of lifting in which the stress is transferred to the leg muscles and joints which are well able to withstand it. The general rule is to keep the back as upright as possible with the normal spinal curves whether lifting loads, picking up children, digging, carrying heavy objects, driving a car or merely sitting at a desk.

Exercise and health

Human communities that depend on hunting, gathering or non-mechanized agriculture indulge in exercise as an essential part of daily life. Today, many people in industrialized socie- ties have sedentary occupations and little cause for exercise in obtaining food and shelter. There is a good deal of circumstantial evidence to suggest that lack of exercise is a contributory factor in many of the common ailments of industrialized communities, such as coronary heart disease (p. 79). In Britain, one man in five is likely to have symptoms of coronary heart disease by the age of 65 so any steps, such as regular exercise, that can be taken to avert such illness seem worthwhile.

In a recent study, 16 882 men between the ages of 40 and 64 in sedentary occupations were studied. Their exercise habits were noted carefully and records kept of their state of health. It was found that those who subsequently suffered a coronary heart attack took significantly less vigorous exercise than those who remained free from heart disease.

The precise reasons why exercise should reduce the susceptibility to heart disease are not known, but it is most likely that regular vigorous activity increases the supply of blood to the heart muscle either by increasing the diameter of the coronary arteries or by causing them to develop more branches. There is also evidence to suggest that athletes metabolize the fats in their blood plasma more rapidly than other people and that the level of fats in their blood does not rise with age as it does in the general population. Since the level of fat in the blood may be correlated with the incidence of coronary heart disease this evidence seems to indicate another advantage of exercise.

There is evidence for other long-term effects on the heart of regular exercise. During adolescence, the way in which the heart develops will be influenced by the sort of exercise a person takes. Regular 'steady state' exercise which produces a pulse rate of 140–150 beats per minute and is continued for 40–60 minutes at a time will develop a heart with large chambers. This will result in a low resting pulse rate.

On the other hand, short-duration heavy work, producing pulse rates of about 180 beats per minute, will thicken up the muscle wall of the heart and improve its blood supply.

In adolescence, programmes of exercise should be designed to include a preponderance of 'steady state' exercise to encourage the development of a large-chambered heart. If the heart muscle thickens before the chambers have enlarged, the heart chambers remain small and the heart can respond to exercise only by a very rapid pulse rate.

Exercise also helps to prevent obesity, although careful feeding is the best method of controlling this condition.

The immediate effects of exercise are to increase the flow of blood through the muscles, thus removing the waste products of metabolism. Contractions of the body muscles also help to return lymph and venous blood to the heart (p. 83). In addition to the improved circulation, increased heartbeat and ventilation of the lungs are beneficial and the improved appetite resulting from exercise probably aids digestion.

Practical Work

Experiment 1 **The structure of bone**

Obtain two small bones, e.g. limb bones from a chicken. Place one of them in a test-tube or beaker, cover it with dilute hydrochloric acid and leave it for 24 hours, during which time the acid will dissolve most of the mineral salts in the bone. After 24 hours pour away the acid, wash the bone thoroughly with water and then try to bend it.

Take the second bone and hold one end of it in a hot

Bunsen flame, heating it strongly for 2 minutes. At first the bone will char and then glow red as the organic material burns away, but it will retain its shape. Allow the bone to cool and then try crushing the heated end against the bench with the end of a pencil.

Result. Both bones retain their shape after treatment, but the bone whose mineral component had been dissolved in acid is rubbery and flexible because only the organic, fibrous connective tissue is left. The bone that had this fibrous tissue burned away is still hard but very brittle and easily fragmented.

Interpretation. The combination in bone of mineral salts and organic fibres produces a hard, strong and resilient structure.

Questions

1 Construct a diagram similar to Fig. 16.18*a* to show a section through the elbow joint, using Fig. 16.17 for guidance. Show the attachment of the biceps and triceps tendons and state where you would expect to find the principal ligaments.
2 Write a list of the functions of cartilage in the human body (a) during growth and (b) at maturity.
3 Distinguish between ligaments and tendons with respect to their position and their function.
4 What is the principal action of (a) your calf muscle, (b) the muscle in the front of your thigh, and (c) the muscles in your forearm? If you don't already know the answers, try making the muscles contract and feel where the tendons are pulling.
5 Unlike most mammals, man stands upright on his hind-legs. What difference do you think this has made to his skeleton and musculature?

17
Teeth

Teeth are produced from the skin where it covers the upper and lower jaws. The crowns of the teeth break through the skin into the mouth cavity while their roots are enclosed in the bony sockets of the jaws. Human teeth begin their formation in the sixth week of embryonic development and erupt, i.e. grow through the gum, usually by the second year after birth. The first set of twenty deciduous or milk teeth eventually fall out and are replaced by thirty-two permanent teeth, between the ages of six and eighteen.

Structure

The generalized structure of human teeth is best shown in longitudinal section as in Figs. 17.1 and 17.2.

Enamel. This is a hard, brittle, non-living layer up to 2.5 mm thick, 96 per cent of which consists of a mineral comprising chiefly calcium and phosphate arranged in microscopic six-sided prisms. The enamel covers the crown of the tooth, forming a hard biting surface.

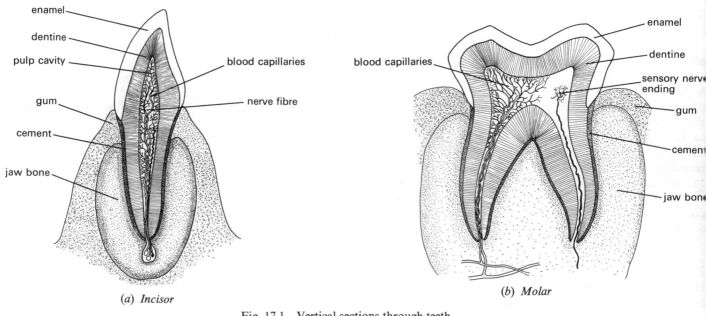

(a) Incisor

(b) Molar

Fig. 17.1 Vertical sections through teeth

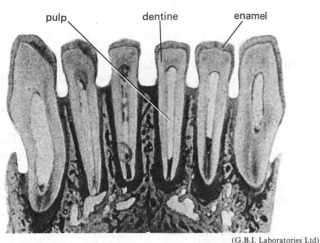

Fig. 17.2 Section through teeth and jaw of cat

(G.B.I. Laboratories Ltd)

Specialization

In many carnivorous reptiles and in the more primitive mammals, the teeth are unspecialized, that is they are all alike in structure, being single sharp pegs which serve to hold the prey while the latter is swallowed whole. In carnivorous mammals, where the food is caught, killed and torn apart, the teeth have to deal with both soft flesh and hard bone. The carnivore's teeth have become adapted to this diversity of functions, with the result that the teeth in different parts of the jaw have different shapes and actions. In a dog, the front teeth, *incisors*, are small and close together; they meet and grip the flesh like a pair of forceps. The long, sharp, pointed canines behind them pass each other, penetrating and holding the prey. The carnassial teeth (last upper premolar and first lower molar) have sharp ridges whose cutting edges pass each other like scissor blades, shearing flesh and cracking bones, while the relatively flat-topped molars meet and crush flesh and bones to a size suitable for swallowing (Fig. 17.4).

Dentine. Dentine is similar to bone in its structure. It is hard but not so brittle as enamel, having a higher proportion of fibrous material. It also has branching strands of living cytoplasm penetrating it. The cells, *odontoblasts,* from which these cytoplasmic strands extend, are able to add more dentine to the inside of the tooth (Fig. 17.3).

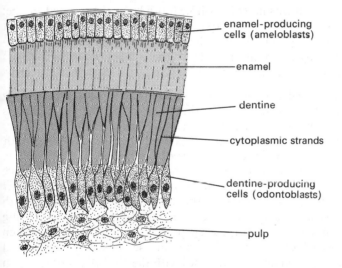

Fig. 17.3 Section through enamel and dentine of unerupted tooth

Pulp. In the centre of the tooth is soft connective tissue called pulp. The pulp contains blood capillaries and sensory nerve endings which may penetrate the dentine. Oxygen and food brought by the blood enable the tooth to live and grow. The nerve endings respond mainly to changes in temperature, but produce only the sensation of pain. The channel in the base of the root through which the blood vessels pass becomes smaller as the tooth reaches full size and restricts the flow of blood. Sufficient blood flows to maintain the life of the tooth but there is not enough to bring about growth.

Root. The root is not set rigidly in the jaw bone but is slung by collagen fibres. This method of suspension may prevent the crushing of the blood vessels and nerve fibres entering the tooth, when biting forces are applied.

Cement is a thin layer of bone-like material covering the dentine at the root of the tooth. The fibres that hold the tooth in the jaw are embedded in the cement at one end and in the jaw bone at the other.

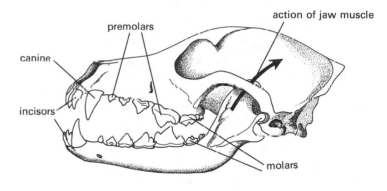

Fig. 17.4 Skull and teeth of dog

Human teeth show less extreme specialization (Fig. 17.5). The four chisel-like incisors in the front of each jaw pass each other and take bites out of solid food. Next to the incisors are two canine teeth, sharp and pointed but little longer than the incisors and much reduced compared with carnivorous mammals or apes. They seem to have a function similar to the incisors. Canines and incisors have single roots. Next come two premolars on each side, with two cusps (blunt points) and usually single roots. The three molar teeth on each side

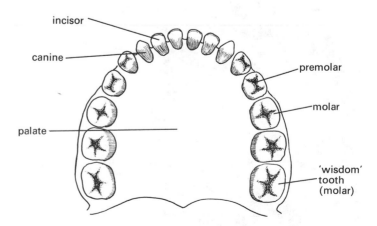

Fig. 17.5 Arrangement of teeth in man's upper jaw

have four cusps and in the upper jaw usually three roots, in the lower jaw two roots. The upper and lower molars and premolars meet, the cusps in one set fitting into the depressions of the other, so crushing the food (Fig. 17.6).

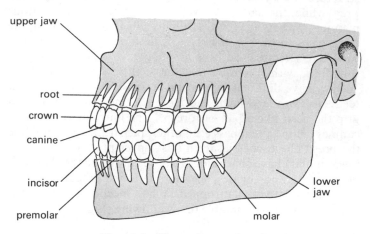

Fig. 17.6   Human jaws and teeth

The deciduous teeth (milk teeth) consist of 4 incisors, 2 canines and 4 premolars in each jaw. As the permanent teeth develop, the roots of the deciduous teeth are resorbed (Figs. 17.7 and 17.8e) so that the teeth eventually fall out quite easily. The position of the deciduous teeth seems to determine the final arrangement of the permanent teeth so the former need to be allowed to complete their natural course of development. Where the deciduous teeth have to be extracted as a result of decay, the permanent teeth may grow with unsatisfactory spacing. The first permanent teeth, i.e. the first molars, erupt at about six years, the second at about twelve and the last or 'wisdom' teeth usually after the seventeenth year or sometimes not at all. The deciduous teeth are usually all replaced between six and twelve years.

Fig. 17.7   Photomicrograph of milk and permanent tooth of kitten

(Gene Cox)

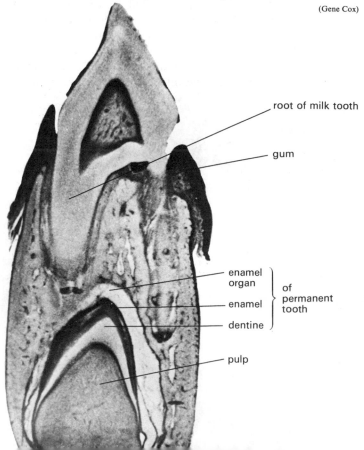

Development

During the development of the embryo, groups of cells in the epithelium of the mouth, overlying the jawbone rudiments, become especially active and give rise to tooth buds. In these, the epithelium thickens and grows into the tissues beneath (Fig. 17.8a). This ingrowth takes on an inverted cup-like form, the inner surface of which secretes enamel and is called the *enamel organ*. The cone of tissue enclosed by the cup is called the *dental papilla* and its outer layers produce dentine. The very elongated cells in the enamel organ become calcified by deposit of calcium phosphate. This process results in the formation of rods of enamel being laid down at right angles to the tooth's surface (17.8b and c).

The outermost cells, the odontoblasts, of the dental papilla form dentine in much the same way as bone is produced (p. 112). A matrix containing collagen fibres forms between the cells and this matrix is then calcified, leaving strands of cytoplasm running from the odontoblasts through fine tubes in the calcified matrix. New dentine is added to the inner surface while the odontoblasts retreat deeper into the pulp. Even before the deciduous tooth erupts, the rudiment of the permanent tooth is forming alongside it in a similar way (Fig. 17.8c).

Experiments in which whole tooth buds, the isolated enamel organ, or the dental papilla have been grafted into different parts of an animal show that the shape of the tooth is determined by the pattern made by the enamel organ as it grows inwards from the epidermis.

Growth and eruption. It is not clear exactly what events bring about the growth of the tooth, but its root elongates and forces the crown through the gum (Fig. 17.8d). At the same time, bone has been formed in the jaw round the base of the tooth and now closes in to hold the root firmly in the socket of bone. Where the enamel organ covers the root it does not produce enamel, but just before it disintegrates it puts down a layer of cement on the root. In this region the *dental sac,* a sheath of connective tissue which has surrounded the developing tooth, enamel organ, dental papilla, etc., forms the collagen fibres which suspend the root in the socket. The ruptured top of the enamel organ fuses with the epithelium of the gum forming a seal around the base of the tooth where it emerges from the gum.

Dental caries and periodontal disease

Caries is the technical name for tooth decay; *periodontal disease* is an infection of the gums and tooth sockets. Caries results in the erosion of the enamel and dentine of the teeth, leading to the formation of cavities. The absence of enamel and the thinner layer of dentine in these cavities results in the tooth being far more sensitive to temperature changes. If the cavities are untreated, the pulp may be invaded by pathogenic bacteria which ultimately cause a painful abscess at the root. Sometimes this can only be cured by extracting the tooth. If bacteria gain access to the circulatory system, they may cause septicaemia (blood poisoning).

Causes of caries. There are several theories to explain the cause of cavities and though all of them involve bacteria, there is no general agreement about how cavities are formed. One theory suggests that the bacterial enzymes act on sugar and starch in the mouth and produce acid, mainly lactic acid, as a by-product. This acid dissolves the calcium salts in the teeth, so forming cavities. A second theory supposes that the enzymes from the bacteria first attack the protein of the enamel and dentine, and a third theory goes on to suggest that the amino acids so formed react in a complex way to combine with calcium ions from the enamel and dentine. All the theories, however, seem to accept that whatever the bacterial activity may be, it takes place in a layer of *plaque* which forms on the teeth.

Plaque. Within a few hours of cleaning the teeth, a coating of saliva containing mucus and other substances forms over the teeth. At first, this layer contains few bacteria, but eventually it is colonized by micro-organisms, even if no food is taken in. These bacteria and their products form a layer of plaque over the teeth. The composition of plaque is 70 per cent bacteria and 30 per cent organic substances which are either produced by the bacteria or deposited from material in the mouth. This organic material helps the bacteria to adhere more securely to the tooth surface.

In this bacterial plaque are produced the enzymes, acids and toxins which might contribute to caries and gum disease. The population of micro-organisms changes as the plaque grows thicker, but perhaps two of the most important bacteria are *Lactobacillus acidophilus* which produces lactic acid, and *Streptococcus mutans*. When the plaque has colonized most of the exposed tooth surface, it begins to spread downwards between the tooth and the gum and so causes gum inflammation or *gingivitis*.

If the bacterial plaque is not removed, it becomes mineralized by the incorporation of the phosphate and carbonate salts of calcium and magnesium. This mineralized plaque, called *calculus* or 'tartar', cannot be removed by normal teeth cleaning but has to be dispersed by scaling at the dentist's.

Refined sugar, sucrose. The intake of refined sugar has long been associated with dental caries and it has now been shown experimentally that sucrose increases the ability of *Streptococcus mutans* to colonize tooth surfaces by forming sticky polysaccharides which stick to the smooth surfaces of the teeth.

Periodontal disease. There is good evidence to connect the degree of plaque formation on teeth and the development of gum disease. The bacterial plaque spreads down the tooth and into the crevice at the junction of tooth and gum. Gingivitis may not result in easily recognizable symptoms but leads at first to bleeding of the gums, bad breath and gum recession in which the gum retreats from the base of the tooth, exposing the cement. 'Getting long in the tooth' is a common expression for gum recession. However it is not a natural consequence of ageing but a result of chronic gingivitis. If treatment or preventative measures for gingivitis are ignored, the bacteria may invade the tooth socket and attack the fibres holding the root in the jaw bone, causing *periodontitis*. The jaw bone between the teeth is also resorbed and consequently the teeth become loose in their sockets and may have to be extracted.

Prevention of caries and periodontal disease

Since bacterial plaque is held to be primarily responsible for both caries and periodontal disease, prevention depends on stopping the development of plaque as far as possible and removing it efficiently when it does form.

Prevention of plaque formation. Plaque forms slowly in the absence of any food in the mouth but it develops rapidly in the

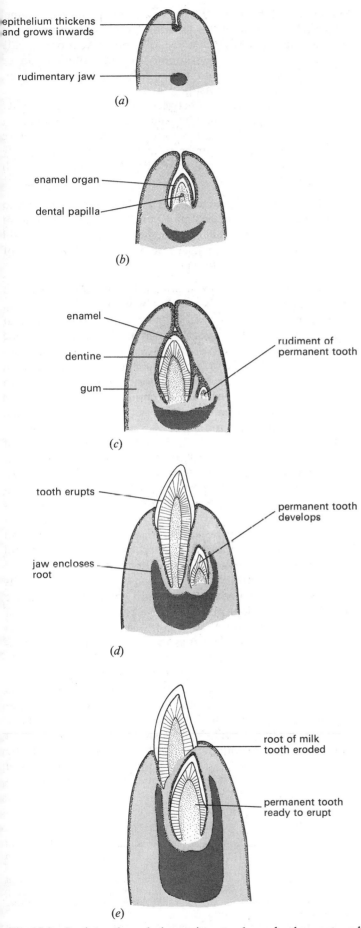

epithelium thickens
and grows inwards

rudimentary jaw

(a)

enamel organ

dental papilla

(b)

enamel

dentine

gum

rudiment of
permanent tooth

(c)

tooth erupts

permanent tooth
develops

jaw encloses
root

(d)

root of milk
tooth eroded

permanent tooth
ready to erupt

(e)

Fig. 17.8 Sections through lower jaw to show development and eruption of tooth

presence of refined sugar, sucrose. The best way to minimize plaque formation is to avoid introducing sucrose into the mouth for as long periods as possible. Sucrose is present in sweets, biscuits, cakes, jam and many soft drinks and the environment most conducive to plaque formation is maintained by a supply of these materials at frequent intervals. It is not the concentration of sucrose which matters, but the constant availability. It is better to eat several sweets at once than to keep introducing them into the mouth one after the other over a long time. But it is better still to avoid them altogether and eat fruit and nuts instead. It is pure sucrose which constitutes the danger; glucose and other sugars occurring naturally in food are not harmful. Workers in sugar plantations may chew the cane constantly and suffer no significant caries but the natural sucrose from the cane is mixed with other cellular contents such as proteins, vitamins and organic salts.

Removal of plaque. Plaque is removed by brushing the teeth with a toothbrush. In cleaning the teeth, it is the thoroughness and not the daily frequency which matters. If the brushing is efficient and removes all the plaque from the tooth surfaces, then once a day is sufficient, but to be efficient the brushing needs to be extended over 3 to 4 minutes, firmly but not roughly executed and to reach all parts of the teeth. No method has proved superior to any other and is seems best to adopt whatever technique is easiest to use, provided it removes the plaque.

One way of checking whether the plaque has been removed is to spread a disclosing agent on the teeth after brushing. The disclosing agent is a harmless dye which, after rinsing the mouth, colours the patches of plaque not removed by the toothbrush. A dentist will advise on the most suitable disclosing agent to use.

The best time to brush the teeth is before going to bed, because during sleep, the salivary flow is reduced and any sucrose in the plaque will be converted to acid. Brushing before meals is also a sound idea; if there is no plaque, the sucrose cannot adhere to the tooth surface. Brushing after meals removes food debris and is better than not brushing at all but the evidence suggests that there is no connection between caries and the amount of food debris left in the mouth.

An effective toothbrush should have a short, straight head with fine nylon bristles in close tufts and be designated medium or soft. Toothpastes make brushing more pleasant and the mild abrasives they contain may help to remove plaque. Additives such as chlorhexidine have not been proved effective in reducing caries but added fluorides do increase resistance to decay.

No toothbrush will remove plaque from between the teeth and so brushing should be supplemented by drawing a waxed thread called 'dental floss', backwards and forwards between the teeth. At one time it was thought that eating apples, raw carrot, celery and other crisp vegetable matter helped to clean the teeth but it is now agreed that these materials do not effectively remove plaque. By replacing sweets and biscuits in the diet, however, they may contribute to dental health.

There is not much evidence to suggest that cleaning the teeth, other than professionally, reduces caries but there is abundant evidence that it does reduce periodontal disease. Since more teeth are lost as a result of gum disease than caries, good dental hygiene is very important.

Application of fluorides. Fluorides taken up by the enamel reduce the susceptibility of teeth to caries. An application of fluoride solution for as little as 2 minutes each year or a weekly rinse with a 0.2 per cent stannous fluoride solution can be beneficial, particularly for children. This treatment, however, needs professional supervision.

There is a wide variation between individuals' susceptibility to caries. Some people may be able to eat sweets, and neglect dental hygiene with relative impunity while others, more conscientious, may still suffer from caries. However, nearly everyone is susceptible to gum disease and this is reason enough for good oral hygiene.

Dental treatment. Regular visits to a dentist will enable him to remove calculus and detect cavities and gum disorders at an early stage. Decayed areas of teeth can be drilled out and plugged with a metallic amalgam, so preventing the advance of decay in the tooth and those next to it.

Fluoridation. Fluoride ions are a fairly common constituent of drinking water occurring naturally in concentrations of up to five parts per million (ppm) or more. It has been shown that in areas where water naturally contained fluoride ions, the incidence of decay was up to 60 per cent less than in areas containing little or no fluoride. Experiments were conducted in some American towns by adding fluoride to drinking water in concentrations of 1 ppm, and the populations of these towns were compared with control areas with little fluoride in the water. A similar reduction in decay was found in the children and no evidence of undesirable side effects. Concentrations of 2 ppm or more, however, tend to cause some degree of mottling. Experimental fluoridation has been carried out in the U.S.A. for over 20 years and in Britain for over 15 years with encouraging results. The way in which fluoride acts is not fully understood, but it is known to be taken up by bones or teeth from the blood, though 95 per cent of it is excreted in the urine; and it is principally effective when the permanent teeth are still developing, having little or no effect in adults.

Opposition to fluoridation has arisen mainly on the grounds that it is a measure forced on all people, giving them no choice in the matter. Biologically it seems a rational adjustment of our environment to meet optimum demands. Teeth seem to need a supply of fluoride just as they need calcium and phosphate, and the best way, it is claimed, of obtaining this supply in continuous small doses is via the drinking water.

Certainly, any adjustment of our environment which affects the health of millions of people needs very careful consideration and though the case for fluoridation seems to have received this study, there are still wide differences of opinion both about the interpretation of the evidence and about the desirability of interfering with the water supplies to achieve medical benefits as distinct from merely making it safe to drink.

Questions

1 What general aspects of the diet of civilized man differ from the diets of other mammals? What effects might these differences have on the way man uses his teeth?

2 An eight-year-old boy pulls out a loose incisor and is alarmed because (a) it has no root and he thinks he has broken it off, and (b) he fears he will have a gap in his front teeth. How would you use your biological knowledge to reassure him?

3 In an erupted tooth, the dentine may continue to increase in thickness but the enamel cannot. Explain the difference.

18
The Sensory System

The sensory system makes an animal aware, though not necessarily in the sense of 'conscious', of conditions and changes both outside and inside its body. In the simpler animals, only very general stimuli such as light or darkness, heat or cold can be perceived by the sensory system. In the higher animals, including man, detailed information about the surroundings, such as distance, size and colours of objects, can be gained as a result of the specialization of the sensory organs and the elaboration of the nervous system.

The *general sensory system* includes organs that are fairly evenly distributed through the dermis of the skin; hence any part of the skin is sensitive to the stimuli of touch, heat, cold and pressure, any of which stimuli may also produce the sensation of pain. Examples of such sense organs are indicated in Fig. 18.1.

It must be emphasized that, in general, a particular sense organ can respond to only one kind of stimulus. That is to say, a sense organ sensitive to touch will not be affected by the stimulus of heat; an organ sensitive to chemicals will not respond to pressure. It is not yet certain just how specific some of the dermal sense organs are in their responses, for the sensory endings that produce the sensation of pain can be activated by a variety of stimuli, such as pressure, heat and cold. Moreover, the extent to which the various sensory endings can be distinguished by their structural appearance in sections is not yet determined. There are three basic types, (a) the *free-ending* type, in which the terminal branches of a sensory nerve cell penetrate the outer tissues of the dermis and possibly into the epidermis, (b) the *hair plexus,* a network of fibres surrounding a hair follicle, and (c) the *encapsulated* type, where a branched or coiled nerve ending is enclosed in a capsule of varying complexity, e.g. *Pacinian* and *Meissner's corpuscles* (Fig. 18.2). There may, however, be physiological differences between these encapsulated endings despite their apparently similar structure. For example, in the pinna of the ear only free endings and hair plexuses can be distinguished, and yet heat, cold, touch and pressure can all be detected there. It may be that one type of ending responds to light pressure, others to temperature changes, etc. It is possible, also, that their position in the dermis may determine the kind of stimulus to which they respond, e.g. the Pacinian corpuscle in the subcutaneous tissue is not likely to be stimulated by a light touch but may be activated by more pronounced pressure on the skin.

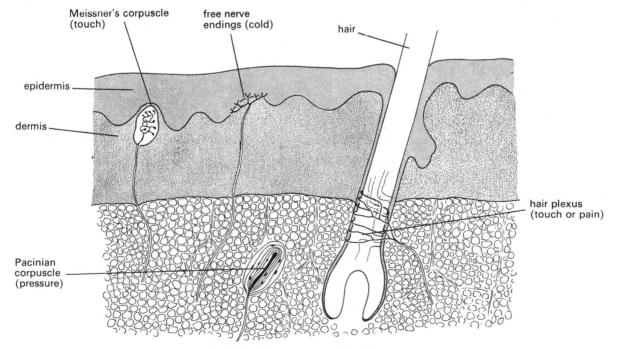

Fig. 18.1   Sense organs of the skin

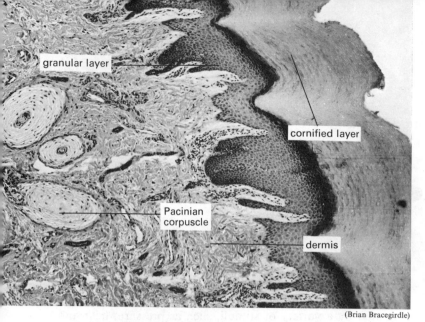

granular layer

cornified layer

Pacinian corpuscle

dermis

(Brian Bracegirdle)

Fig. 18.2 Pacinian corpuscles in human skin

Touch. The encapsulated end organs in the dermis respond to light pressure on the skin, though it is likely that some at least are stimulated by the distortion of the skin rather than by the direct pressure. In the hair-covered areas of skin, the sense of touch also depends on the free nerve endings wrapped round the hair follicles. Any movement of the hair follicle stimulates the nerve ending, the hair acting as a lever.

Heat and cold. Whatever the nature of the receptors that respond to temperature, experiments suggest that there is a difference in either physiology or distribution between those responding to heat and those responding to cold. A cold 'spot' (*see* below) will not respond to heat, or if it does it will produce the sensation of cold. It also appears that the response is made to a change of temperature rather than a steady state, i.e. once the skin ceases to gain or lose heat at a certain rate the receptor ceases to fire off impulses; it is said to be adapted to the new situation (Experiment 4).

Pain. It seems that any kind of stimulus that affects the free nerve endings described above can produce the sensation of pain. However, a pin may elicit a sensation of touch on one area of skin but pain on another. It is unlikely that excessive stimulation of the encapsulated endings can cause pain since, if the sensory fibres passing in the spinal cord from the free endings are severed, pain is prevented while all the other skin sensations are present.

The origin of a painful stimulus can be accurately located even though the stimulated area of skin may contain a number of overlapping free endings whose impulses reach the brain by more than one route.

Although we tend to regard sensations of pain as inconvenient and alarming, they have important biological advantages. By making us respond quickly and automatically by reflex action they tend to remove the affected part from danger. Our response when touching something unexpectedly hot affords a good example. If there were no appreciation of harmful stimuli, untold damage might occur to the tissues. Withdrawal reflexes (p. 148) could be just as effective, however, without necessarily producing the feeling of pain, but association of pain with other sensory information such as the heat and light of a naked flame allows a conditioned reflex (*see* p. 150) to be established, or a store of information to be built up, so reducing the chances of hazardous encounters in the future. Where pain occurs without producing a reflex action,

as in toothache, it serves as a warning that all is not well in that region and advice or treatment should be sought.

As might be expected, however, the significance of pain is not so straightforward as has been suggested. There is plenty of experimental evidence and everyday experience to indicate that our psychological state determines the intensity of pain we feel from any one stimulus. A person wholly preoccupied with some activity may be quite unaware of injuries received until his attention is called to them. In fact, it appears that we tend to experience the degree of pain which we expect to feel, or have learned to feel. Analgesic drugs, hypnosis, self-imposed mental states and many other effects can influence our experience of pain.

Distribution of sensory endings. Certain regions of the skin have a greater concentration of a particular type of sense organ. In general, the hairy regions of the skin have mainly hair follicle plexuses while in hairless regions, e.g. lips and fingertips, encapsulated end organs predominate. The fingertips have a large number of touch organs, making them particularly sensitive to touch. The front of the upper arm is sensitive to heat and cold probably as a result of the large numbers of those sense organs present. Some areas of skin have relatively few sense organs and can be pricked or burned in certain places without any sensation being felt. In the different regions of the body there is also a difference in the sensitivity to any one type of stimulus. In some areas, a light stimulus will produce an appreciable nerve impulse while in other areas a stronger stimulus is needed. In this respect, the tongue, nose and lips are most sensitive to touch, i.e. respond to weak stimuli, while the shin, sole of the foot and back of the forearm are the least sensitive (Experiments 1 and 2). The arms can detect changes of temperature of just over 0.2 °C while the fingers need a change of 0.5–1.0 °C to produce a sensation. In a newborn baby, the heat-sensitive endings are not fully functional, making the baby very vulnerable to injuries from heat, e.g. hot bath-water.

When the skin is explored with fine bristles or finely pointed hot or cold instruments it appears that areas sensitive to a particular stimulus are arranged in discrete 'spots', i.e. small areas of skin which will detect (say) touch, while the area next to it will not. Similar heat and cold spots can be mapped out. The spots do not correspond to single receptors since many different receptors must be affected by even the smallest stimulus. In some cases, the areas mapped are not even consistent from one day to the next. The density of the spots, however, varies with the sensitivity of the region tested. The physiological condition of the skin also affects the distribution of these spots, e.g. there is a more uniform sensitivity to heat and cold in an inflamed area; the spots have merged or 'vanished', perhaps as a result of the vasodilation that accompanies the reddening of the skin.

Internal receptors. Many internal organs and connective tissues have free nerve endings in them. In some cases they respond to stretching; for example, the alimentary canal if distended may produce a sensation of pain which is not produced by pinching or cutting. The inflation of the lungs is controlled to some extent by a reflex in which stretch receptors play a part (p. 89) and the emptying of the bladder (p. 94) is probably initiated by stretch receptors in its walls. In the aorta are sense organs that help to regulate the blood pressure (p. 82) and in the carotid arteries there are chemoreceptors that respond to changes in oxygen concentration. In certain regions of the brain, too, there is sensory apparatus that responds to changes in the osmotic pressure (p. 155), carbon dioxide concentration (p. 89) and temperature (p. 98) of the blood.

The response of these receptors to changes in the internal environment enables corrections to be made by the body, and so keeps the blood and body fluids at optimum conditions for the vital chemical reactions of life to take place rapidly and predictably.

Proprioceptors. Proprioceptors are internal sense organs which occur most frequently in muscles. For the most part they are sensory endings embedded in a specialized group of muscle fibres called *muscle spindles* (Fig. 18.3). The spindles fire off

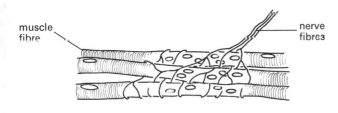

muscle fibre — nerve fibres

Fig. 18.3   Stretch receptor in muscle

impulses when stretched either by the extension of the muscle around them or by contraction of their own fibres. The muscle spindle by feeding back sensory impulses into the spinal cord affects the motor impulses which are bringing about contraction, and so controls the movement of limbs. After a period of learning, the sensory information about the tension of muscles that reaches the brain from the proprioceptors enables an individual to know (consciously or otherwise) the precise orientation of his limbs at any moment, an essential requirement for co-ordinated activity. One can put food into the mouth, for example, without having to watch the hand all the time.

Information to the brain

Stimulation and conduction of impulses. The sense organs are connected to the brain or spinal cord by nerve fibres. When the sense organ receives an appropriate stimulus it sets off a burst of electrical impulses in the nerve fibre supplying it. The impulses travel along the nerve fibre to the spinal cord and on to the brain, sometimes producing an automatic or reflex action, or recording an impression by which the person feels the nature of the stimulus and where it was applied.

Sense organs of one kind, and those in a definite area, are connected principally but not exclusively with one particular region of the brain. It is the region of the brain to which the impulse comes that gives rise to the knowledge about the nature of the stimulus and where it was received. For example, if the region of the brain receiving impulses from pain nerve endings were eliminated or its activity suppressed by drugs, no amount of stimulation of the pain sensory endings would produce any sensation of pain at all, even though impulses were being fired off and travelling as far as the brain. On the other hand, if a region of the brain dealing with impulses from

sense organs in the leg is stimulated by any means, e.g. a weak electric current applied directly to the appropriate part of the brain, the sensations so produced seem to have come from the leg. If a limb has been amputated the nerves from the stump may still send impulses to the region of the brain that formerly received them from the limb, and pain is felt as if the limb were still there.

Another important consideration is the fact that the impulses transmitted along the nerve fibres are all exactly the same in quality. It is not the sensations that are carried but simply a surge of electrical energy, which is the same whether it is a heat organ or touch ending that sets off the impulse. Only in the brain can the stimulus be identified, according to the region of the brain which the impulse enters. For example, if the nerves from the arm and leg were changed over just before they entered the brain, stubbing one's toe would produce a sensation of pain in the arm or hand (Experiment 3).

Intensity of sensation. A strong stimulus usually produces a more pronounced sensation than a weak stimulus. This is probably the result of (a) a more rapid sequence of impulses fired off from the receptor, (b) the stimulation of a greater number of sensory organs in the area, and (c) the stimulation of a number of sensory organs that do not respond at all unless the stimulation is intense. Vigorous stimulation does not have any effect on the quality or intensity of the nerve impulses travelling in the sensory fibres, but increases the total number of impulses reaching the brain (Fig. 19.4, p. 147).

Interpretation. It will be appreciated that an enormous amount of sensory information is being constantly fed in to the nervous system. All this sensory data enables the organism to adjust itself to changes taking place internally and externally, so that in the first instance it maintains a constant and optimum internal environment for its metabolism, and in the second case can behave in an appropriate manner for the survival of itself and its species. Much of the sensory information never reaches conscious levels, e.g. changes in blood pressure or carbon dioxide content; the adjustments are made entirely on a reflex basis. Those sensory impulses which do reach consciousness produce sensations.

It seems that the sense organs on the whole respond to changes in conditions. As soon as conditions settle down, the sensations and probably the impulses cease or return to a low level. For example, we are unaware of the tactile stimulus of our own clothing once we have dressed; we become accustomed to unfamiliar smells after a time though a newcomer will notice them at once.

There is a fairly accurate location of the source of skin sensation. Touch is precisely located, heat and cold with less precision. The ability to locate the source of stimulation depends on memorizing the muscular movements needed, on previous occasions, to reach it.

We often tend to attribute our source of information to one particular sense organ, though in most cases we are interpreting the sum effect of a whole range of sensory data. Texture, for example, is appreciated by sense of touch, temperature (i.e. loss or gain of heat from the fingers when touching) and even the sound which is heard when running the fingers over an object. If one of these sources of information is lacking, our judgement is likely to be faulty. Information from the pressure receptors of the buttocks is of importance to a pilot controlling an aircraft or a motorist controlling his car, although normally it is assumed that the eyes and semicircular canals are the sole sources of information about position and movement.

The special senses

Sight, hearing and balance, smell and taste are called the special senses. The relevant sense organs each consist of a great concentration of cells that are sensitive to one kind of stimulus. These sensory cells may be associated with structures that direct the stimulus on to the sensory region.

Taste. The sense of taste is conferred by groups of sensory cells that are stimulated by chemicals. The receptors are grouped into about 9 000 taste buds (Fig. 18.4) containing both sensory

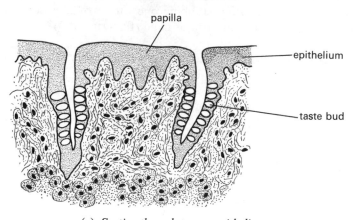

(a) Section through tongue epithelium

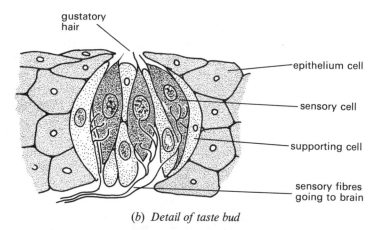

(b) Detail of taste bud

Fig. 18.4 Taste receptors in tongue

cells and supporting cells embedded in the epithelium round the base of the papillae on the tongue. Taste buds are also found in the soft palate, the epiglottis, the opening of the oesophagus and, at least in children, the cheek lining.

Only chemicals soluble in water can affect the taste buds, by dissolving in the moisture of the mouth. Their solutions enter the pores of the taste buds and stimulate the sensory cells, probably affecting the cytoplasmic filaments (*gustatory hairs*) projecting from their outer end. Although all the taste buds appear to be identical in structure, they are not equally sensitive to the chemicals described as sweet, sour, salt and bitter (the only tastes we can discriminate). Most taste buds appear to respond to all four classes of chemical but to differing extents.

For example, one taste bud may make its maximum response to salts, a lesser response to sour, and weak responses to sweet or bitter substances. The different types of taste bud are unevenly distributed over the tongue so that some parts of the tongue are more sensitive than others to a particular chemical.

The means by which the sensory cells are activated by chemicals is not known, but when the cells are stimulated by the appropriate solution, impulses are fired off in nerve fibres that pass to the medulla of the brain. Combinations of chemicals will affect the different taste buds simultaneously and so, according to the type and proportions of taste buds stimulated, a fairly wide range of discrimination is possible, over and above the four basic tastes. Lemonade, for example, will stimulate sweet and sour receptors simultaneously and its taste will be judged accordingly.

The fact that only four tastes can be distinguished indicates the limited importance of the sense of taste compared with the other senses. Few behaviour patterns are likely to be initiated by taste stimuli, which seem primarily to serve for discrimination of acceptable and undesirable food.

The wide variety of flavours attributed to food result from the simultaneous stimulation of taste buds of the tongue and olfactory (smell) organs in the nasal cavity, the latter organs being affected by the vapours emanating from food in the mouth. When the nasal cavity is congested, as with a heavy cold, the sense of flavour is lost although taste is unaffected, and the sufferer may realize the extent to which flavour depends on smell. The limited discriminatory power of taste can also be demonstrated by placing solutions or pieces of food on the extended tongue while the nostrils are pinched and chewing is forbidden. In these circumstances it is more difficult to distinguish between the taste of apple, turnip and onion, whose flavour and texture usually make them easy to recognize. It is also observed that, unlike most sensory organs, there is a long interval between application of the stimulus and appreciation of the sensation.

The tongue is also sensitive to touch, heat, cold and pain, and much of our information about food and our reactions to

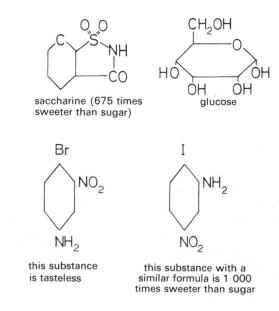

saccharine (675 times sweeter than sugar)

glucose

this substance is tasteless

this substance with a similar formula is 1 000 times sweeter than sugar

Fig. 18.5 Taste and chemical composition (it is difficult to see any connection between the formula of a substance and its taste)

it depends on the texture as well as the taste of the food. Hot food is more easily tasted than cold and, in addition, has more flavour.

The relationship between a particular chemical and its taste has not been elucidated, although it is true that acid solutions are sour-tasting and that chlorides, sulphates and nitrates of certain metals, particularly sodium, are salty. Different substances that taste sweet, however, often seem to bear no relationship to each other in their chemical structure (Fig. 18.5).

Smell. The olfactory organs, sensitive to smell, are two small patches of epithelium located in the upper regions of the nasal cavity in narrow crevices on each side. The several million receptors are not grouped into buds as are the taste organs, but distributed more or less evenly between the supporting cells. The sensitive cells (Fig. 18.6) are derived from the cell bodies

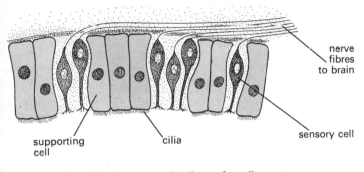

Fig. 18.6   Sensory epithelium of smell receptor

of bipolar nerve cells (p. 146), a short fibre (dendron) projecting outwards and terminating in sensory filaments in the nasal epithelium and a longer fibre (axon) running into the forebrain. Tubular nasal glands secrete a fluid which moistens and flushes the surface of the sensory epithelium. During ordinary breathing, the main stream of air passes below the olfactory organs and only swirls or eddies of air reach them. In sniffing, however, the air is directed upwards on to the sensitive surfaces.

The olfactory cells, like those of taste buds, respond to chemical stimulation, though the chemicals must be volatile (i.e. easily vaporized) at ordinary temperatures, and in most cases soluble in fat solvents, to produce any sensation of smell. These two conditions apply mainly to organic compounds, though inorganic gases can be detected, for example chlorine, ammonia, hydrogen sulphide. Although it is often considered that our sense of smell is poor compared with that of other mammals, we can nevertheless recognize an enormous number of chemicals in extremely low concentrations; with one chemical at least, it is estimated that a concentration of one molecule per 5 000 molecules of air can be detected. In general, about 3 000 times as much material is needed to elicit a sense of taste as is necessary to give a sensation of smell. Far too many different odours can be distinguished for it to be likely that there is one kind of receptor for each type of substance, and it is suggested that discrimination depends on a small number of different types of receptor being stimulated in varying proportions.

The sense of smell is readily fatigued, so that after a few minutes' exposure to a new smell it is no longer perceived, although other observers on arrival will detect it at once. The fatigue may be due to the sensory cells failing to set off nervous impulses, or to the suppression of impulses arriving in the

central nervous system from the olfactory area. The impulses pass via complicated nerve plexuses to the forebrain and cerebral cortex, and in vertebrates as a whole may be responsible for initiating complex behaviour patterns related to food seeking, mating or marking out territory.

Sight. The eyes are the organs of sight. They are spherical organs housed in deep depressions of the skull, called orbits. They are attached to the wall of the orbit by six muscles which can also move the eyeball (Fig. 18.7). The structure is best seen in a horizontal section, as shown in Fig. 18.8.

Hearing. *See* p. 139.

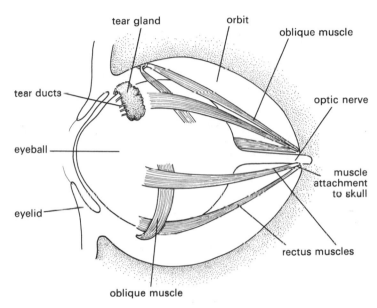

Fig. 18.7   Muscles of left eye (side view)

Structure and functions of parts of the eye

Eyelids. These can cover and so protect the eye. Closing the eyelids can be a voluntary or a reflex action to protect the cornea from damage. Regular blinking serves to distribute fluid over the surface of the eye and prevent drying. Modified sebaceous glands (*see* p. 97) secrete an oil at the margins of the eyelids.

Conjunctiva. This is a thin epithelium which lines the inside of the eyelids, the front of the sclera and is continuous with the epithelium of the cornea.

Tear gland. The tear gland is housed in the upper part of the orbit above the eyeball, and its ducts open under the top eyelid (Fig. 18.7). It secretes a solution of sodium chloride and sodium hydrogencarbonate (bicarbonate) that keeps the exposed surfaces of the conjunctiva and cornea moist and washes away dust and other particles. An enzyme, *lysozyme*, is present in tear fluid, and has a destructive action on bacteria. Tear fluid normally evaporates from the eye as fast as it is secreted but some may be drained into the nasal cavity through the *lachrymal duct* (Fig. 10.3) which leads from the corner of the eye nearest the nose.

Eye muscles. These muscles are attached to the sclera at one end and to the wall of the orbit at the other (Fig. 18.7). Their

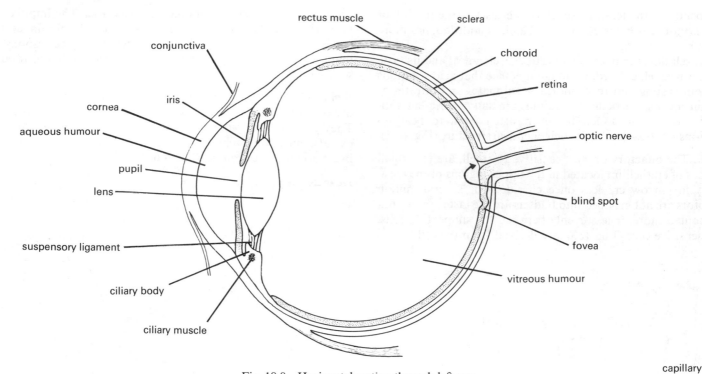

Fig. 18.8   Horizontal section through left eye

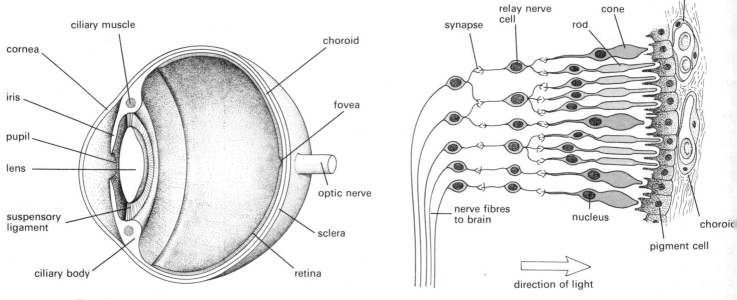

Fig. 18.9   Vertical section through left eye

Fig. 18.10   Structure of the retina

co-ordinated contractions can make the eye move from side to side and up and down. The muscles are so co-ordinated by the brain that they move both eyes together in the same direction, and by reflex action can fixate on moving objects, i.e. follow the path of a moving object without conscious effort on the part of the observer.

Sclera. The sclera is a tough, non-elastic fibrous coating on the outside of the eyeball. It opposes the outward force of the eye fluids (*humours*) and maintains the shape of the eyeball.

Cornea. This is the transparent disc in the front part of the sclera. Light passing through the curved surface of the cornea is refracted and the rays begin to converge. There are free nerve endings in the cornea which, if stimulated, cause reflex blinking, tear secretion and produce sensations of pain.

Choroid. The choroid is a layer of tissue lining the inside of the sclera. It contains a network of blood vessels supplying food and oxygen to the eye and particularly to the retinal cells. It is also deeply pigmented, the black pigment reducing the reflection of light within the eye.

Aqueous and vitreous humours. The aqueous humour occupies the anterior chamber of the eye between the cornea and the lens. It is a watery solution, having a composition similar to blood plasma with dissolved salts and glucose, though there is more sodium and chloride and less urea than in plasma. Aqueous humour contains dissolved oxygen and supplies the lens and cornea, which contain no blood vessels, with nutrients and oxygen. The humour is secreted by the ciliary body and probably drains into a circular canal which runs around the junction of sclera and cornea, and which itself empties into the venous system. The pressure of the aqueous humour, some 25-30 mm of mercury, maintains the shape of the cornea and keeps the lens stretched against its natural elasticity.

The jelly-like vitreous humour is a protein gel filling the space between the retina and lens. It helps to maintain the shape of the eye. Both fluids play a part in refracting the light which enters the eye.

The lens. The lens continues the refraction of light which begins at the cornea and produces an image on the retina. It is made of transparent, ribbon-like fibres and living epithelial cells arranged in concentric layers like the scales of an onion. The material in the centre of the lens has a greater refractive power than that at the edges, and this property enables it to produce a sharper image than could a simple glass lens. The lens is held in position by the fibres of the suspensory ligament which radiate from its edge and attach it to the ciliary body (Fig. 18.9). The shape of the lens can be altered by the contraction or relaxation of the muscles in the ciliary body.

Ciliary body. This is the thickened edge of the choroid in the region around the lens. It contains blood vessels and muscle fibres, some of which run in a circular direction, that is, parallel to the outer edge of the lens. These muscles control the curvature of the lens during accommodation (*see* below). The ciliary body also secretes aqueous humour.

Iris. The iris consists of an opaque disc of tissue. It is continuous at its outer edges with the choroid. In the centre is a hole, the pupil, through which passes the light that will produce an image on the retina. The contraction or relaxation of opposing sets of circular and radial involuntary (unstriated) muscle fibres in the iris increases or decreases the size of the pupil, so controlling the amount of light entering the eye. The iris contains blood vessels and sometimes a pigment layer that determines what is usually called the 'colour' of the eyes. Blue eyes have no special pigment, the colour being produced by a combination of the black inner surface of the iris, the blood capillaries and the white outer layers.

Retina. The retina is a layer of cells which respond to light. There are two kinds of light sensitive cell called, according to their shape, *rods* and *cones* (Fig. 18.10). There are about 7 million cones and 12 million rods, the cones having a density of about 6 000 per mm^2 and the rods 150 000 per mm^2 over the general surface of the retina. Only the cones can discriminate coloured light but they need a stronger stimulus than the rods. It follows that colour discrimination is only possible in high light intensities. The rods and cones are connected to the brain by nerve fibres though, since the optic nerve contains only about 800 000 fibres, many of the receptor cells must feed their impulses into the same fibre.

As a result of the development of the retina from an outgrowth of the brain, the nerve fibres from the rods and cones lie on the inner surface of the retina. Thus light entering the eye has to pass through or between these fibres before it can stimulate the receptors.

Some detail about the mechanism of the rods but little about the cones is known. The rods contain a pigment, *visual purple* or *rhodopsin*. This is formed from two chemicals, *opsin* and *retinene*, the latter being derived from vitamin A. It is known that light bleaches this pigment, and the present theory supposes that bleaching is a result of rhodopsin splitting into opsin and retinene. This chemical decomposition in some way starts a nerve impulse in the nerve fibre supplying the rod. The rhodopsin is then resynthesized, involving an expenditure of energy by respiration.

The rods are extremely sensitive and it is thought that one quantum of light (the smallest unit of energy) will decompose one molecule of rhodopsin and that, in some parts of the retina, from 4 to 14 quanta falling on an area containing 500 rods will just succeed in producing a sensation of vision on most occasions. When a dark night sky is just visible, every rod receptor is receiving on average one quantum per minute.

Blind spot. The nerve fibres from the rods and cones pass across the front of the retina and all leave the eye at one point to form the optic nerve, which passes through the skull to the brain. At the point where the optic nerve passes through the retina there are no light receptors, so leaving a non-sensitive disc, the blind spot, about 1.5 mm across. If part of an image falls in this region, no impression is recorded in the brain (Experiment 6). We are not normally aware of this 'blank' in our vision because (a) it never coincides with an image on which we are concentrating, (b) it is compensated by the use of two eyes scanning the same field, and (c) the eyes are constantly making small movements so that the image is not projected on to the same part of the retina for more than a fraction of a second.

Fovea. The fovea is a small depression, 500 μm across, in the centre of the retina. It contains no rods but the cone density is about 12 500 per mm^2. There are no overlying capillaries, and the great concentration of light-sensitive cells makes it the region of the retina where greatest discrimination is possible. In addition, each cone is connected to a separate nerve fibre and, although cross-linkages occur later, a detailed pattern of impulses corresponding to the retinal image can be sent to the brain. When an observer concentrates on an object or part of an object, its image is thrown on to the fovea. Only in this region is there detailed appreciation of form and colour. Since the fovea contains only cones, it is not very sensitive to low light intensities.

Control of light intensity. When the circular muscles of the iris contract, the size of the pupil is reduced and less light is admitted. Contraction of the radial muscles widens the pupil, so admitting more light. This is a reflex action set off by changes in the light intensity. In poor light the pupils are wide open; in bright light the pupils are contracted. In this way the retina is protected from damage by light of high intensity, and in poor light the wider aperture of the pupil helps to increase the brightness of the image. The eyes are linked by nervous paths so that each makes the same adjustment, no matter which eye is stimulated, and the adjustment takes about five seconds to complete.

Seeing in the dark. No creature can see in total darkness, but the sensitivity in low light intensities varies from one animal to the next. The sensitivity of the eye is increased in poor light intensity partly by widening the pupil, but more important are changes that take place in the retina. After half an hour in the dark the eye will respond to light intensities 10 000 times less bright than when light-adapted. This may be the result of the greater concentration of rhodopsin in the rods during darkness.

The fovea contains only cones, which respond only to high light intensities. Thus concentrating on a poorly lit object, to focus its image on the fovea, is a less effective way of studying it than by looking to one side of it. This action throws the image on to a part of the retina containing many more rods than cones, the rods being more easily stimulated. Less detail can be seen but a more distinct outline is appreciated.

Image formation and vision. Light from an external object enters the eye. The curved surfaces of the cornea, the lens and the humours refract the light and focus it so that 'points' of light from the object are represented as corresponding points of light on the retina. The image thrown on to the retina is real, upside-down and smaller than the object (Figs. 18.11 and 18.12). Although the image is inverted (Experiment 5) the brain forms an upright impression of the object or, at least, the observer interprets correctly the position of external objects with respect to himself. Experiments have been conducted in which a person wears glasses that produce an upright image on the retina. Although this at first gives the impression that external objects are upside down, this sensation wears off and the experimenter gets used to interpreting the sensory information in the same way as before, reporting vision to be normal. When the spectacles are removed and the retinal image restored to its usual inverted position, the visual field is, at first, reported as upside-down.

The light-sensitive cells of the retina are stimulated by the light falling on them, and impulses are fired off in the nerve fibres which pass along the optic nerve to the brain where, as a result, an impression is formed of the shape, size and colour of the object. The nervous impulses travelling in the optic nerve reach a relay centre in the brain, after which some pass to the *oculomotor centre* in the midbrain. Here are initiated the automatic adjustments to the eyes, e.g. co-ordination of the eye muscles for following a moving object with the eyes, accommodation, pupil size and reflex blinking. Further fibres carry impulses to the cerebral cortex (p. 155) where the nerve impulses are interpreted and related to the object producing them.

The accuracy of the impression in the brain of the image depends on how numerous and how closely packed are the light-receiving cells of the retina, since each one can only record the presence or absence of a point of light and, in the case of cones, its colour. If there were only ten such cells, the image of a house projected on to five of them would record an impression of its size, the fact that it was differently coloured at the top and bottom and a vague representation of its shape, but no detail of windows, doors or fabric.

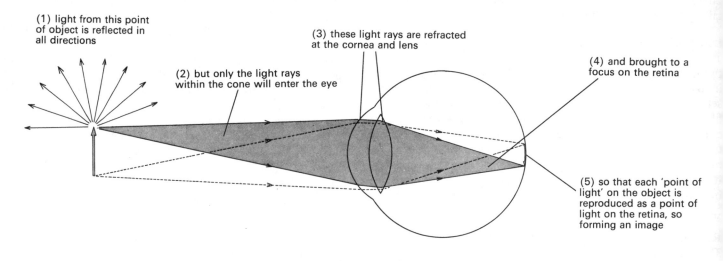

(1) light from this point of object is reflected in all directions

(2) but only the light rays within the cone will enter the eye

(3) these light rays are refracted at the cornea and lens

(4) and brought to a focus on the retina

(5) so that each 'point of light' on the object is reproduced as a point of light on the retina, so forming an image

Fig. 18.11   Image formation on the retina (shown graphically)

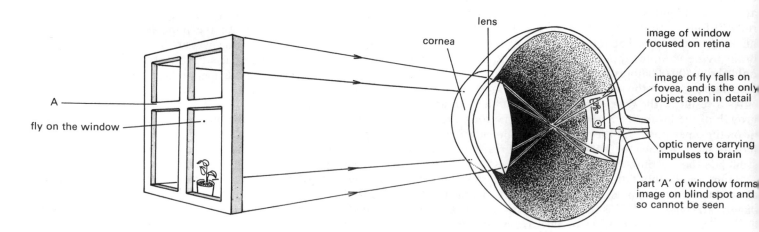

lens

cornea

image of window focused on retina

image of fly falls on fovea, and is the only object seen in detail

A

fly on the window

optic nerve carrying impulses to brain

part 'A' of window forms image on blind spot and so cannot be seen

Fig. 18.12   Image formation in the eye

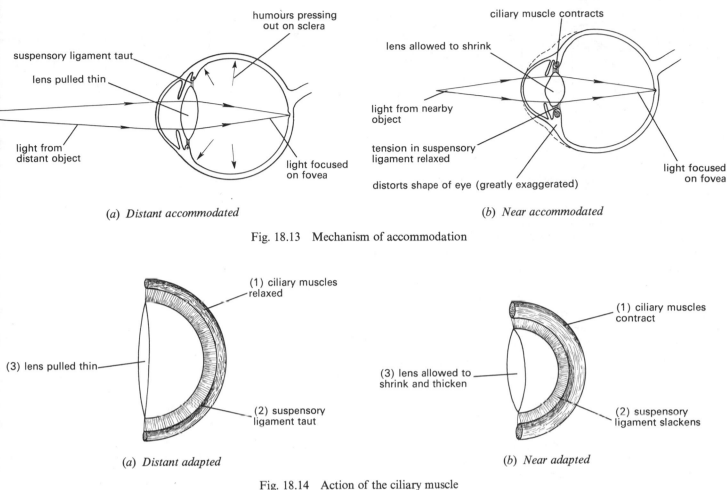

Fig. 18.13   Mechanism of accommodation

(a) Distant adapted

(b) Near adapted

Fig. 18.14   Action of the ciliary muscle

Accommodation is the adjustments made in the eye to focus on near or distant objects. With a rigid lens of definite focal length and at a fixed distance from a screen, it is possible to obtain a sharply focused image of an object only if it is at a certain distance from the lens. The focal length of the lens in the eye can be altered by making it thicker or thinner. In this way, light from objects from about 25 cm distant to the limits of visibility can be brought to a focus. This ability of the eye to alter its focal length is called accommodation.

The majority of the refraction that brings about image formation takes place at the surface of the cornea, with the lens contributing only about one quarter of the total refraction. The lens is therefore mainly concerned with accommodation. A person with a cataract (opaque lens) can have the lens removed and, with the aid of spectacles, still focus a clear image on the retina.

The lens is surrounded by an elastic capsule and tends to change its shape, becoming thicker in the centre, but the aqueous humour pushing outwards on the cornea maintains a tension in the suspensory ligament which stretches the lens into a thinner shape. Thus, when the eye is at rest, the lens is thin, has a long focal length and is adapted for seeing distant objects (Fig. 18.13a). When a nearby object is to be observed, the ciliary muscles running round the ciliary body contract and so reduce its diameter. The ciliary body holds the suspensory ligaments, pulling on the margins of the lens, so any reduction in the diameter of the ciliary body reduces the tension in the suspensory ligament and allows the lens to shrink, becoming thicker (Fig. 18.14). A thicker lens has a shorter focal length,

and light from a close object can be brought to a focus (Fig. 18.13b). Relaxation of the ciliary muscles allows the fluid pressure acting on the cornea and sclera to pull the lens back to its thin shape. When the eye is focused on a near object, the pupil is also contracted. Since this allows only the centre of the lens to be used, it sharpens the image.

Colour vision. The mechanism by which we appreciate colour is not yet fully understood. One of the most straightforward theories that fits many of the observed facts suggests that there are three types of cone in the retina with their maximum sensitivity in the red, blue and green parts of the spectrum respectively. These respond maximally only to one particular wavelength of light, so that according to the kind of cell and the numbers stimulated, the brain receives an impression of colour. Light that stimulates the red-sensitive cones we describe as red light. If red and green-sensitive cones are stimulated simultaneously we describe the sensation as yellow; when all three types of cone are stimulated, we describe the sensation as white. Amongst the mammals only the primates, that is the lemurs, monkeys, apes and man, are thought to be able to distinguish colours. The others see only in black, white and shades of grey.

Colour blindness. About 8 per cent of men and 0.4 per cent of women suffer from one or other forms of colour blindness. Only rarely is this the total inability to distinguish colours from shades of grey with equal light intensity. More often it is the failure to discriminate between red, brown and green. (*See* p. 180 for an account of the inheritance of colour blindness.)

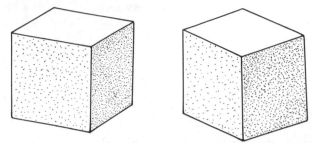

(a) *Left eye sees this view* (b) *Right eye sees this view*

Fig. 18.15 Cube as seen by left and right eyes

Stereoscopic vision. Each eye forms its own image of an object under observation, so that two sets of impulses are sent to the brain. Normally the brain correlates these so that we gain a single impression of the object. Since each eye 'sees' a slightly different aspect of the same object (Fig. 18.15) the combination of these two images produces the impression of solidarity based on the three-dimensional properties of the object.

If the eyes are not aligned normally or if the centres of the brain dealing with sight impressions are dulled, for example with alcohol, the two sensory impressions from the eyes are not properly correlated and we 'see double' (Experiment 8).

Judgement of distance. For the eyes to focus an image of a nearby object they must be turned slightly inwards, directed towards the object. The eye muscles that control this movement have in their tissues sensory receptors which respond to the stretching of the muscles. Impulses reaching the brain from these receptors indicate the extent to which the eyes are converging, and so give an impression of the distance of the object. The stereoscopic vision described above also helps to judge distance. It is very difficult to estimate distance using only one eye, though other information such as the relative size of an object and its apparent movement against the background (parallax) also contribute to our judgement of distance, and these factors do not depend on binocular vision.

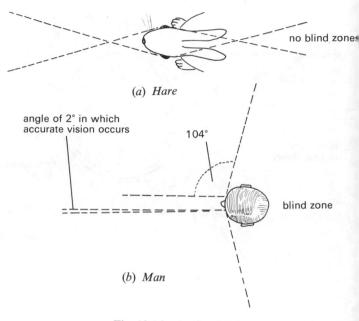

(a) *Hare*

(b) *Man*

Fig. 18.16 Angle of vision

Field of vision. If the eyes and head are held stationary, a man can see objects within an angle of about 200° from his face. The shape of the face and nose will influence this field in different individuals. Only objects that subtend an angle of about 2° at the eye will form an image on the fovea and so be observed in accurate detail (Fig. 18.16). This is a considerably narrower range of accurate vision than most people imagine, and means, for example, that only about one letter at a time in any word on this page can be studied in detail.

Eye defects. The causes and corrections of long and short sight are explained diagrammatically in Fig. 18.17. As one gets older, the lens loses some of its elasticity and hence its power to accommodate. The near point (shortest distance from the eye where vision is still perfect) for a 20-year-old is about 250 mm but more like 500 mm for a 40-year-old.

(a) *Long sight*

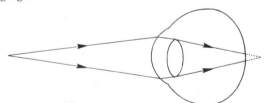

Long sight is caused by small or 'short' eyeballs. Light from a close object would be brought to a focus behind the retina, so the image on the retina is blurred

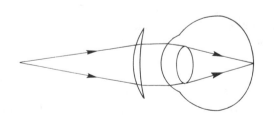

Long sight can be corrected by wearing converging lenses

(b) *Short sight*

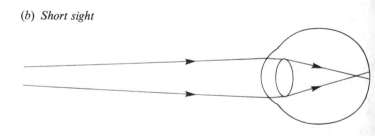

Short sight is usually caused by large or elongated eyeballs. Light from a distant object is focused in front of the retina, so the image on the retina is blurred

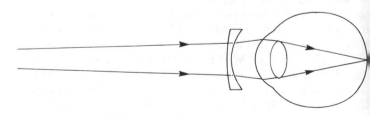

Short sight can be corrected by wearing diverging lenses

Fig. 18.17 Long and short sight

Astigmatism. This occurs when the curvature of the cornea and lens is not uniform in all planes. If, for example, the curvature from top to bottom is greater than that from side to side, it is not possible for the eye to focus both horizontal and vertical lines at the same distance from the eye (Fig. 18.18*a*). This defect is corrected by using cylindrical lenses (Fig. 18.18*b*) which effectively refract the light in one plane only.

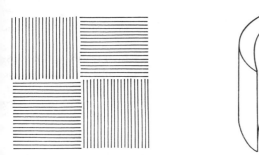

(*a*) *The astigmatic eye cannot focus the vertical and the horizontal lines at the same time*

(*b*) *Example of a cylindrical lens*

Fig. 18.8   Astigmatism

The ear (Fig. 18.19)

The ear contains receptors sensitive to sound vibrations in the air between frequencies of 20 Hz and 25 000 Hz, the precise range varying with age. (The unit of frequency is the hertz, symbol Hz. A frequency of 10 cycles per second is called 10 Hz.)

Outer ear. This is a tube opening on the side of the head and leading inwards to the ear drum. Its lining of skin contains sebaceous and *ceruminous glands.* The latter, which may be modified sweat glands, secrete wax. At the outer end of this tube there is an extension of skin and cartilage, the pinna, which in some mammals helps to concentrate and direct the vibrations into the ear and assists in judging the direction from which the sound came. Its function, if any, in man is not very clear. A membrane of skin and fine collagen fibres is stretched across the innermost end of the outer ear, closing it off completely. This is called the *ear drum.* A muscle, the *tensor tympani,* running from the ear drum to the wall of the middle ear maintains a tension in the ear drum by pulling it inwards.

Middle ear. The middle ear is an air-filled cavity in the skull. It communicates with the back of the nasal cavity (nasopharynx) through a narrow tube, the Eustachian tube. Three small bones, or *ossicles,* in the middle ear link the ear drum to a small opening in the skull, the *oval window,* which leads to the inner ear.

Inner ear. The inner ear is filled with a fluid, *perilymph,* and contains a coiled tube, the *cochlea,* with sensory endings in it. It is here that the sound vibrations are converted to nervous impulses.

Eustachian tube (Figs. 10.3 and 18.19). Air pressure in the middle ear is usually the same as atmospheric pressure. If changes take place in the pressure outside the ear drum, for example when gaining height rapidly in an aircraft, the pressure is equalized by the opening of the Eustachian tube to admit more air to or release air from the middle ear. Normally the Eustachian tubes are closed by a muscle and are opened only in swallowing or yawning, when a 'popping' sound may be heard in the ears. Violent nose-blowing may sometimes force air or mucus up the Eustachian tubes into the middle ear, resulting in temporary deafness or earache.

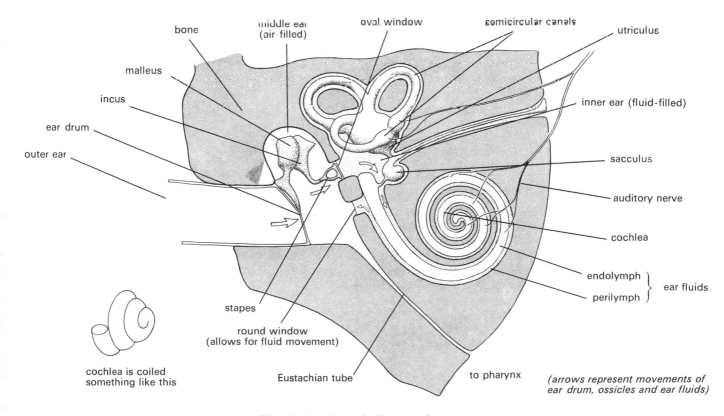

Fig. 18.19   Schematic diagram of the ear

Hearing. The vibrations in the air that constitute sound waves enter the outer ear and set the ear drum into vibration. The tiny displacements of the ear drum are transmitted through the three ossicles, which act as levers (Fig. 18.20), and cause the innermost of them, the *stapes*, to vibrate against the oval window. The greater area of the ear drum, 85 mm², compared with the oval window, 3.2 mm², and the leverage of the ossicles, cause an increase of about 22 times in the force of vibrations that reach the inner ear. The stapedial muscle tends to pull the stapes away from the oval window and, by means of a reflex action, damps down any violent oscillations of the ear ossicles produced by loud noises.

The oscillations of the stapes, acting like a miniature piston, set the fluids of the inner ear and cochlea into vibration. A membrane containing sensory endings runs the length of the cochlea, and when these endings are stimulated by vibrations,

perilymph of the inner ear these are conducted to the perilymph of the scala vestibuli; they are transmitted across the inner tube, or *cochlear duct* as it is termed, at right angles to its long axis and so reach the scala tympani and round window. The floor of the cochlear duct consists of the *basilar membrane* which contains transverse fibres. The roof of the cochlear duct is membranous and thin. Resting on the basilar membrane is a single layer of sensory cells, about 30 000 of them, with fine cytoplasmic hairs on their free, upper edge. These hairs are embedded in a gelatinous ribbon, the *tectorial membrane*. The hair cells and their supporting tissues are called the *organ of Corti*.

The distortion of the cochlear duct which results from pressure differences in the upper and lower compartments of the cochlea are shown diagrammatically in Fig. 18.22, and can be visualized as causing the tectorial membrane to give a tug

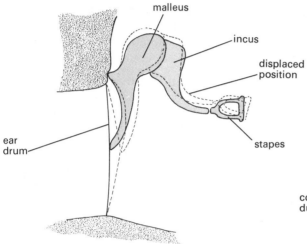

Fig. 18.20   Movement of the ear ossicles in transmitting sound

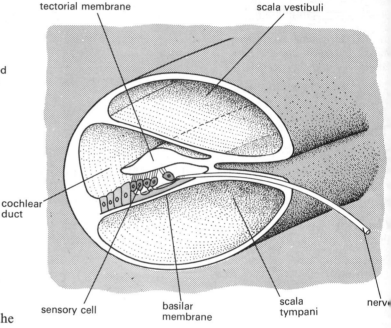

Fig. 18.21   Section through cochlea

they fire off impulses which travel in the auditory nerve to the brain. When these nervous impulses reach the brain they are interpreted as sound, the quality, pitch and loudness of the sound being determined by the way in which the vibrations affect the cochlea.

Cochlea. The cochlea can be visualized as a tube of triangular cross-section enclosed within a cylindrical tube (Fig. 18.21) so that the outer tube is divided into upper and lower compartments by the inner tube. (*Note*: the terms 'upper' and 'lower' refer to the diagrams in this book, rather than to the real anatomical position.) The upper compartment or *scala vestibuli* opens to the perilymph in contact with the oval window, while the lower compartment or *scala tympani* communicates with the round window. Since fluids are not compressible, any change in pressure in the upper compartment will be transmitted at once to the lower compartment across the inner tube. The changes in pressure in the lower compartment will be relieved by the membrane of the round window bulging in or out. The upper and lower compartments do communicate at the tip of the cochlea by a small hole, the *helicotrema*, but this is too small to permit rapid movement of fluid during vibrations. The inner tube is distorted by alterations in the pressures of perilymph in the upper and lower compartments.

When the stapedial movements induce vibrations in the

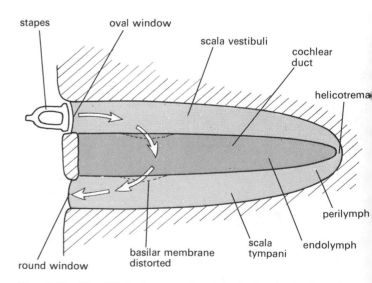

Fig. 18.22   Simplified diagram of cochlea in longitudinal section to show effect of sound vibration

on the hair cells. This is most probably the stimulus that induces the hair cells to fire off a nervous impulse in the nerve fibres connected to them.

Determination of pitch. It was once thought that the transverse fibres or 'auditory strings' of the basilar membrane were responsible by virtue of their differing length and tension for an appreciation of pitch, i.e. high or low notes. There are about 24 000 of these strings, ranging in length from about 60 μm near the base of the cochlea to 500 μm at the tip, giving about $2\frac{1}{2}$ strings per tone. If a group of strings were able to resonate (vibrate) in response to only one particular frequency, then only the sensitive hair cells resting on these fibres would be stimulated by a single note of that pitch, i.e. one part of the cochlea would be stimulated by a high note and another part by a low note. The brain, by detecting which section of the cochlea had been stimulated, would be able to determine the relative pitch of the note.

Something like this is known to happen, but the role of the basilar fibres is not clear since they do not appear to be under tension. Experiments show that for sounds of low pitch (frequency up to 60 hertz or cycles per second), the upper end of the basilar membrane vibrates as a whole. Above 60 Hz, however, the region of maximum response of the cochlea becomes more localized, shifting down the cochlea as the frequency rises. Between 300 and 2 000 Hz the localized region of response moves even more rapidly down the cochlea, but above 2 000 Hz observation becomes too difficult. It has also been shown that the region of cochlea responding at one time to a certain note produces a pattern of electrical activity in a particular zone of the cerebral cortex. It is on these lines that an understanding of the ability to distinguish pitch seems to be unfolding.

Sensitivity. The sensitivity of the ear is least with sounds of low frequency, e.g. 100 Hz. This may have the advantage that the low-frequency sounds of the body, e.g. muscle contractions, are not constantly picked up and transmitted. Since the movements of the ear drum are very small at some frequencies it seems that the maximum sensitivity of the ear is very high, but it is known to fall off steadily with increasing age. Children can usually detect sounds of 30 000 Hz, and this ability decreases by about 80 Hz every six months after reaching maturity. The brain is remarkable in its ability to single out sounds that a person wants to hear and suppressing or ignoring a large proportion of all others.

Sense of direction of sound. When the sound from a single source is perceived by both ears, the sound will be heard more loudly in one ear than the other, and also very slightly earlier. The fact that the two ears are stimulated to different extents enables the animal to estimate the direction from which the sound came (Experiment 9). Most mammals can also move their ear pinnae to a favourable position for receiving the sound, and so obtain a more accurate bearing. A source of sound that is equidistant from both ears is difficult to locate, since it can be below eye-level, directly above or behind the head and still stimulate both ears equally (Experiment 10). A dog can locate the position of a sound in one of thirty-two positions all around it, while man is accurate in the perception of only one out of eight possible sources; i.e. the dog can distinguish sounds only 11° apart while man can rarely distinguish between sounds less than 45° apart (Fig. 18.23).

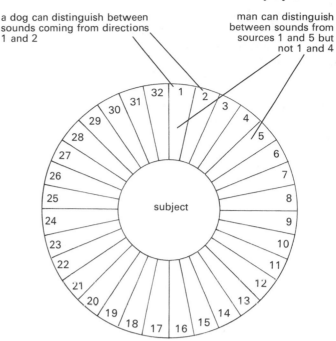

Fig. 18.23 Discrimination of sources of sound

Speech. A large proportion of the sounds we produce during speech, particularly those sounds of low frequency, are transmitted through the bones of the skull to the inner ear and give us the impression of qualities of vibrancy and depth in our voices which are not credited to us by our listeners, who hear only the airborne sounds. Tape-recordings of one's voice are usually disappointingly flat and toneless for this reason.

The complicated co-ordination of lips, tongue and larynx during speech depends on accurate feedback of information via the ears, so that delicate adjustments can be made according to the sounds we hear ourselves making. For example, in singing a note, the first sound produced may need to be adjusted to the correct pitch as a result of the sensory feedback which indicates it to be above or below the pitch of the note required. It follows that totally deaf people will not learn naturally to speak in the usual way, because they simply cannot hear the sounds they are making and so learn to make the necessary corrections. Other sensory information, such as vibrations detected by the fingertips, has to be used instead. Such deaf people are occasionally described as 'dumb', suggesting incorrectly that they lack the equipment for producing sounds.

Deafness. Deafness can be caused by long exposure to a high level of noise, drugs, ear infections or deposition of bone in the oval window. In the latter case, the membrane of the oval window is invaded by bone, so fusing the stapes to the skull and preventing the transmission of sound via the ear drum and ossicles. Such deaf people can still hear sounds transmitted through the skull, e.g. a ticking watch pressed to the temple, and the condition can be helped up to a point by amplification of sounds by a 'deaf aid' or by surgery in which the stapes is freed or removed altogether and replaced by a plastic strut.

Damage to the cochlea and auditory nerve, which can be caused by loud noises, produces incurable deafness. Infections of the middle ear often produce fluids which burst the ear drum in escaping. Similar breaks or perforations can be produced by violent changes of pressure. Small perforations usually heal, but the thickening produced by scar tissue may impair the hearing. Experiments with cats show that a 1 mm hole destroys hearing for frequencies below 100 Hz but does not affect sounds of above 1 000 Hz.

We tend to be rather impatient with deaf people compared with our sympathetic attitude to the blind. This behaviour is quite irrational; deaf people need as much patience and understanding as the blind, perhaps even more, since their primary means of communicating with other people is cut off.

Balance

The semicircular canals, utriculus and sacculus are organs used in maintaining balance and posture (Fig. 18.24), the former responding mainly to changes in direction of movement, the two latter to changes in posture. The principle on which they all work involves the displacement during movement of gelatinous plates, which pull on sensitive, cytoplasmic hairs so initiating nerve impulses.

As a result of these pulses, reflex actions occur in which the tone of the body muscles is adjusted to maintain the body in a stable position. For example, if a moving vehicle suddenly stops, standing passengers are thrown forward; the reflex contraction of the muscles of the legs will tend to correct for this temporary upset of posture.

In the sacculus, the macula and gelatinous plates are more or less vertical, but possibly do not function as organs of balance in mammals, though it is thought that they play some part in hearing at low frequencies.

Semicircular canals. The membranous ducts of the semicircular canals are each about 15 mm long and enclosed in corresponding but wider ducts in the bone of the skull. The space between the canals and the bone contains perilymph, while the canals are filled with endolymph. In the swelling or *ampulla* at the end of each canal is a raised mound of sensory and supporting cells, the *crista*. The tufts of hairs from the sensory cells of the crista are embedded in a gelatinous mass called a *cupula* which extends most of the way across the ampulla (Fig. 18.25a). A rotation of the semicircular canal in

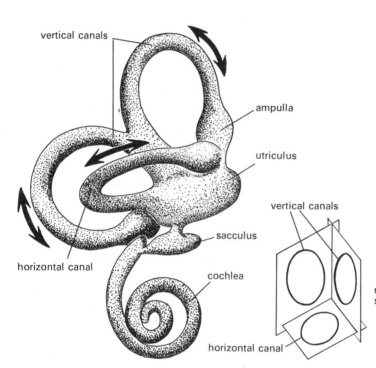

Fig. 18.24   Semicircular canals (arrows show the direction of rotation that has maximum stimulatory effect on each canal)

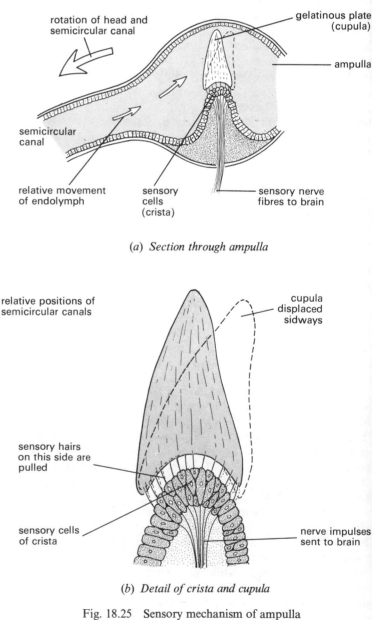

(a) *Section through ampulla*

(b) *Detail of crista and cupula*

Fig. 18.25   Sensory mechanism of ampulla

Utriculus and sacculus. The utriculus is a sac filled with *endolymph*. On its floor is an area of sensory hair cells with their supporting cells; this is called the *sensory macula*. The hairs of the sensory cells are embedded in a gelatinous plate, containing chalky granules called *otoliths* which increase its density. The gelatinous plate is not quite horizontal and so pulls on the hairs of the sensory macula causing a steady stream of impulses to reach the brain. Any change of posture will tend to displace the gelatinous plate and it will exert more or less pull on the hair cells, causing more or less rapid pulses to be fired off in the nerve.

its own plane causes the endolymph to exert more pressure on one side of the cupula than the other. The fluid tends to lag behind the movement of its enclosing canals and, although the canals are probably too narrow for it actually to flow, a difference in pressure as little as 0.05 mmHg (in fish) is sufficient to produce a movement of the cupula.

The cupula on being displaced to one side pulls on the hair cells (Fig. 18.25*b*) and alters the pattern of nervous discharge originating from them. Rotation in one direction causes a greater frequency of discharge, while rotation in the other direction reduces the frequency of the discharge pattern. Each semicircular canal responds most strongly to rotations in its own plane.

The reflex actions resulting from the stimulus of the semicircular canals involve movements of the eyes and muscular adjustments to keep the body suitably orientated during movement.

Much of our information about posture and movement is derived from our eyes and muscle stretch receptors, as well as from the semicircular canals and utriculus. Any conflict in this information may produce dizziness. Motion sickness is often caused by constant rotational movements about a horizontal axis, e.g. swinging round corners in a car on a winding road.

Practical Work

SKIN: Experiment 1   Spatial discrimination

A pair of compasses or a simple apparatus such as is shown in Fig. 18.26 can be used. The distance apart of the compass points or pins is measured, and starting at about 2 cm apart, the experimenter touches the two points simultaneously on parts of the skin of a 'volunteer' whose eyes are closed. In the more sensitive regions of the skin, the two pin-pricks are felt as separate stimuli. Elsewhere, e.g. the back of the hand or the neck, a single stimulus is felt, perhaps because there are fewer touch endings. By reducing the distance between the points from time to time, the degree of sensitivity of different regions of the skin can be mapped out.

It is best to vary the stimulus, using sometimes one point and sometimes two so that the subject does not know in advance which is to be used.

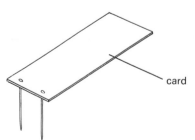

Fig. 18.26   Apparatus for applying double or single stimulus

Experiment 2   Sensitivity to touch

A patch of skin on the back of the wrist is marked with regular dots, using a rubber stamp such as is illustrated in Fig. 18.27. A similar pattern is stamped on a piece of paper so that the results can be recorded. Held by a pair of forceps or stuck to a wooden handle, a bristle such as a horse hair (Fig. 18.27) is pressed on the skin at each point marked by a dot, with enough force just to bend the bristle. The subject, who must not watch the experiment, states when he can feel the stimulus. A third person, with a duplicate set of marks on paper, indicates the positive or negative result of each stimulus, which can finally be expressed as a percentage. Using the same technique on different parts of the skin the relative concentration of touch organs can be estimated, though the sensitive 'spots' do not correspond to single nerve-endings.

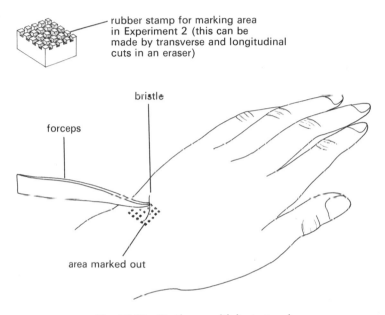

Fig. 18.27   Testing sensitivity to touch

Experiment 3   Location of the source of stimulation

If a dried pea or marble is rolled about on a table between the crossed tips of the first and second fingers, an impression of two solid objects is received in the brain. The eyes should be closed while doing this so that only sensations of touch are received. Normally these regions of the fingers are stimulated simultaneously only by two separate objects, and it is this impression that has been learned by the brain.

Experiment 4   Sensitivity to temperature

Obtain three jars or beakers of about the same size and fill one with cold water (10–15 °C), one with hot water (40–45 °C) and the third with warm water (about 25 °C). Place the first finger of the left hand in the cold water and the first finger of the right hand in the hot water and leave both fingers immersed for at least one minute. After this time, remove the fingers from the hot and cold water and dip them *alternately* in and out of the warm water. The finger which has been in cold water will give the sensation of warmth while the other finger will register cold.

The mechanism of temperature sensitivity is not well understood but the result of this experiment suggests that the receptors respond not so much to the actual temperature as to the *change* of temperature. The cold finger registers an increase while the warm finger registers a decrease in temperature.

EYES: Experiment 5   **Inversion of the image**

If the apparatus shown in Fig. 18.28 is held close to the eye and the pin observed by looking through the pin-hole, an upright silhouette of the pin's head is seen. The apparatus is now reversed so that the pin is nearer to the eye, and moved until the pin-head can be seen against the outline of the pin-hole. In this case, an upright and enlarged shadow is cast on to the retina, and the brain makes the usual correction so that the impression gained is of the pin-head upside down.

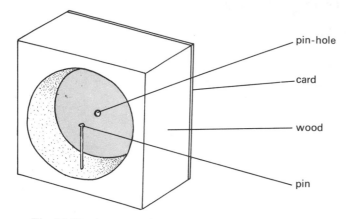

pin-hole

card

wood

pin

Fig. 18.28   Apparatus for showing inversion of the image

Experiment 6   **The blind spot**

Hold the book about 60 cm away. Close the left eye and concentrate on the cross with the right eye. Slowly bring the book closer to the face. When the image of the dot falls on the blind spot it will seem to disappear.

Experiment 7   **To find which eye is used more**

A pencil is held at arm's length in line with a distant object. First one eye is closed and opened and then the other. With one the pencil will seem to jump sideways. If the pencil 'jumps' when the right eye is closed, it means that the right eye was dominant in lining up the pencil.

Experiment 8   **The double image**

If a nearby object is observed, and a finger pressed against the lower lid of one eye so as to displace the eye-ball slightly, an impression of two separate images will result, one formed in each eye.

EARS: Experiment 9   **Location of sound** (1)

Two large funnels, held in clamps, are connected to lengths of rubber tubing which can be inserted into the ears of the sub-ject. The subject holds the tubes in his ears so that only sounds entering the funnels will reach the ear-drums. The subject is blindfolded and the two funnels crossed over so that the one leading to the left ear is pointing to the right and vice versa. When sounds are made on the right of the subject, he thinks they are coming from the left. By altering the position of the funnels, without the subject's knowledge, interesting results can be obtained.

Experiment 10   **Location of sound** (2)

A ticking clock is held, in turn, above, behind, and in front of a blindfolded subject, so that it is always equidistant from both ears. The subject is asked to indicate its position. These results are then compared with the number of successes scored when the clock is held in similar positions but to the sides of the subject.

TONGUE: Experiment 11   **Sensitivity to taste**

Solutions of sucrose (sweet), sodium chloride (salt), citric acid (sour) and quinine (bitter) are prepared. The subject puts out his tongue and the experimenter places a drop of one of the solutions at one point of the tongue using a glass rod or pipette. Without withdrawing the tongue, the subject tries to identify the taste. The various solutions are applied in turn to all parts of the tongue, washing the glass rod or pipette between each application. In this way it may be possible to determine (a) which regions of the tongue are most sensitive to a particular group of chemicals, and (b) the minimum concentration needed to produce a sensation of taste.

Questions

1   Most animals have a distinct head end and tail end. Why do you think the main sensory organs are confined to the head end?
2   Chemicals such as sugar and saccharine both taste sweet and yet they are chemically quite different. Middle C on the piano has a frequency of 264 Hz whereas D has a frequency of 297 Hz. The difference is small and yet the two notes are easily distinguished.
   What are the properties of the sense organs concerned which make for poor discrimination of chemicals and precise discrimination of sounds?
3   In what functional way does a sensory cell in the retina differ from a sensory cell in the cochlea?
4   An eye defect known as 'cataract' results in the lens becoming opaque. To relieve the condition, the lens can be removed completely. Make a diagram to show how an eye without a lens could, with the aid of spectacles, form an image on the retina. What disadvantage would result from such an operation?
5   In poor light, an object can be seen more clearly in silhouette by looking to one side of it than by looking at it directly. Explain this phenomenon.
6   A person whose ear ossicles are ineffective can often hear a ticking watch pressed against his head better than he can if it is held close to his ear. Explain this effect.
7   On board a ship which is pitching and rolling it is fairly easy to maintain an upright posture when standing still. When walking, however, it is very difficult to maintain balance. Suggest reasons why this should be so.

19

Co-ordination

The various physiological processes in living animals have been described so far as if they were quite separate functions of the body, the total result of which produces a living organism. In fact, although this is true in a limited sense, all these processes are very closely linked and dependent on each other. The digestion of food, for example, would be of little value without a blood stream to absorb and distribute the products; release of energy in a contracting muscle would quickly cease if the lungs failed to supply oxygen via the circulatory system.

The working together of these systems is no haphazard process. The timing and location of one set of activities is closely related to the others. Some examples may give a clearer idea of this. During locomotion, while the muscles that pull the leg forward are contracting, the antagonistic muscles are relaxed without the walker's having to think consciously about it. During exercise, when the muscles need to lose excess carbon dioxide and obtain more glucose and oxygen, the breathing rate is automatically increased and the heart beats faster, so sending a greater volume of oxygenated blood to the muscles. When eating a meal, the position of the food is recorded by the eyes and as a result of this information the arms are moved to the right place to take it up, not by trial and error but with precision and accuracy. As the food is raised to the mouth, the latter opens to receive it at just the right moment. Chewing movements commence and saliva is secreted. At the moment of swallowing, many actions happen at the same time, as described on p. 62. In the stomach, the gastric glands begin to secrete enzymes which will digest the food when it arrives.

In the sequences described above, many bodily functions come into action at just the right moment, with the result that no unnecessary movements are made and enzymes are not wasted by being secreted when no food is present. The linking together in time and space of these and other activities is called co-ordination. Without co-ordination, the bodily activities would be thrown into chaos and disorder. Food might pass undigested through the alimentary canal for lack of enzyme secretion, even assuming it negotiated the hazard of the windpipe in the absence of unco-ordinated swallowing; extensor and flexor muscles of limbs might contract simultaneously instead of alternately; a runner would collapse after a few yards through lack of an increased blood supply to his muscles.

The activities of the organs and systems of the body are not only closely related to each other and the overall pattern of activity within the body, but to changes outside the body. In response to environmental changes the mammal makes adjustments that tend to maintain its internal conditions, e.g. its temperature, its posture, and the composition of its body fluids, and also reacts by patterns of behaviour that favour its survival, e.g. it moves towards food and away from danger. Our elaborate sense organs receive stimuli from the outside world and convert these into nerve impulses which are transmitted to the brain. As a result, these impulses may cause alterations in the pattern of activity of the organs in the body.

Co-ordination is brought about by the nervous system and the endocrine system. The former is a series of conducting tissues running to all parts of the body (Fig. 19.1), while the latter comprises a number of glands in the body which produce chemicals that are circulated in the bloodstream and stimulate certain organs when they reach them.

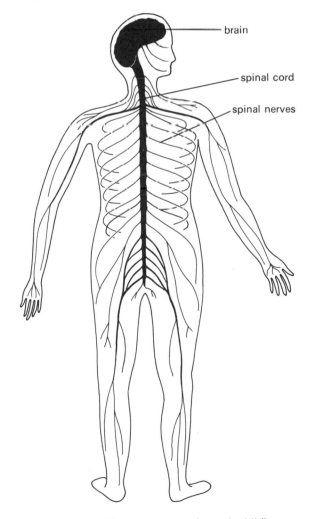

Fig. 19.1   Nervous system of man ($\times 1/14$)

The nervous system

Nerve cells. The basic units of the nervous system are nerve cells or *neurones*. Although they vary greatly in structure they may be visualized generally as consisting of a cell body, i.e. a central nucleus in a cytoplasmic mass, from which branch numerous filaments or *dendrites* (Fig. 19.2). Often one of these filaments is very long, and is called an *axon* if it conducts impulses away from the cell body and a *dendron* if the impulses are carried towards the cell body; in more general terms it is simply called a nerve fibre. In mammals the cell bodies are mostly confined to the brain or spinal cord (Fig. 19.3) while their fibres extend the whole distance to the organ being supplied. The fibre, consequently, is sometimes very long; e.g. from the spinal cord to the foot the fibre could be over a metre long, though only 1–20 μm in diameter. The fibre contains cytoplasm in the form of a viscous solution and in many cases is itself enclosed in a sheath of fatty material, the *myelin sheath,* which is formed by distinct cells, *Schwann cells,* wrapped several times around the fibre. Between the Schwann cells, which extend 0.3–1.5 mm along the fibre, are short zones of exposed axon called *nodes of Ranvier.* The myelin sheath has an important insulating effect, causing the impulse to

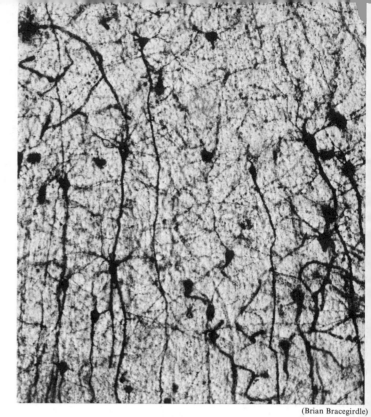

(Brian Bracegirdle)

Fig. 19.3   Multipolar neurones in brain cortex

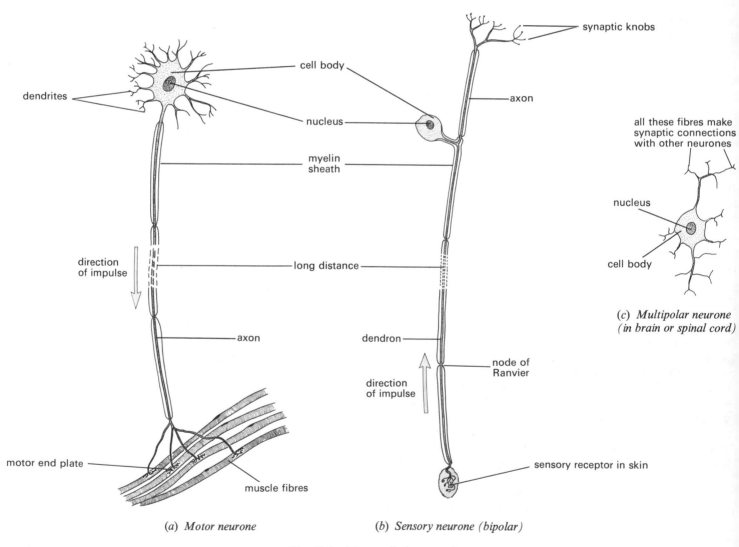

(a) *Motor neurone*   (b) *Sensory neurone (bipolar)*

(c) *Multipolar neurone (in brain or spinal cord)*

Fig. 19.2   Nerve cells (neurones)

ravel rapidly from one node to the next, greatly increasing the peed of conduction.

The nature of the conduction along a nerve fibre is not comparable with electrical conduction along a wire. In the latter here is a flow of electrons along the wire, the rate of flow depending on the voltage difference between the ends of the wire. In the nerve fibre a difference of potential in the region of '0 millivolts is built up between the inside and outside of the ibre, the inside being negative. It is thought that a stimulus applied to a sense organ causes a temporary reversal of this potential difference, so that the fibre is discharged along its ength. The rate at which this wave of discharge travels varies between 1 metre and 120 metres per second, according to the liameter of the fibre and the presence or absence of the thick nyelin sheath formed by the Schwann cells. Once the nerve mpulse has passed down the fibre, the potential difference has to be restored again, probably by means of energy released n the respiration of the nerve cell. A good blood supply bringing fresh supplies of glucose and oxygen is essential to normal nervous conduction.

The nerve cell is ready for conduction again in a period of ime ranging from 1/500 to 1/1 000 of a second. This is such a short interval that even a very brief stimulus will give rise to a series of electrical discharges at rates usually between 20 and 100 per second. A stimulus below a certain strength, i.e. below the *threshold of response,* will produce no impulse, but once the threshold is exceeded the impulse so initiated will travel to the end of the nerve fibre without diminishing in intensity. In fact, the intensity of the impulse depends only on the potential difference between the inside and outside of the fibre and bears no relationship to the intensity of the stimulus. A strong stimulus will, however, produce a more rapid burst of impulses than a weak stimulus (Fig. 19.4) and in this way the central nervous system can distinguish between stimuli of varying intensity.

Although impulses may be initiated by heat, light, touch, etc. in the respective sense organs, there is no difference in the quality of the nervous impulse travelling in the fibres. If one could 'tune in' to the optic nerve from the eye or the auditory nerve from the ear, one would detect only rapid bursts of

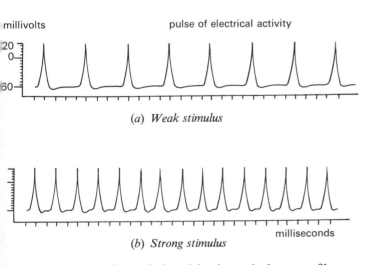

(a) Weak stimulus

(b) Strong stimulus

milliseconds

Fig. 19.4 Pattern of electrical activity in a single nerve fibre as measured by sensitive recording apparatus. (*Note*—there is no difference in amplitude (strength) of the electrical discharge; only the frequency changes)

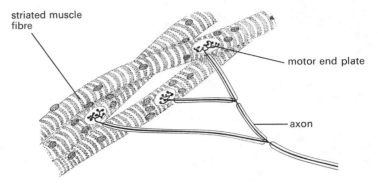

striated muscle fibre

motor end plate

axon

Fig. 19.5 Motor nerve ending (one nerve fibre may branch to supply 100 muscle fibres; in an eye muscle, however, each muscle fibre has its own nerve fibre giving very precise control)

electrical activity. It is the response of the region of the brain at which the impulses arrive that enables us to distinguish the type of stimulus. If the auditory and optic nerves could be transposed so that impulses from the eye reached the part of the brain normally served by the ear and vice versa, a light shone in the eye would give the sensation of noise and a shout in the ear would cause the subject to see flashes of light.

Motor ending and synapses. A motor nerve fibre, i.e. one carrying an impulse from the central nervous system to a muscle or gland, branches repeatedly in the muscle it is supplying, each branch terminating in a *motor end plate* (Figs. 19.5 and 19.7) on a single muscle fibre. When a burst of impulses reaches the motor end plate they cause the muscle fibres to contract.

A sensory nerve cell carrying an impulse from a sense organ to the central nervous system passes its impulse on to another nerve cell across a *synapse* (Fig. 19.6). At the synapse there is

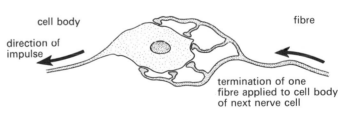

cell body

fibre

direction of impulse

termination of one fibre applied to cell body of next nerve cell

Fig. 19.6 Schematic diagram of synapse

no cytoplasmic connection between the nerve cells, so leaving a 'gap' across which the nerve impulse has to 'jump'. The 'jump' occurs by the production, at the termination of one nerve fibre, of a chemical that stimulates the next nerve cell in line. Although a synapse offers a barrier to the passage of an impulse, e.g. a single impulse is very unlikely to get across, it does enable one fibre to form connections with many other nerve cells and so produce correspondingly complex reactions. If a direct connection were made between all the nerve fibres of the body, the activation of one fibre would cause simultaneous discharge in the entire nervous system!

On some cells of the spinal cord there are as many as 2 000 synaptic terminations, and it is probable that only the simultaneous arrival of impulses at many of these terminations will set off a fresh impulse in the cell.

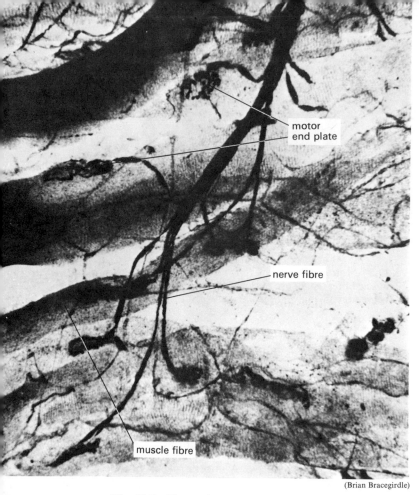

motor
end plate

nerve fibre

muscle fibre

(Brian Bracegirdle)

Fig. 19.7   Photomicrograph of motor end plate

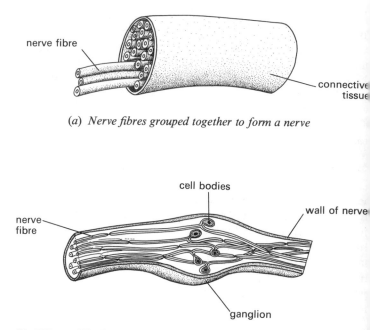

nerve fibre

connective
tissue

(a) *Nerve fibres grouped together to form a nerve*

cell bodies

nerve
fibre

wall of nerve

ganglion

(b) *When cell bodies occur outside the brain and spinal cord they produce a bulge (ganglion)*

Fig. 19.8   Structure of a nerve

The nervous system. The thousands of nerve cells are organized into a nervous system. The cell bodies are grouped largely into the *central nervous system,* i.e. the brain and spinal cord, and the fibres are arranged in bundles with connective tissue to form nerves (Fig. 19.8) which are clearly visible during dissection. The *cranial nerves* leave the brain through holes in the skull, while the *spinal nerves* leave the spinal cord between adjacent vertebrae and usually carry both sensory and motor fibres. From between the vertebrae of the neck emerge nerves which supply the diaphragm and the skin and muscle of the neck and arms. The nerves from the thoracic region of the spinal cord supply the skin and muscles of the thorax, while those from the lumbar and sacral regions go to the legs and also supply the skin and muscle of the abdomen.

Each spinal nerve contains both sensory and motor fibres carrying impulses towards and away from the spinal cord, and also fibres of different diameter. Narrow fibres conduct more slowly than wider ones, with the result that impulses generated in one region will travel at different rates and arrive in the central nervous system at different times.

Reflex. One of the patterns of co-ordination that is simplest to explain in terms of nervous conduction is the reflex. A reflex action is a quick, automatic response to a particular stimulus. The response does not require conscious control and in some cases cannot be influenced by the conscious will. A *spinal reflex* is one that need not involve the brain for its successful completion. Coughing, sneezing and blinking can all be reflex actions. The path traversed by the nerve impulse during a reflex action is called a *reflex arc,* and such a path (Fig. 19.9) is described below for the withdrawal reflex that results from inadvertently touching something hot.

The sensory endings in the skin of the hand are stimulated by the heat, and set off a stream of nerve impulses which travel in the sensory fibres running up the arm in a nerve to the spinal cord in the neck. For simplicity, only one of these fibres will be considered. In the spinal cord, the sensory fibre makes a synapse with a short *relay neurone.* The volley of nerve impulses crosses this synapse, passes along the relay neurone and traverses a further synaptic connection with the dendrites and cell body of a motor neurone (Fig. 19.10). The motor fibre carries the impulses, in the same spinal nerve, to the biceps muscle of the arm. The muscle contracts, flexes the elbow and

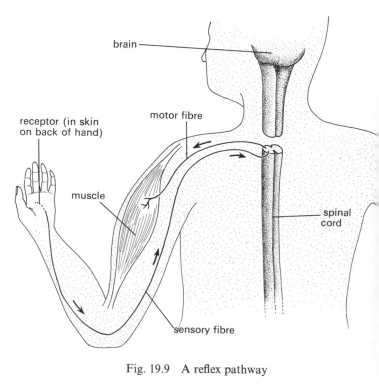

brain

motor fibre

receptor (in skin
on back of hand)

muscle

spinal
cord

sensory fibre

Fig. 19.9   A reflex pathway

148

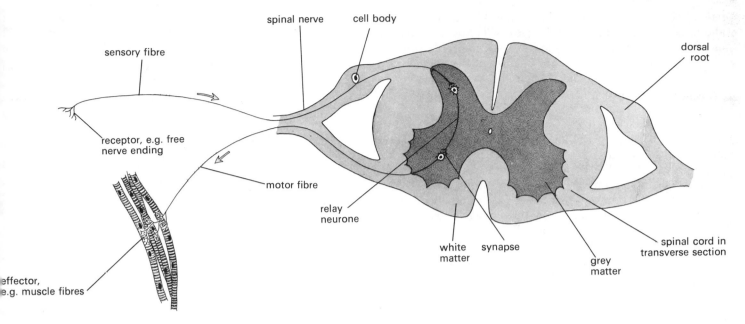

Fig. 19.10   One of the simplest connections for a reflex action

withdraws the hand from the hot object (Fig. 19.11). This prompt withdrawal prevents serious damage to the tissues of the fingers, and many human reflexes have this protective function.

Although, theoretically, the brain is not necessary for this reaction, the relay neurones will make synaptic connections with sensory fibres running to the brain, and impulses reaching the brain by this path will make the person aware of the heat of the stimulus and give rise to a sensation of pain. Motor impulses may consequently be sent from the brain and add to or modify the pattern of reflex response, e.g. cause a cry of pain. Moreover, the reflex can be suppressed by the brain: a hot object which if touched unexpectedly would produce a reflex withdrawal can nevertheless be deliberately touched or grasped.

The sensory data fed into the brain, namely the heat and

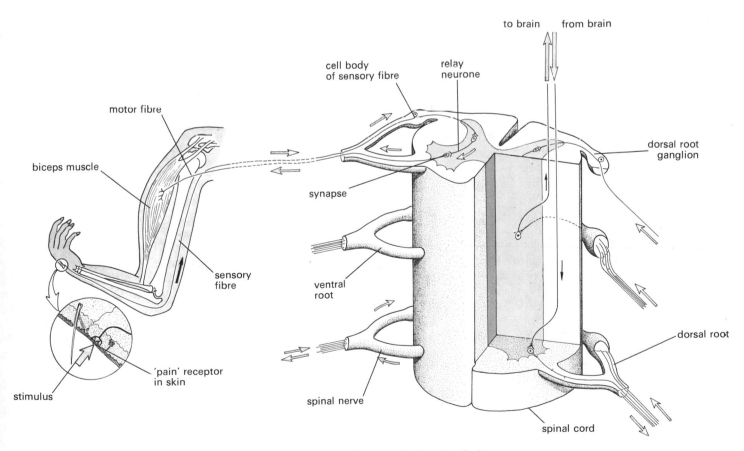

Fig. 19.11   The reflex arc (withdrawal reflex)

pain arising from the stimulation of the skin and information about the object coming from the eyes, will be associated in the higher centres of the brain such as the cerebral cortex in a memory store, and so reduce the chances of the same hazardous situation arising again. When the same object is encountered in the future it will be recognized as likely to be hot and contact will be avoided.

An experiment with frogs shows the automatic nature of the spinal reflex. If a frog's brain is destroyed or the spinal cord cut behind the head, and a drop of acid placed on the skin, the hind-leg will still move to the affected area as if to remove the cause of the stimulus. The nervous pathway is still intact and functional. If an injury severs a man's spinal cord some spinal reflexes are retained below the damaged area, but in a normal individual, all reflexes are influenced to some extent by the activities of the brain.

Reflex actions are rarely as simple as the description of the withdrawal reflex above would make it seem. They usually involve much more sensory data and a far more complex response by many sets of muscles. Coughing, for example, is a reflex initiated by the irritation of the trachea by a foreign particle and involves precise co-ordination of the contraction of the abdominal muscles and temporary closure of the glottis to produce the explosive bursts of exhalation which tend to dislodge the particle. In the withdrawal reflex described for the hand, further co-ordination is required to ensure that when the biceps muscle is suddenly contracted, its antagonistic muscle, the triceps, is relaxed. Synaptic connections via the relay neurone with the motor nerve cells supplying the triceps suppress nervous impulses which might normally pass to the triceps via the fibres of these cells. In particular, they suppress the contraction of the triceps, which would normally follow from the stimulation of the stretch receptors when the muscle is extended by the sudden contraction of the biceps. This, incidentally, is a good example of synaptic connections that inhibit rather than excite their connecting neurones.

Other examples of reflex actions are sneezing, in response to the irritation of the nasal mucous membrane; ejaculation of semen at the climax of sexual intercourse; secretion of saliva in response to taste stimuli on the tongue; contraction of the iris diaphragm in response to intense illumination; and the many responses under the control of the autonomic nervous system described on p. 151. In some cases the reflex pathways lie principally in the brain, e.g. iris diaphragm response and salivation, but the reflex arc involved is basically the same as in the spinal cord.

Conditioned reflex. The conditioned reflex is one way in which animals and perhaps man may learn. The Russian biologist, Pavlov, carried out many experiments on the conditioned reflex in dogs, and since one of them is something of a classic, it is described here. If a dog tastes or smells food, the salivary gland secretes saliva as a result of an inborn reflex, i.e. the dog does not have to learn this behaviour. If a bell is rung, no salivation occurs; but if a bell is rung at the same time as food is presented on a number of occasions, eventually the ringing of the bell alone will cause salivation. The appropriate stimulus of taste has been replaced or supplemented by an inappropriate stimulus of sound and the dog has been conditioned to respond to a new stimulus. Our guess is that, in some way, new nervous pathways have been established in the brain, perhaps by forming fresh synapses between neurones

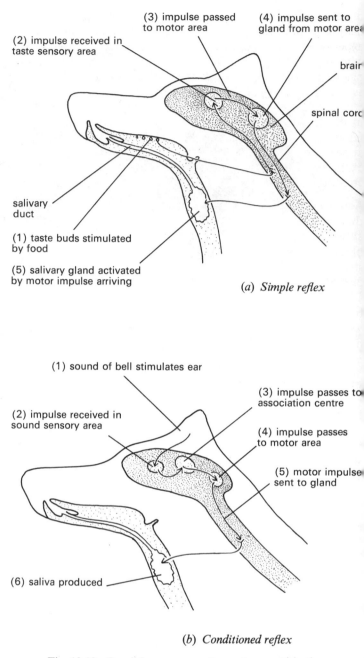

(a) *Simple reflex*

(b) *Conditioned reflex*

Fig. 19.12   Possible nervous pathway for conditioning

or facilitating the path of impulses across existing synapses. Fig. 19.12 shows this in pictorial form but our knowledge of what really happens is very scant. The conditioned reflex established in the laboratory cannot readily be extended to explain behaviour in the natural life of the animal. The dog in the experiment has to be trained to stand still throughout the experiment and all other sources of stimuli must be eliminated, whereas in its normal life the animal would be receiving a wide variety of stimuli and selecting information from them while constantly responding to internal and external changes.

Establishment of conditioned reflexes may be the basis of training of animals, the conditioning being achieved sometimes by reward and sometimes by punishment. To what extent conditioned reflexes as apparently simple as these play a part in human behaviour is difficult to say. We learn to walk, to swim, to ride bicycles and a great many other complex patterns of activity, which we carry out more or less efficiently without having to think consciously about what we are doing. If an experienced car driver rides as a passenger with another driver who approaches hazards at speed and pulls up rather late, the passenger may find his right foot pressing hard on the floor, as if to apply the foot-brake. You may have done similar things, e.g. switched off the light on leaving a room leaving the family in darkness, or wound up your watch automatically when taking it off in the middle of the day. These have all the appearances of conditioned reflexes and there are many similar examples, but it is misleading to think of learning as isolated conditioned reflexes.

Autonomic nervous system. The part of the nervous system that co-ordinates the internal and largely involuntary bodily activities such as digestion, vasoconstriction, heartbeat and blood pressure, is called the autonomic nervous system. The structure of its neurones and their system of connections to the organs is slightly different from that of the rest of the nervous system. The final nerve fibres supplying the organs do not have a thick myelin sheath and are thus sometimes called unmedullated. In addition, the cell bodies of these motor fibres do not lie in the spinal cord but are enclosed in ganglia outside it. The autonomic nervous system is further subdivided into the *sympathetic* and *parasympathetic* systems. In general, impulses in the sympathetic nervous system prepare an animal for activity, e.g. they speed up the heart and breathing rate and divert blood from the alimentary canal to the muscles, while the parasympathetic system is concerned with conservation of the animal's resources, as in feeding and sleeping. Most organs of the body receive fibres from both the sympathetic and parasympathetic nervous systems and impulses in these fibres produce opposite, i.e. antagonistic, effects. For example, impulses in the sympathetic fibres supplying the heart make it beat faster, whereas stimulation by the parasympathetic fibres slows it down. The final synapses of the motor fibres in the sympathetic system occur in the ganglia, but in the parasympathetic system the final synapses are in the organ being supplied. Fig. 19.13 shows a few of the organs that receive sympathetic and parasympathetic fibres and indicates the function of these fibres. It is not possible to generalize about the effects of the two sets of fibres and say that one always enhances while the other inhibits the organ's activity. For example, although the parasympathetic fibres reduce the number of heart contractions, they increase the rate of peristaltic contractions in the alimentary canal.

Structure and function of the central nervous system

The spinal cord. The spinal cord consists of a great number of nerve cells, both fibres and cell bodies, grouped into a cylindrical mass, running from the brain to the second lumbar vertebra. It is enclosed in two fibrous membranes, the *meninges*, and protected by the bone of the spinal column. From

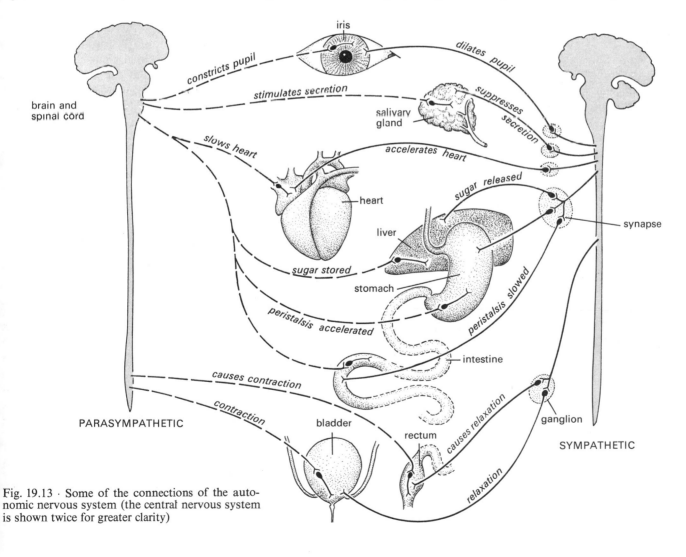

Fig. 19.13 · Some of the connections of the autonomic nervous system (the central nervous system is shown twice for greater clarity)

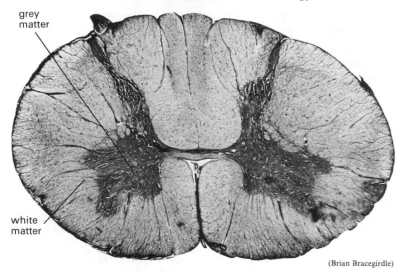

Fig. 19.14 Section through spinal cord

(Brian Bracegirdle)

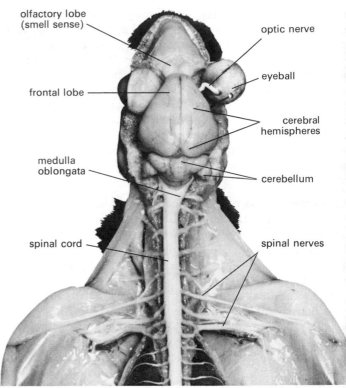

(Dissection by Gerrard and Haig Ltd)

Fig. 19.15 Dissection of the brain and spinal cord of a rabbit (seen from above)

between the vertebrae, spinal nerves emerge and run to all parts of the body. The fibres of these nerves may be concerned with spinal reflexes, or may carry sensory impulses to the brain or motor impulses from the brain to the muscles and other effector organs of the body. A central canal containing *cerebrospinal fluid* runs through the centre of the spinal cord.

The nerve cell bodies are grouped in the centre of the cord making a roughly H-shaped region of *grey matter* when seen in transverse section (Fig. 19.14). Outside this is the *white matter* consisting of nerve fibres running up and down the cord or passing out to the spinal nerves. The spinal cord is concerned with the spinal reflex actions described above, and the conduction of nervous impulses from one region of the spinal cord

to another and to and from the brain (*see* Fig. 19.11). Most of the sensory information from the skin and muscles reaches the brain by way of the spinal cord, and all the 'commands' from the brain to the muscles are conveyed in motor fibres through the spinal cord and out into the spinal nerves.

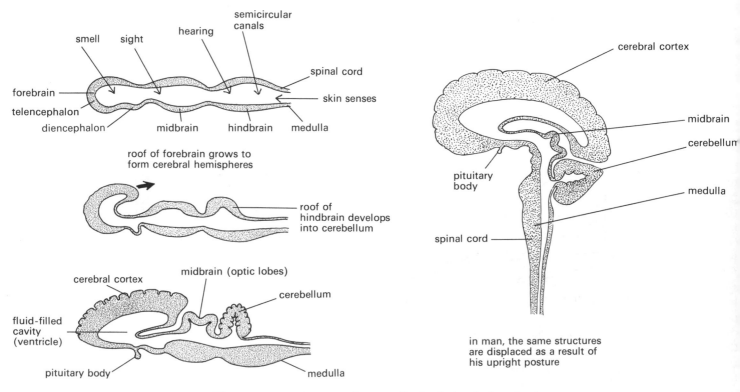

Fig. 19.16 Development of mammalian brain (vertical sections)

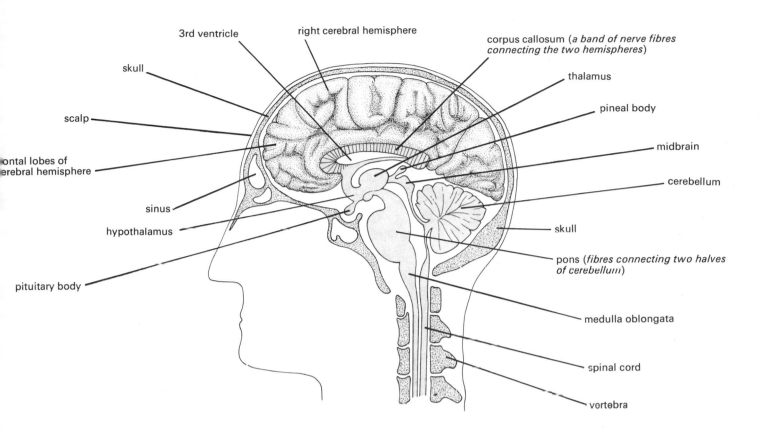

Fig. 19.17 Section through head to show brain

The brain. It seems likely that during evolution the increasing effectiveness and specialization of the sensory organs of the head, particularly the eyes, ears and nose, led to more and more sensory fibres entering the front part of the spinal cord. Consequently, this region has enlarged and developed to form the brain of the vertebrate animals. It consists of some 15 000 million neurones.

The brain is thus an enlarged, specialized, front region of the spinal cord (Fig. 19.15). Like the spinal cord it is basically cylindrical with a central canal containing cerebrospinal fluid. The nerve fibres constituting the white matter lie outside the central grey matter which consists of cell bodies. Twelve pairs of sensory and motor nerves enter and leave the brain, though not in the regular sequence seen in the spinal cord. The complicated structure of the brain is probably best understood by tracing in a simplified form its development in the embryo from the neural tube, the rudimentary central nervous system (Fig. 19.16). The anterior part of this tube enlarges in such a way that three regions or *vesicles* are distinguishable, the *fore-, mid-* and *hindbrain*. The enlarged regions of the cerebrospinal canal in these vesicles are called *ventricles* and when the brain is fully developed they may communicate by only narrow ducts. In the course of development two regions can be distinguished in the forebrain, the *telencephalon* in front and the *diencephalon* behind it.

The roof of the telencephalon grows out on each side to form the cerebral hemispheres which enlarge to such an extent that they come to overlie the whole of the rest of the brain

(Fig. 19.17). Outgrowths from the sides of the diencephalon form the *optic vesicles* which contribute to the retina of the eyes. Internally, the side walls of the diencephalon thicken to form the *thalami*, while a downgrowth from the ventral surface fuses with an upgrowth from the roof of the developing mouth and forms the *pituitary body*. The pituitary body retains its connection with the floor of the diencephalon or *hypothalamus*. The roof of the thalamencephalon, which remains thin and vascular, secretes cerebrospinal fluid into the third ventricle. It is called the *anterior choroid plexus*. The roof of the midbrain thickens to form the *optic lobes* while in the floor is a tract of fibres linking the thalami with the hindbrain. The anterior part of the roof of the hindbrain enlarges greatly to form the *cerebellum* while the posterior portion remains thin, vascular and non-nervous forming the *posterior choroid plexus*, which secretes cerebrospinal fluid into the fourth ventricle. The floor and sides of the hindbrain thicken to form the *medulla*.

In the primitive (and hypothetical) brain the primary vesicles merely accept sensory impulses and send out the appropriate motor responses, i.e. a reflex associated with a particular sense organ. The forebrain, for example, receives sensory information from the organs of smell, the midbrain from the eyes, and the hindbrain from the ears and semicircular canals. The structures such as the cerebral hemispheres, thalamus, optic lobes and cerebellum are not, however, principally concerned with one particular sense organ but are *association centres*, receiving information from a variety of sources and then

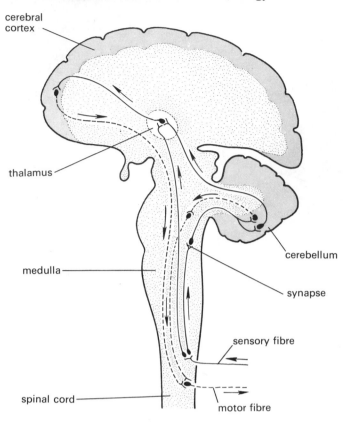

Fig. 19.18   Some of the main sensory and motor pathways

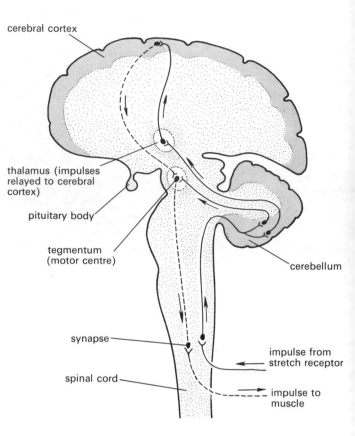

Fig. 19.19   Some of the nervous pathways involving the cerebellum and tegmentum

relaying impulses to other regions of the brain (Fig. 19.18) to produce a greater flexibility of behaviour.

If the nervous system were nothing more than a system of direct pathways from sensory organs to effectors, (a) the number of different possible responses would be very limited, and (b) they would always be the same in a given situation. An animal would respond to the smell of food by approaching it irrespective of whether it was hungry or not. A jackal would approach a carcass in response to its smell regardless of the sensory data from its eyes indicating that a lion was in possession. These are purely hypothetical illustrations, but a set of unalterable nerve circuits would produce a set of unalterable responses and sensory information from different sources could not effectively interact.

The jackal's brain will, in fact, receive sensory data from nose, eyes and stomach indicating, though not necessarily in the conscious sense, food, danger and hunger. These impulses are received in the primary sense centres of the fore-, mid- and hindbrain but are relayed to association centres where they may suppress or reinforce each other to produce a response with maximum survival value. Stored information from memory centres will also reach the association centres, and the outcome will not be automatic and unnecessary flight from the lion or uncontrollable and hazardous approach to the food, but a delaying action until the combination of stimuli produces a different behaviour pattern.

Knowledge of the function of different parts of the brain comes from a variety of sources; electrical stimulation of small areas of the exposed brain during operations for removal of brain tumours, for instance, may produce motor response if a motor area is stimulated or a recognizable sensation if a sensory area is stimulated; detailed anatomical studies reveal the nervous connections between the sense organs, the spinal cord, effectors and association centres so that functions may be inferred from these connections; sensitive electrical measuring instruments can detect the bursts of electrical activity that occur in localized areas of the brain when parts of the body are moved or stimulated in some way; accidental damage (in man) and experimental brain lesions (in animals) indicate to some extent, the function of the part of the brain removed according to the activities that the animal can no longer perform normally. All these methods have their defects; stimulation of only a small area of the brain at its surface is a quite abnormal state of affairs, and removal of one part of the brain interferes with so many nervous pathways that it is difficult to tell whether the new behaviour observed is a result of the region removed or the other centres affected by its removal.

Medulla. The medulla is largely concerned with the automatic adjustment of bodily functions, e.g. heart and breathing rates, blood pressure and temperature regulation, and is the primary sense centre for taste, hearing, balance and posture; i.e. the sensory fibres from the tongue, the cochlea, the semicircular canals, some touch receptors and some muscle spindles make their first synapse here. The medulla receives sensory information from internal organs by way of the *vagus nerve* and, after synaptic connections in the tissue of the medulla, motor impulses are fired off, also in the vagus, to the heart, diaphragm, etc. Rhythmical discharges also arise from it which influence the rhythmical changes in the body, e.g. the breathing rhythm.

Although most of these actions are under reflex control via the medulla, the latter is influenced by higher centres in the brain, particularly the hypothalamus. A situation involving excitement or emotion is likely to be interpreted first by the cerebral cortex which will then directly or indirectly influence the regulatory centres in the medulla, quickening the heartbeat, increasing the breathing rate, releasing more glucose into the blood stream, and so on. Similarly, most of the sensory impulses reaching the synapses in the medulla will be relayed to the higher brain centres. The impulses from the semicircular canals, for example, are passed on to the cerebellum and cerebral cortex. Relaying the information to the cerebral cortex enables the individual to become aware of what is happening as well as making reflex adjustments at the level of the medulla. A great many fibres pass through the medulla without making any synaptic connections on their way to or from the brain.

The cerebellum. The cerebellum receives, predominantly, sensory fibres from the stretch receptors of the muscles, semicircular canals, utriculus and sacculus. These fibres may proceed directly from the sense organ or the spinal cord to the cerebellum or via synapses in the medulla or other association areas. Outgoing fibres pass, not directly to effector organs, but to motor centres in the *tegmentum* (floor of the midbrain) and medulla or to the cerebral cortex via the thalamus (Fig. 19.19). This pattern of connections and the experimental results of removing parts of the cerebellum suggest that the cerebellum exercises control over posture, balance and, in particular, the finely co-ordinated patterns of muscular activity. Although the reflex responses may be co-ordinated in the cerebellum, the large tract of fibres that runs into it from the cerebral cortex indicates that the cerebellum probably translates the 'commands' from this higher centre into positive action by the muscles.

Unlike the spinal cord, there is a layer of nerve-cell bodies on the outside of the cerebellum, the *cerebellar cortex,* the surface of which is greatly increased by deep folds. In this cortex the incoming impulses in only a few fibres are enabled to make connections with a vast number of outgoing fibres via relay neurones and the densely branching dendrites of the *Purkinje cells* at the head of the outward-going fibres. In this way, the impulses are amplified and spread over a wide range of outgoing fibres so that a small, localized sensory impulse could produce a powerful and widespread response.

Without the cerebellum, movement would be jerky, violent and spasmodic instead of smooth and controlled, as if the cerebral cortex were commanding a pattern of activity but without the means of controlling its detailed execution. For instance, if one reaches for a glass of water, the initial act of extending the arm may be swift and inaccurately directed, but as the hand nears its objective the action slows down, the aim is more precise and finally, a slow, positive muscular action grips the glass. Without cerebellar control, the arm may overshoot the mark, the fingers close too late or too weakly. In this kind of action the feedback of information from the stretch receptors to the cerebellum is of great importance, indicating the position of the limb and the speed with which it is moving and, in conjunction with visual information, correcting any errors of judgement as fast as they arise.

The cerebellum probably damps down the oscillations that arise when the stretch receptors of antagonistic muscles are stimulated, e.g. when the biceps contracts, the stretch receptors of the triceps are extended and these initiate a reflex which would shorten the triceps and thus extend the biceps, whose stretch receptors would produce reflex contraction, and so on.

Hypothalamus. The hypothalamus is formed from a thickening of the walls in the lower region of the diencephalon. Part of the hypothalamus extends downwards to contribute to the pituitary body. It receives fibres from the cerebral cortex and sends impulses back to the cerebral hemispheres and to the tegmentum. The hypothalamus influences a great variety of bodily activities concerned with maintaining a constant internal environment and with finding and digesting food. Much of its motor activity is brought about by the secretion of hormones from the pituitary body. For example, it is in the hypothalamus that the osmoreceptors are situated. These detect changes in the concentration of the blood passing through the hypothalamus and cause the pituitary body to release more or less ADH which, in turn, makes the kidney reabsorb more or less water from the urine (p. 94). The temperature of the blood is also monitored in the hypothalamus, and impulses are sent out that result in vasoconstriction or vasodilation and sweating, according to whether the blood temperature is too low or too high. There are, however, other centres in the brain which play a part in temperature control.

The hypothalamus is the brain centre for the parasympathetic nervous system and accordingly plays a part in controlling blood pressure, heart rate and peristaltic movements in the alimentary canal.

Cerebral hemispheres. These enormous outgrowths of the roof of the forebrain have a cortex of nerve cells, deeply folded and grooved in such a way as to increase the total surface. In this cortex a tremendous number of possibilities arise for the interconnection of sensory, motor and relay fibres. Nearly all impulses from sense organs are relayed to the cerebral cortex which is thus in possession of all the relevant information about events in the environment and to some extent within the organism. It seems likely that in the course of learning certain nervous pathways become established between the various sensory centres, so that complex patterns of nervous activity build up and leave a 'memory store'. From all the sensory input and memory store the cortex calculates the best course of action, i.e. that with the greatest immediate or long-term survival value, and sends out appropriate motor impulses either directly to the spinal cord or via the hypothalamus and tegmentum.

In a general sense, the pattern of behaviour for the whole animal is decided by the cerebral hemispheres, and the detailed execution is carried out by lower centres in the brain. Motor impulses start in the cortex, may be relayed to the tegmentum, translated by the cerebellum and pass down the spinal cord. Even at this level, the connection in the spinal cord will ultimately determine the pattern of movement by, for example, a limb. There are, however, fibres running from the motor areas of the cortex, which pass through the brain and down the spinal cord without making any synapses until they are about to leave the spinal cord.

Experiments in which the cortex is stimulated by fine electrodes, or in which electrical activity is detected in the cortex when a sense organ is stimulated, show that there is a certain localization of function in the cortex as indicated in Fig. 19.20. A particular region of the cochlea when stimulated would produce activity in a precise area of the cortex, and similarly a particular group of retinal cells is ultimately connected with a specific area of the cortex, but the interconnections between these areas are, in a way, more important than this localization. Some regions of the cortex can be removed without serious loss of the function with which they are concerned.

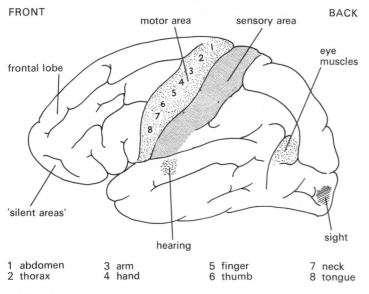

FRONT　　　　　　　　　　　　　　　　　BACK

motor area　　sensory area

eye muscles

frontal lobe

'silent areas'

hearing　　　　　　　　　　　sight

| 1 abdomen | 3 arm | 5 finger | 7 neck |
| 2 thorax | 4 hand | 6 thumb | 8 tongue |

Fig. 19.20　Localization of areas in the left cerebral hemisphere

Consciousness is probably the outcome of activity in the cortex, but we are able to suppress from consciousness a great deal of the sensory information which pours constantly into the cerebral hemispheres and single out for attention only those aspects on which we want to concentrate. One can listen to a single conversation in the midst of a crowded room where everyone is talking.

A complex group of neurones called the *reticular formation* in the floor of the midbrain appears to be able to 'switch' the cortex on or off. During sleep, sensory information is still being relayed to the cortex but without reaching consciousness. On waking, the reticular formation arouses the cortex and the sensory input becomes meaningful sensations. It seems that the reticular formation can alert the cortex during wakefulness as well, to make a person 'sit up and take notice'.

The hypothalamus and medulla at the time of birth probably have built-in nerve circuits which maintain the heartbeat, blood pressure, etc. These are inborn, or inherited, patterns of nervous activity. The cerebral cortex starts life as a blank slate but with vast possibilities of incredibly complex connections. The cortex thus acquires its characteristic circuitry and activities as a result of learning during the lifetime of the individual.

Prefrontal lobes. The most anterior portion of the cerebral cortex (the 'silent area') does not produce any movement or sensation when stimulated experimentally and does not appear to be associated with any specific part of the body. Cases of severe anxiety neurosis are sometimes alleviated by severing the tracts of fibres running from these prefrontal lobes to the rest of the brain. From this and other evidence, it is suggested that this area has something to do with self-restraint, the inhibition of natural drives, perhaps even the 'conscience', which distinguish man from other mammals.

Functions of the brain. To sum up:

1　The brain receives impulses from all the sensory organs of the body.
2　As a result of these sensory impulses it sends off motor impulses to the glands and muscles causing them to function accordingly.
3　In its association centres it correlates the various stimuli from the different sense organs.
4　The association centres and motor areas co-ordinate bodily activities so that the mechanisms and chemical reactions of the body work efficiently together.
5　It stores information so that behaviour can be modified according to past experience.

The endocrine system

Co-ordination is also effected by chemicals called hormones, secreted from the endocrine glands (Fig. 19.21). These glands have no ducts or openings. The chemicals they produce enter the blood stream as it passes through the glands and they are circulated all over the body. When the hormones reach particular parts of the body they cause certain changes to take place. Their effects are much slower and more general than nerve action and they control rather long-term changes such as rate of growth, rate of activity and sexual maturity. When they pass through the liver, the hormones are converted to relatively

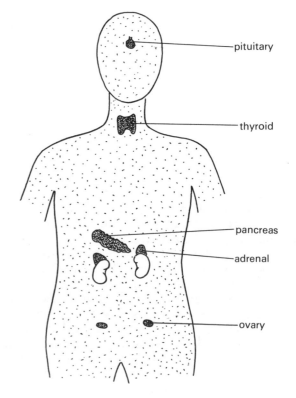

pituitary

thyroid

pancreas

adrenal

ovary

Fig. 19.21　Position of endocrine glands in the body

inactive compounds which are excreted, in due course, by the kidneys (hence the tests on urine for the hormonal products of pregnancy). The liver in this way limits the duration of a hormonal response which might otherwise persist indefinitely.

Thyroid. The thyroid gland is in the neck, in front of the windpipe. It produces a hormone, *thyroxine,* which in young animals controls the rate of growth and development. In tadpoles, for example, thyroxine brings about metamorphosis. Feeding tadpoles on thyroxine induces early metamorphosis. In adult humans thyroxine controls the rate of chemical activity, particularly respiration: too little tends to lead to overweight and sluggish activity; too much can cause thinness and over-activity. Deficiency of the thyroid in infancy causes a certain type of mental deficiency called *cretinism,* which can be cured in the early stages by administering thyroxine.

Adrenal. The adrenal glands are situated just above the kidneys. The outer layer of the adrenal body, the cortex, produces several hormones, including *cortisone,* one of whose functions is to accelerate the conversion of proteins to glucose (p. 67). Secretion by the adrenal cortex is stimulated by certain pituitary hormones.

The inner zone, the medulla, of the adrenal gland is stimulated by the nervous system and produces *adrenaline.* When the sense organs of the animal transmit to the brain impulses associated with danger or other situations needing vigorous action, motor impulses are relayed to the adrenal medulla which releases adrenaline into the blood. When this reaches the heart it quickens the heartbeat. In other regions it diverts blood from the alimentary canal and the skin to the muscles; it makes the pupils dilate and speeds up the rate of breathing and oxidation of carbohydrates. All these changes would increase the animal's efficiency in a situation that might demand vigorous activity in running away or putting up a fight. In ourselves, they do the same but, together with the nervous system, they produce also the sensation of fear: thumping heart, hollow feeling in the stomach, pale face, etc. In humans, adrenaline may be secreted in many situations which promote anxiety or excitement, and not only in the face of danger.

The conditions that cause a release of extra adrenaline will already have stimulated the sympathetic nervous system (p. 151) and the sensations described above cannot be ascribed solely to one or the other, except in the sense that the sympathetic nervous system produces a rapid and immediate response while adrenaline secretion acts more slowly and over a longer period.

Pancreas. As well as containing cells that secrete digestive juices, the pancreas contains endocrine cells, which control the use of sugar in the body. The hormone is called *insulin;* it determines how much sugar is converted to glycogen and how much is oxidized for energy.

Insulin (a) accelerates the rate at which blood sugar is converted to glycogen in the liver (p. 69), (b) promotes the uptake of glucose from the blood by the body cells, and (c) increases protein synthesis in some cells. The failure of the pancreas to produce sufficient insulin leads to *diabetes.* The diabetic cannot effectively regulate the blood sugar level. It may rise to above 160 mg/100 cm^3 and so be excreted in the urine, or fall to below 40 mg/100 cm^3 leading eventually to convulsions and coma. The diabetic condition can be corrected by regular injections of insulin.

Reproductive organs. The ovary produces several hormones called *oestrogens* of which oestradiol and oestrone are the most potent. These oestrogens (a) control the development of the secondary sexual characters at puberty (*see* p. 108), (b) cause the lining of the uterus to thicken just before an ovum is released, and (c), in some mammals at least, oestradiol brings the female 'on heat', i.e. prepares her to accept the male. Progesterone, the hormone produced from the corpus luteum (p. 103) after ovulation, promotes the further thickening and vascularization of the uterus. Progesterone also prevents the uterus from contracting until the baby is due to be born.

Testosterone is the male sex hormone, produced by the testis. It promotes the development of the masculine secondary sexual characters.

Duodenum. The presence of food stimulates the lining of the duodenum to produce a hormone, *secretin,* which on reaching the pancreas in the blood stream, initiates the production of pancreatic enzymes. In this way, the enzymes are secreted only when food is present.

Pituitary. The pituitary gland is an outgrowth from the base of the forebrain (Figs. 19.16 and 19.17). It releases into the blood several different hormones. Some of them appear to have a direct effect on the organ systems of the body. For example, *antidiuretic hormone* (ADH) controls the amount of water reabsorbed into the blood by the kidneys (*see* p. 94). *Growth hormone* influences the growth of bone and other tissues. Injection of growth hormone in experimental animals causes them to grow larger and to continue growing for longer than usual. Growth, however, is affected by other endocrine glands as well, in particular the thyroid and pancreas, and the growth hormone may exert its influence through these glands rather than directly on the tissues.

In fact, the majority of the pituitary hormones do act upon and regulate the activity of the other endocrine glands to such an extent that the pituitary is sometimes called the 'master gland'. It is a pituitary hormone which, acting on the ovary, causes the Graafian follicle to develop and secrete its own hormone, oestrogen. Another pituitary hormone stimulates the thyroid gland to grow and to produce thyroxine, and a third acts on the cortex of the adrenal gland and promotes the production of cortisone.

Homeostasis

The foregoing account shows how the hormones co-ordinate the organs of the body to meet various contingencies (e.g. adrenaline), to produce rhythmic patterns of activity (e.g. the sex hormones), and to maintain control over long-term processes such as the rate of growth (thyroid and pituitary). It can also be seen that they fulfil a homeostatic function in regulating the composition of the internal environment (*see* p. 92). If the blood sugar level rises, the pancreas is stimulated to secrete insulin which increases the amount of glucose removed from the blood and stored as glycogen in the muscles and liver. A fall in the blood sugar level suppresses the production of insulin from the pancreas. An increase in the osmotic potential of the blood results in the release of ADH from the pituitary gland and the consequent reabsorption of water from the kidney tubules.

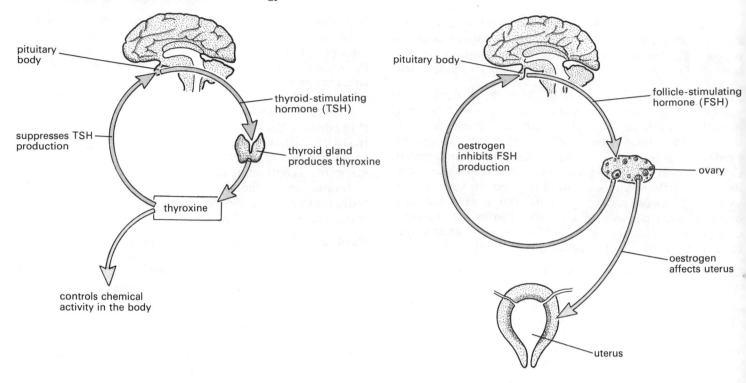

Fig. 19.22   Feedback

Interaction and feedback

For effective control, two opposing systems are needed. A car needs an accelerator and brakes, a muscle must have its antagonistic partner (p. 119). The hormones too have antagonistic effects. Adrenaline promotes the release of sugar into the blood while insulin has the opposite effect. Oestrogen stimulates the growth of the follicle while progesterone suppresses it. A fine adjustment of the balance of these antagonistic hormones helps to maintain the controlled growth, development and activity of the organisms in constantly changing conditions.

Such a balance is maintained partly by the 'feedback' effect of hormones, i.e. a system whereby 'information' is 'fed back' to a source 'telling it' about events in the body and so enabling it to adjust its output accordingly. A pituitary hormone stimulates the thyroid to produce thyroxine but thyroxine production is kept in check by the fact that when thyroxine reaches the pituitary via the circulation, production of thyroid-stimulating hormone is suppressed. The feedback of thyroxine to the pituitary regulates the output of the latter. The ovarian follicles are stimulated to produce oestrogen by a pituitary hormone, but when the oestrogen in the blood reaches a certain level it suppresses the secretion of follicle-stimulating hormone by the pituitary. A delay in the feedback effect leads to rhythmic changes. For example, it may take two weeks for the level of oestrogen in the blood to affect the pituitary, by which time the uterus lining has thickened and the ovum has been released from the follicle. The output of follicle-stimulating hormone is diminished as a result of increasing oestrogen and this in turn reduces the output of oestrogen from the ovary which, in the absence of fertilization and the development of the corpus luteum, leads to the breakdown of the uterine lining, characteristic of menstruation (Fig. 19.22).

Questions

1 List the differences between control by hormones and control by the nervous system.
2 Trace by diagram or description the possible reflex arc involved in (a) sneezing, (b) blinking. Do not attempt to describe the effector systems in detail and treat the brain as simply an enlarged region of the spinal cord.
3 All nervous impulses, whether from the eyes, ears, tongue or skin are basically the same. This implies that the information reaching the brain is little more than a rapid series of electrical pulses of identical strength. How then is it possible for us to distinguish between light and sound, heat and touch?
4 It is possible to train a dog to seek food concealed behind one of several identical doors by flashing a light over the appropriate door. Suggest a nervous pathway by which this behaviour is established.
5 Study Fig. 19.13 and then suggest why stimulation of the sympathetic nervous system should lead to greater efficiency in a situation that demands rapid and vigorous action.

20
Chromosomes and Heredity

Most living organisms start their existence as <u>a single cell</u>, a *zygote* (fertilized egg, p. 100). This single cell divides into two cells, four, eight and so on to produce eventually the millions of cells which make up the new organism.

If the new cells all behaved in the same way, they would produce only a mass of structureless tissue. The cells, however, as they develop, become different from each other in structure and function. Therefore, in the processes which turn a zygote into an organism there must be forces directing the cells to determine that some become muscle, some skin, some bone or blood, and these cells must be directed into groups in the right order and in the right place to produce tissues, organs and ultimately the complete, integrated, co-ordinated organism.

Moreover, a zygote does not produce just any organism. It will produce one which resembles the parents from whom the zygote was derived. The zygotes of a human and a cat may look identical, a nucleus surrounded by a little cytoplasm, but they will develop in quite different ways. The cat zygote will produce a cat and not a man. A mouse zygote will produce a mouse and not a rat. The study of the mechanism by which the characteristics of the parents are handed on to the offspring is known as genetics.

The zygote of a bird develops into a chick inside the egg without any outside interference other than incubation. It follows therefore, that the 'instructions' for building a bird from a single-celled zygote must reside somewhere inside the zygote. What is more, the 'instructions' must be present in the two gametes which fuse to form the zygote. They could be in the cytoplasm, the nucleus or both.

When one examines the gametes of most animals, the egg usually has a relatively large volume of cytoplasm associated with its nucleus. The male gamete, on the other hand, consists of little more than a nucleus with a very thin layer of cytoplasm round it, and a tail. However, there is nothing to suggest that the male's contribution to the 'instructions' or *genotype* of the zygote is any less than the female's so it looks as if the bulk of the genotype for building a cat or a man resides in the nucleus.

The next question is, can the 'instructions' be seen or studied in some way? One would not expect to see printed directions but there might be structures to be seen which would give some idea about the nature of the 'instructions'. Thus, a study of the nucleus would seem to be the most profitable course, particularly at a time when the nucleus is dividing because the genetic information, the genotype, must be handed on intact and undiminished to each cell. For example, if the two cells resulting from the first division of a frog's zygote are separated,

each cell can develop into a complete frog. This is true of cells even at the 4- and 8-celled stage. Thus the 'frog-building instructions' are intact and complete in each of these cells after cell division.

Thus, if one could observe a structure or structures, reproduced exactly in the nucleus and shared equally between the two nuclei at cell division, this might give a clue to the site of the genetic information. The next section, consequently, examines the events in the nucleus at cell division in some detail.

Cell division

In the early stages of growth and development of an organism, all the cells are actively dividing to produce new tissues and organs. Later, particularly when the cells become specialized, this power of division is lost and only a limited number of unspecialized cells retain the power of division, e.g. the cells of the germinative layer in the skin which produce new epidermis. In those cells that continue to divide, the sequence of events leading to cell division is basically the same. Firstly, the nucleus divides into two and then the whole cell divides,

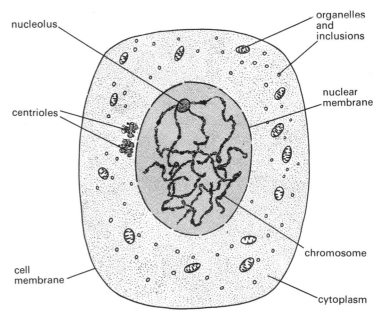

Fig. 20.1   Cell at early prophase

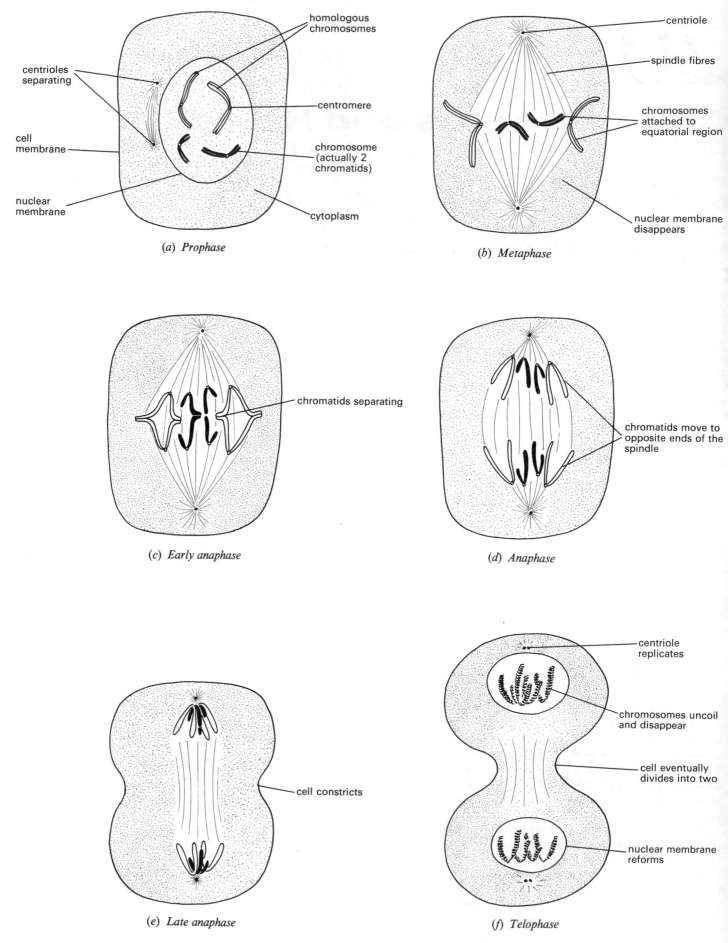

homologous
chromosomes

centrioles
separating

centromere

cell
membrane

chromosome
(actually 2
chromatids)

nuclear
membrane

cytoplasm

(a) Prophase

centriole

spindle fibres

chromosomes
attached to
equatorial region

nuclear membrane
disappears

(b) Metaphase

chromatids separating

(c) Early anaphase

chromatids move to
opposite ends of the
spindle

(d) Anaphase

cell constricts

(e) Late anaphase

centriole
replicates

chromosomes uncoil
and disappear

cell eventually
divides into two

nuclear membrane
reforms

(f) Telophase

Fig. 20.2   Mitosis

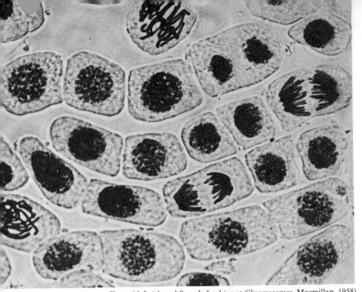

Fig. 20.3 Cell division in the root tip of a plant

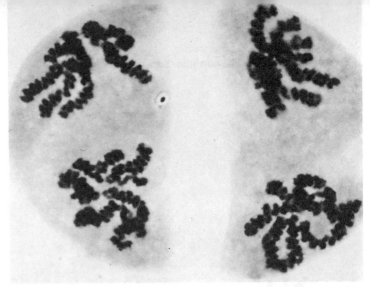

Fig. 20.4 Plant chromosomes at telophase of meiosis (p. 171) showing coiling

separating each nucleus in a unit of cytoplasm, so that two cells now exist where previously there was only one. Both cells may then enlarge to the size of the parent cell. Such cell division and enlargement gives rise to growth.

The detailed sequence of events which takes place when the nucleus of a cell divides has been worked out over the last eighty years and is called *mitosis.*

Mitosis   P M A T

Prior to division, the nucleus of the cell enlarges and in the nucleus there appear a definite number of fine, coiled, thread-like structures called *chromosomes* (Fig. 20.1). The behaviour of these chromosomes during cell division is usually described as a series of stages, prophase, metaphase, etc., though, in fact, the events occur in a smoothly continuous pattern and do not occupy equal periods of time (*see* Fig. 20.2).

1 **Prophase.** The chromosomes become more pronounced (that is, they react more readily to stains and chemical fixatives). They shorten and thicken (Fig. 20.9*a*), probably by coiling like a helical spring, but with the coils so close to each other that they are not visible at low magnifications (Figs. 20.4 and 20.5). The nuclear membrane dissolves, leaving the chromosomes suspended in the cytoplasm, and at the same time the one or more *nucleoli* disappear.

2 **Metaphase.** In the cells of animals and some of the simpler plants there is a pair of minute bodies called the *centrioles* which lie just outside the nucleus. At this stage they move away from each other and migrate to opposite ends of the cell. From each centriole there radiate what appear to be cytoplasmic fibres which meet and join near the centre of the cell. This system of 'fibres' makes a web-like structure called the *spindle* (Fig. 20.2*b*) and the chromosomes become attached by their *centromeres* (Fig. 20.5) to the equatorial region of the spindle. By this time it is apparent that each chromosome consists of two parallel strands, called *chromatids* (Fig. 20.9*b*), joined in one particular region, the *centromere*. In forming two chromatids, the chromosome *replicates*; that is, it reproduces an exact copy of itself but the two identical chromatids remain in contact along their length. This replication has already occurred at prophase but is more evident during metaphase.

3 **Anaphase.** The two chromatids now separate at the centromere and begin to migrate in opposite directions towards either end of the spindle (Fig. 20.9*c*). Experiments show that the spindle fibres play some part in separating the chromatids. The appearance is that of the chromatids first repelling each other at the centromere and then being pulled entirely apart by the shortening spindle fibres, although such a mechanism has not yet been verified.

4 **Telophase.** The chromatids, now chromosomes, collect together at the opposite ends of the spindle (Fig. 20.9*d*) and become less distinct, probably by becoming uncoiled and therefore thinner. The one or more nucleoli reappear, and a nuclear membrane forms round each group of daughter chromosomes so that there are now two nuclei present in the cell. At this point in animal cells, the cytoplasm between the two nuclei constricts, and two cells are formed. Both may retain the ability to divide, or one or both may become specialized and lose their reproductive capacity.

From a study of mitosis it seems very likely that the chromosomes are the site of the genetic instructions, since they reproduce themselves when they form chromatids and the chromatids are shared equally between the cells by the events of mitosis. A further study of chromosomes provides more evidence that they carry genetic information.

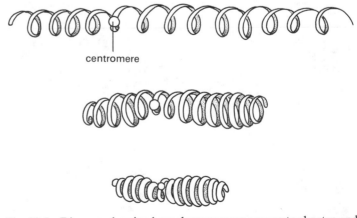

centromere

Fig. 20.5 Diagram showing how chromosomes appear to shorten and thicken during prophase

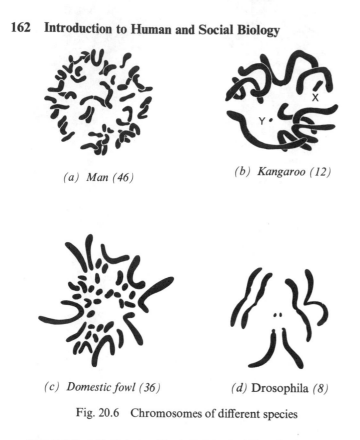

(a) Man (46)   *(b) Kangaroo (12)*

(c) Domestic fowl (36)   *(d) Drosophila (8)*

Fig. 20.6   Chromosomes of different species

(From C. C. Hurst, *The Mechanism of Creative Evolution*, Cambridge University Press, 1933)

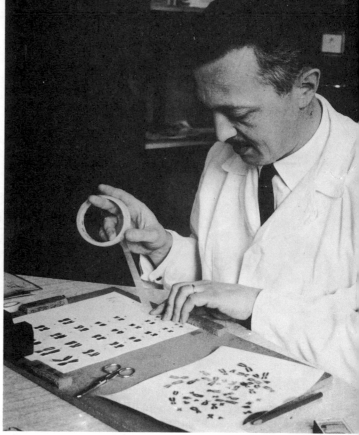

(World Health)

Fig. 20.7   Studying human chromosomes. A member of a team of scientists under Professor Jerôme Lejeune at the Institut de Progénèse, Paris, identifies and prepares pictures of human chromosomes

Chromosomes

Chromosomes are so called because they take up certain basic stains very readily (*chromos* = colour, *soma* = body), but they can also be observed by phase contrast microscopy in the unstained nuclei of dividing, living cells. When the cell is not dividing, the chromosomes cannot be seen in the nucleus, even after staining. Nevertheless, it is thought that they persist as fine, invisible threads, isolated patches of which still respond to dyes and show up as flakes or granules of deeply staining material. The chromosomes consist of protein and a substance called *deoxyribonucleic acid* (DNA: *see* p. 166), but the exact relationship between these two components in forming the chromosome is not known.

Counts of chromosomes show that there is a definite number in each cell of any one species of plant or animal: e.g. mouse, 40; crayfish, 200; rye, 14; fruit fly (*Drosophila*), 8; and man, 46 (*see* also Fig. 20.6). This confirms our expectation that the chromosomes determine the difference between one species and another. It can also be seen (Fig. 20.8) that the chromosomes exist in pairs, although not actually joined together, each pair

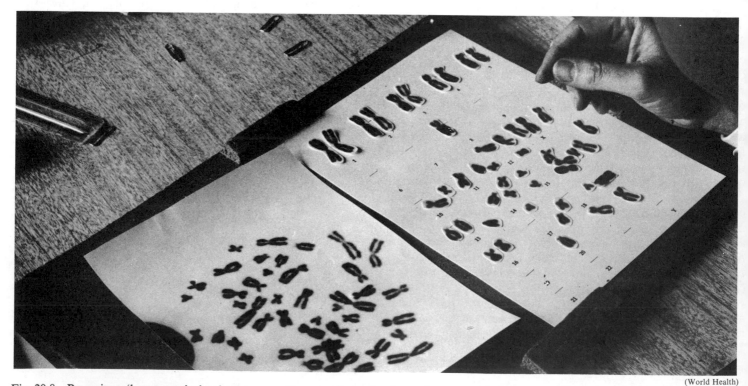

(World Health)

Fig. 20.8   Preparing a 'karyogram': the chromosome silhouettes from the photomicrograph on the left are cut out and arranged in order on the right-hand chart

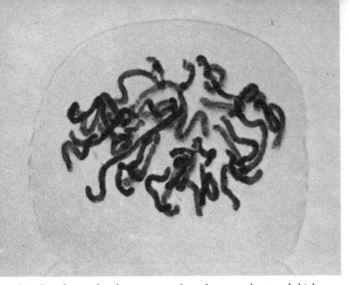

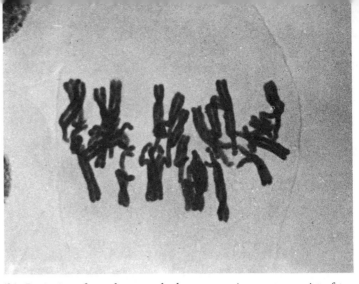

(a) Prophase; the chromosomes have become short and thick

(b) Beginning of anaphase; each chromosome is seen to consist of two chromatids which are attached to the equator of the spindle and are beginning to separate

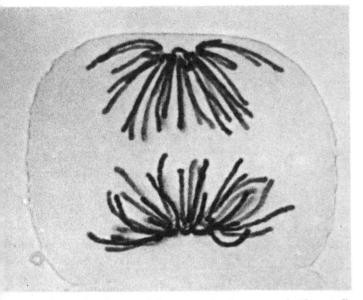

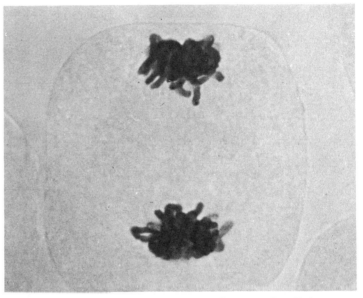

(c) Anaphase; the chromatids have completely separated. The spindle is not visible in this photograph

(d) Telophase; the chromosomes are becoming less distinct

Fig. 20.9   Stages in mitosis in a plant root cell

(From McLeish and Snoad, *Looking at Chromosomes*, Macmillan, 1958)

having a characteristic length and, during anaphase, a characteristic shape (Fig. 20.9c) governed by the position of the centromere at which the chromatids are pulled apart; e.g. a V shape if the centromere is central, or a $\sqrt{}$ shape if it is close to one end. In other words, human cell nuclei contain 23 pairs of chromosomes, mouse cells 20 pairs and so on, one member of each pair having been derived from the male and one from the female parent. The members of each pair are called *homologous chromosomes*, and the total number of chromosomes in each cell is called the *diploid number*.

Although the constituent chemicals of the cytoplasm of a cell are constantly being broken down and rebuilt from fresh material, the chemicals of the chromosomes remain remarkably stable. Other investigations show that during cell division, no protoplasmic material is shared so exactly as that of the chromosomes in the nucleus. Such evidence points again to the chromosomes as the main source of the chemical information which determines that a cell should become like its parent cell, and that in their development, the cells of the organism will endow the animal or plant with all the characteristics of its

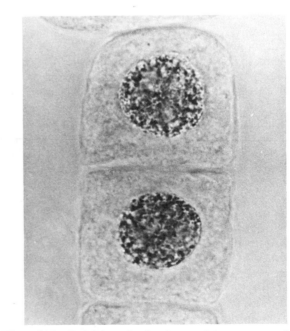

(e) The end of cell division; the daughter nuclei are separated by a new cell wall

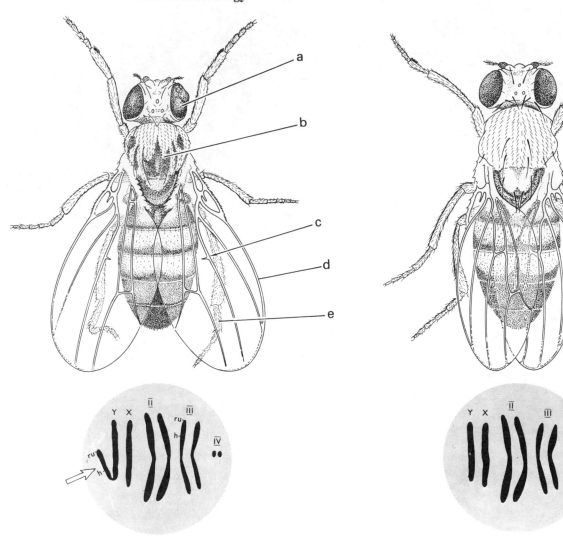

(After Muller, *Journal of Genetics*, 1930

Fig. 20.10 Effects of a chromosome mutation in *Drosophila*. The cells of the fruit fly on the left have an extra segment of chromosome no. 3 which has become attached to the Y chromosome. As a result, this fly has (*a*) mis-shapen eyes, (*b*) dark patterned thorax, (*c*) imperfect cross veins, (*d*) broad wings, (*e*) incurved hind legs. The normal fly is shown on the right

species. Although the supporting evidence is very sketchily outlined here, the hereditary material must almost certainly lie on the chromosomes of the nucleus and be passed on to each daughter cell by the process of mitosis. In a similar way the nuclei of the sperm and egg carry a set of chromosomes from the male and female parent, and these chromosomes determine that the zygote grows and develops to an animal or plant of the same species as the parents, reproducing to quite a minute degree, individual characteristics of both parents.

The fruit fly, *Drosophila melanogaster,* which has four pairs of chromosomes in its nuclei is, for various reasons, a suitable subject for study. By breeding many hundreds of flies through many generations, geneticists have become very familiar with the detailed anatomy of the fly and the appearance of its chromosomes. It has been observed on many occasions that some unexpected change in the external appearance of a fly is associated with a change in the chromosome pattern (*see* Fig. 20.10). This chromosome aberration must take place at an early stage in the development of the fly for it to affect so many parts of the body, or it may have occurred in one of the gametes from which the zygote was formed.

Cells from the salivary glands of *Drosophila* and other flies have very large chromosomes called giant chromosomes, on which bands can be seen (Fig. 20.12). The size, shape and position of these bands is quite consistent and characteristic for any pair of chromosomes. If, due to some accident in replication, one or other of the bands is lost, there is a corresponding malformation in the adult fly (Fig. 20.11). Although the bands can be seen on only these rather unusual giant chromosomes, it is thought that they represent the site of genes or gene activity on all the chromosomes in the body.

Genes. A gene is a theoretical unit of inheritance, theoretical in the sense that the word was coined long before chromosome structure was investigated in detail or the DNA theory of inheritance put forward. The gene is one of the 'words' in the genetic 'instructions' (*see* p. 159). For example one gene will specify whether the cat is to have black fur or white fur. Another gene will determine whether the fur is long or short. Today the gene is thought to consist of a group of chemicals situated on the chromosome.

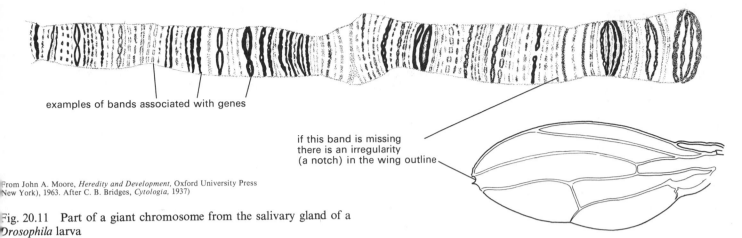

examples of bands associated with genes

if this band is missing
there is an irregularity
(a notch) in the wing outline

From John A. Moore, *Heredity and Development*, Oxford University Press
New York), 1963. After C. B. Bridges, *Cytologia*, 1937)

Fig. 20.11　Part of a giant chromosome from the salivary gland of a
Drosophila larva

Gene function

The picture that emerges from this and other evidence is that
the genes which determine the characteristics of the organism
are somehow arranged in line down the chromosome. These
genes control the production of enzymes, which in turn
determine what functions go on in a cell, and eventually in the
organs and entire organism. If anything happens to a gene it
will affect the organism, e.g. in mice there is a gene which
determines that the coat will be coloured. If this gene is missing,
the mouse will be without pigment; it will be white with pink
eyes. In this case, as in many others, more than one gene will
in fact play a part in determining the characteristic.

The number of genes in man is not known but it could be
about 1 000 per chromosome. At mitosis, each chromosome,
and therefore each of any of the genes it carries, is exactly
reproduced.

Two problems arise from this account. Since every cell in the
body carries an identical set of chromosomes and since cell
structure and function are determined by the genes on the
chromosomes, why is not every cell of the body identical?
Furthermore, what possible part can a gene for brown eyes
play when it is in the nucleus of a cell lining the stomach wall?
Briefly, when we follow the development of a particular cell, it
seems that the way in which one of its genes will affect the cell
depends not only on the gene itself but also on the physiology
of the cell, which in turn is related to its particular position in
the body. For example, the chemical environment in a certain
cell in the scalp allows the gene for black hair to operate in a
particular way. Just what the same gene does in another part
of the body is not certain, its action may simply be suppressed,
but it is known that most genes have more than one effect, and
the characteristic by which they are recognized is not necessarily their most important function; e.g. the genes responsible
for producing colour in the scales of one kind of onion also
confer a resistance to fungus disease because they determine
the presence of certain chemicals which act as a fungicide. The
colour, however, is the more obvious characteristic. The gene
in *Drosophila* which produces the effect of diminutive wings
also reduces the expectation of life to half that of normal flies.
The wing characteristic is the more immediately obvious effect
but the effect on life span may be far more important and
damaging to the species. The idea that the expression of a gene
depends to some extent on the physiology of the cell and the

situation in which it finds itself is illustrated by the experimental work with certain amphibian embryos. If a piece of
tissue, which would normally become skin, is taken from the
abdomen and grafted into a region overlying the developing
eye, the graft will be incorporated into the eye as a lens. It has
the same chromosomes and genes, but its new position has
altered its fate. This effect is by no means true of all animals
and is certainly not the case in insects in which the fate of
individual cells seems to be determined at a very early stage in
development and is not affected by moving the cells to a new
situation.

Fig. 20.12　Four giant chromosomes from a cell in the salivary gland
of the midge larva, *Chironomus tentans*, showing transverse banding
(magnification approx ×350)

(Courtesy of Professor Wolfgang Beerman, Max Planck Institute, Tübingen, from *Sci. Amer.*, April 1964)

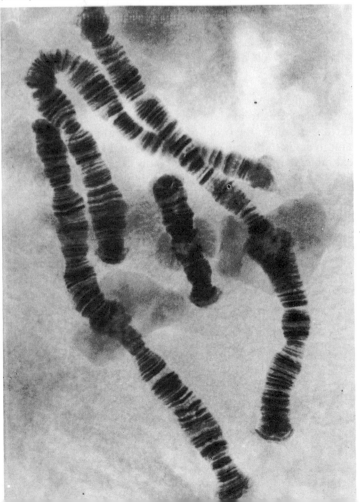

How genes work

The role of DNA. It was mentioned earlier (p. 162) that chromosomes consist of protein and a nucleic acid, deoxyribonucleic acid (DNA). Although the precise relationship between the DNA and the protein is not known, the structure of DNA has been intensively studied. This chemical consists of long molecules coiled in a double helix. The strands of the helix are chains of sugars and phosphates, the sugar being a 5-carbon compound, *deoxyribose*. The two helices in a DNA strand are linked together by cross-bridges made by pairs of organic nitrogenous bases joined to the sugar molecules (Figs. 20.13 and 20.14). Although there are only four principal kinds of base in the DNA molecule, *adenine, cytosine, thymine* and *guanine*, it is thought that the sequence of these bases is the important factor in heredity, and that a gene may consist of a particular sequence of up to 1 000 base pairs in a DNA molecule.

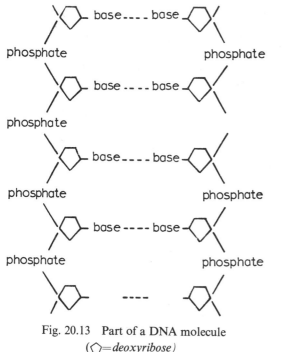

Fig. 20.13   Part of a DNA molecule
($\bigcirc$ = *deoxyribose*)

The different sequence of bases *along the length* of the DNA molecule seems to act like a code, instructing the cell to make certain proteins, the order of bases indicating the sequence of amino acids to be joined up in order to make the protein. For example, the sequence CAA (cytosine–adenine–adenine) specifies the amino acid *valine*; three thymines in a row, TTT, specify *lysine,* while AAT specifies *leucine.* So the sequence of bases CAA–TTT–AAT would direct the cell to link up the amino acids valine–lysine–leucine to make the appropriate peptide, and in a similar way proteins are formed (*see* p. 17).

The role of RNA. Cell proteins are not made by the nucleus but by the ribosomes in the cytoplasm. The coded information in the nuclear DNA must somehow be transposed to the cytoplasm. This transfer is carried out by a nucleic acid, *ribonucleic acid* (RNA), which differs slightly in composition from DNA. Each part of the DNA that is active in the chromosomes builds up a replica of itself in RNA. These lengths of RNA, called *messenger RNA,* become detached from the chromosomes, leave the nucleus through the nuclear pores and become attached to ribosomes (Fig. 20.15*a* and *b*).

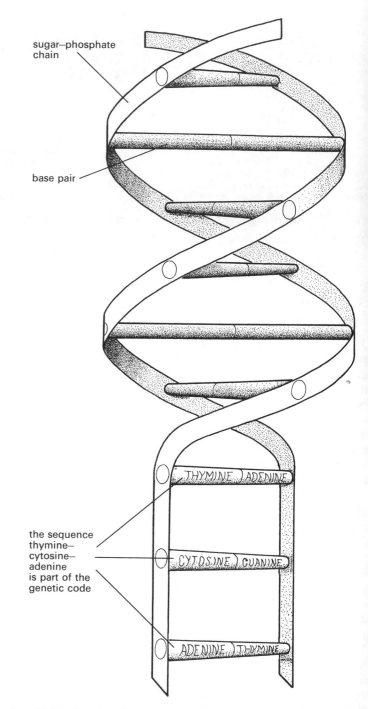

Fig. 20.14   The drawing shows schematically part of a DNA molecule; the lower part is shown uncoiled to emphasize the position of the base pairs

In the cytoplasm there are many amino acids and some of these become attached to a second kind of RNA called *transfer RNA*. Three of the bases on each molecule of transfer RNA correspond to one of the groups of three bases on the messenger RNA. The amino acid molecules attached to the transfer RNA will eventually encounter a ribosome to which is attached a strand of messenger RNA. If the section of messenger RNA attached to the ribosome has the three bases that correspond to those on the transfer RNA, the latter will combine temporarily with the messenger RNA. As the mes-

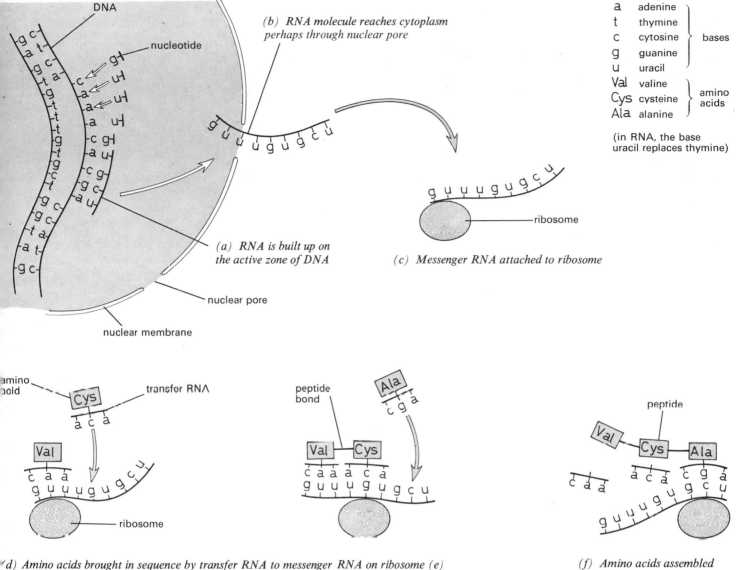

(b) *RNA molecule reaches cytoplasm perhaps through nuclear pore*

a	adenine	
t	thymine	
c	cytosine	bases
g	guanine	
u	uracil	
Val	valine	
Cys	cysteine	amino acids
Ala	alanine	

(in RNA, the base uracil replaces thymine)

(a) *RNA is built up on the active zone of DNA*

(c) *Messenger RNA attached to ribosome*

(d) *Amino acids brought in sequence by transfer RNA to messenger RNA on ribosome* (e)

(f) *Amino acids assembled to make peptide molecule*

Fig. 20.15   The role of DNA and RNA

senger RNA moves along the ribosome, the triplets of bases will be presented in turn, and each triplet will allow its corresponding transfer RNA to attach itself, bringing an amino acid with it. The amino acids are linked together by peptide bonds (*see* p. 17) in the correct sequence to make polypeptides and proteins (Fig. 20.15 *d–f*).

Most of the proteins made are enzymes which direct the pattern of chemical activity in the cell. Thus DNA, by determining the kinds of enzyme formed in the cell, will control the cell's activities. This in turn will affect the nature of the cell, the organ of which it is a part and eventually the organism as a whole. A change in the sequence of bases in the DNA molecule will result in a different order of amino acids and, hence, a different and probably ineffective enzyme. This will usually act adversely on the metabolism of the cell.

A rat with coloured fur has a gene that controls the production of the enzyme *tyrosinase*. This enzyme converts *tyrosine*, a colourless amino acid, to *melanin*, a black pigment. An albino

rat has no gene for tyrosinase production, and consequently no pigment is formed from the tyrosine in its body (*see* p. 169).

Normal humans have a gene that controls the production in the blood of an enzyme that accelerates the breakdown of a chemical, *alcapton*. Persons having no gene for the enzyme excrete in the urine unchanged alcapton which darkens on exposure to the air. This relatively harmless effect is associated with pigmentation in other parts of the body and, later, with arthritis. The condition is inherited as a recessive factor (p. 175). This is a rather peculiar example of the mechanism of inheritance, but if a gene controlled the production of an enzyme essential in a much earlier stage of a series of vital reactions, the absence of the gene could have devastating effects even to the extent of causing premature death. Conversely, since normal physiology is the result of hundreds of chemical changes catalysed by hundreds of enzymes, it is not surprising that characteristics such as intelligence, stature and activity come under the influence of many genes.

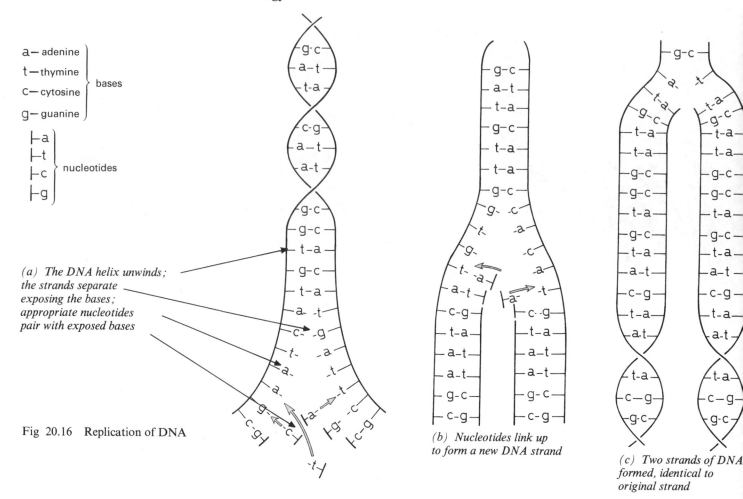

a—adenine
t—thymine } bases
c—cytosine
g—guanine

├a
├t } nucleotides
├c
├g

(a) The DNA helix unwinds; the strands separate exposing the bases; appropriate nucleotides pair with exposed bases

Fig 20.16 Replication of DNA

(b) Nucleotides link up to form a new DNA strand

(c) Two strands of DNA formed, identical to original strand

Replication of genes. When a chromosome forms two chromatids prior to cell division, its constituent DNA also replicates. It is thought that the component strands of each double helix unwind, exposing the organic bases. In the nucleoplasm are the corresponding bases attached to sugar and phosphate molecules. This combination of organic base, sugar and phosphate is called a _nucleotide_. The bases on the appropriate nucleotides become attached to the exposed bases of the separated DNA strands, and so build up a new molecule of DNA with exactly the same sequence of bases as the original partner. In this way the genetic code is preserved intact to be passed on with the chromosomes to the new cell (Fig. 20.16).

Mutations

A mutation is a spontaneous change in a gene or a chromosome which may produce an alteration in the characteristic under its control. Fig. 20.10 shows a chromosome mutation. A fairly frequent form of mental deficiency known as Down's syndrome (mongolism) results from a chromosome mutation in which the ovum carries an extra chromosome, so that the child has 47 chromosomes in his cells instead of 46.

A mutation in a single cell may not be very important in heredity, but if the cell is a gamete mother cell, a gamete or a zygote, the entire organism arising from this cell may be affected. Since the mutant form of the gene is inherited in the usual way, the mutation will persist in subsequent generations.

On the whole, genes are stable structures because DNA is a stable chemical, but once in a hundred thousand replications or more a gene may mutate.

Gene mutations occur when a section of the DNA in a chromosome is not copied exactly at cell division. For example, part of the haemoglobin molecule consists of a sequence of eight amino acids:

valine—histidine—leucine—threonine—proline
—_glutamic acid_—glutamic acid—lysine

This order will have been determined by the sequence of the four bases on part of a DNA strand (_see_ p. 167). In persons suffering from a disease called sickle cell anaemia one of the DNA bases has not been correctly paired prior to the cell division that formed the gamete from which the individual developed. As a result, the sixth amino acid directed into the haemoglobin fragment depicted above is _valine_ instead of glutamic acid. This small difference so alters the properties of the haemoglobin that in low concentrations of oxygen it becomes relatively insoluble and forms rod-like particles which distort and eventually destroy the red blood cells. The production of the 'faulty' DNA is a mutation, and since this DNA will faithfully reproduce itself in all the cells of the body, including the sex cells, the mutated gene will be passed on to the offspring. This is an example of a harmful mutation which is heritable.

Harmful mutations. Consider the sequence of bio-chemical reactions which occur in cells of the liver (Fig. 20.17).

The letters 'a', 'b' and 'c' represent enzymes which control the reactions indicated by the arrows. Each enzyme is a protein and is built up from amino acids according to the pattern determined by the base sequence of DNA in a gene. Mutations

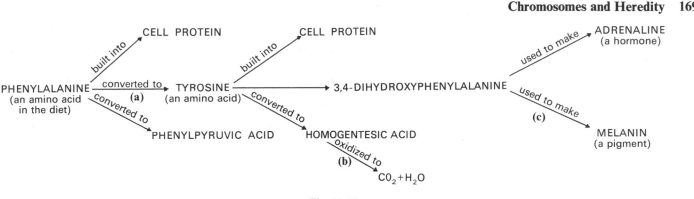

Fig. 20.17

may occur in the genes which result in the failure to produce one or other of these enzymes.

If enzyme 'a' is lacking, tyrosine cannot be made from phenylalanine. Since tyrosine is available from the normal diet this does not matter, but blocking this pathway leads to excessive production of phenylpyruvic acid. This compound collects in the cerebrospinal fluid and is thought to cause the brain damage leading to mental retardation characteristic of the disease *phenylketonuria*.

If there is no enzyme 'b', homogentesic acid (alcapton) is not oxidized to carbon dioxide and water but excreted unchanged in the urine which darkens on exposure to air, a symptom of *alcaptonuria*. Alcapton also collects in the cartilage of the joints causing a form of arthritis.

In the absence of enzyme 'c', the production of melanin from 3,4-dihydroxyphenylalanine is not possible, in which case the person will be an albino, lacking pigment in his skin, hair, and eyes.

As mentioned on p. 162, the chromosomes in the nucleus occur in pairs, one chromosome of each pair having come from the male parent and the other from the female parent. It follows, therefore, that since they are located on the chromosomes, the genes also occur in pairs. If a person inherits a mutated gene from only one parent, it is likely that its effects will be masked by the corresponding normal gene from the other parent, and the harmful condition will not appear in the individual. The mutant gene is then said to be *recessive* to the normal gene, and the normal gene is *dominant* to the mutated form (*see also* p. 175). The clinical conditions described above will therefore appear only if an individual inherits two mutated recessive genes, one from each parent.

Most mutations that produce an observable effect seem to be harmful if not actually lethal. This is not surprising, since any change in a well- but delicately balanced organism is likely to upset its physiology. Most mutations, however, are recessive and so in the presence of a normal gene do not usually produce obvious symptoms. In humans there occurs a form of dwarfism known as *achondroplastic dwarfism*, in which the limb bones do not grow normally. This condition arises as a result of a dominant mutation having a frequency of about 1 in 20 000, though 80 per cent of such dwarfs may die in their first year.

Although the majority of mutations are potentially harmful, there is a small number that are beneficial, either at the time when they occur or at a later date when the population carrying them encounters changing conditions. The beneficial mutations thus tend to be preserved in a population because they confer some advantage on the organisms. It is from such beneficial or neutral mutations that variations arise in populations and, in the course of evolution, give rise to new species.

Mutation in bacteria. Mutations can occur whenever DNA is reproducing itself, an event which takes place prior to cell division. Some bacteria can divide every twenty-five minutes, and it follows that there is a very high chance of mutations occurring per unit of time. One such mutation produces a resistance to specific drugs and occurs about once in every thousand million cell divisions. This seems very infrequent but a colony of ten bacteria could produce a population of that order in four or five hours, and it is likely that a thriving colony will contain several individuals resistant to, say, penicillin. In the 'normal' environment the mutation may have no advantage, but in the presence of penicillin all but the mutants will be destroyed. The progeny of the surviving mutants will inherit the resistance to penicillin and in this way a population of resistant bacteria can soon become established. For this reason, the widespread use of antibiotics is discouraged.

Mutation rate. One cannot predict when a gene is going to mutate but the frequency of its occurrence can be determined in some cases; for example in achondroplastic dwarfism it is possibly as high as one mutation in 20 000, compared with one in 100 000 for many genes. The rate of mutation is characteristic of particular genes in particular species, but the frequencies are such that in a human ejaculate of, say, 200 million sperms, there are likely to be a considerable number of nuclei bearing gene and chromosome mutations.

Exposure to radioactivity, X-rays and ultraviolet radiation is known to increase the rate of gene and chromosome mutation.

Radiation and mutations. The cause of mutation is not known, but exposure to X-radiation, gamma radiation, ultraviolet light, etc., is known to cause an increase in the mutation rate in experimental animals such as fruit flies and mice. The artificially induced mutations are the same as those that occur naturally, but the frequency with which they occur is greatly increased.

There is a fairly constant background of radiation on the Earth's surface as a result of cosmic rays. Individuals also receive radiation from X-rays used in medicine, television tubes and luminous watch dials. Workers in atomic power stations and other people handling radioactive materials in industry or research may receive additional radiation. The radioactive fall-out from atomic explosions has increased the background radiation.

It is of obvious importance to assess the effect of any increase in radiation on the health of individuals and, as a result of mutations in their reproductive cells, the health of their children.

There is, so far, insufficient information to determine the

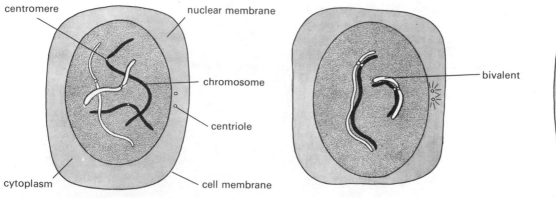

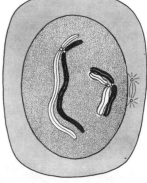

PROPHASE

(a) *The diploid number of chromosomes appear*

(b) *Homologous chromosomes pair with each other, shorten and thicken*

(c) *Replication has occurred and the chroma tids become visible*

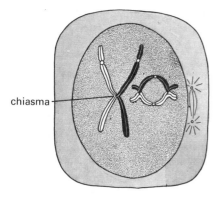

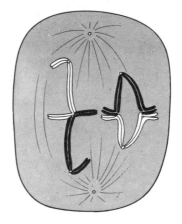

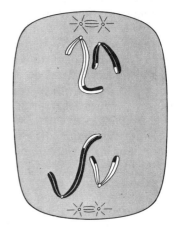

(d) *Homologous chromosomes move apart except at the chiasmata where chromatids have exchanged portions*

ANAPHASE

(e) *A spindle forms and homologous chromosomes move to opposite ends taking exchanged portions with them*

(f) *Homologous chromosomes separated bu not enclosed in nuclear membranes*

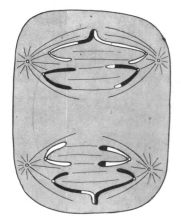

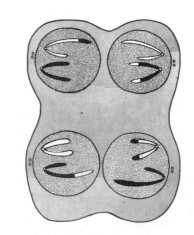

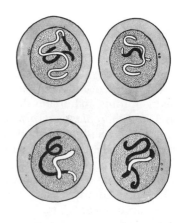

SECOND MEIOTIC DIVISION

(g) *Spindles form at right angles to the first one and the chromatids separate*

TELOPHASE

(h) *Four nuclei appear, each enclosing the haploid number of chromosomes*

(i) *Cytoplasm divides to form four gametes*

Fig. 20.18   Meiosis in a gamete-forming cell

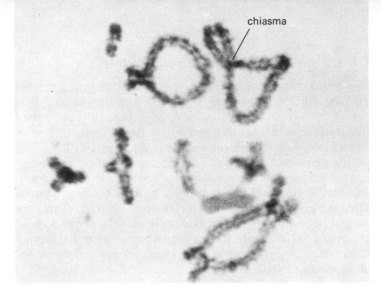

(From colour slide set, *Meiosis in Chorthippus brunneus*, published by Harris Biological Supplies Ltd)

Fig. 20.19 Meiosis in grasshopper testis (late prophase)

correlation between the radiation dose and the mutation rate in man. The maximum safe dose in respect of direct effects on the individual such as leukaemia is still a matter of controversy. Nevertheless it is probably safe to say that any increase in the mutation rate is likely to have harmful effects on the population. Consequently, the exposure of individuals to the hazards of radiation is limited, though somewhat arbitrarily, by law.

Variation

The exact replication of chromosomes and genes and their equal distribution between cells at mitosis produces conformity; the organism breeds true to type, e.g. a sheep reproduces sheep and not goats or cows. Nevertheless, the offspring will differ in many respects from its brothers and sisters and from its parents. It is possible for two black mice to have some white babies as well as black ones. A child of blood group O could be born to a mother of blood group B and a father of group A.

The variations in question must arise in the first instance from neutral or beneficial mutations, but the appearance and distribution of the varieties in the population will depend on how the parental chromosomes and genes are rearranged in the offspring. For example, in a white mouse the absence of a gene for pigment is the result of a mutation, but the numbers of white mice appearing in a population will depend on the frequency with which a sperm carrying the mutated gene fertilizes an ovum with the same gene. The distribution of genes in the gametes is a direct result of the way in which the chromosomes separate at the cell division that leads to gamete formation. This sequence of chromosome separation is called meiosis.

Meiosis

Cells in the reproductive organs which are going to form gametes, either sperms or ova, undergo a series of mitotic divisions resulting, in the case of sperms, in a vast increase of numbers. The final divisions, however, which give rise to mature gametes are not mitotic. Instead of producing cells with 46 chromosomes in man, they form gametes with only 23 chromosomes. When, at fertilization, there is a fusion of the two gametes, the resulting zygote contains the diploid number of 46 chromosomes, and this number is present in all the cells of the offspring. The halving of the chromosome number which occurs at gamete formation, ultimately maintains the diploid number of chromosomes characteristic of the species. If gametes were produced by mitosis, a human egg and sperm would each contain 46 chromosomes and when they fused at fertilization would give rise to a zygote with 92 chromosomes. The gametes from the resulting organism would in turn give rise to offspring with 184 chromosomes and so on.

1 **Prophase.** In meiosis, the chromosomes appear in the nucleus (i.e. they appear when the cell is fixed and stained or observed by phase contrast microscopy) in much the same way as described for mitosis, but although it is reasonably certain that two chromatids are present in each chromosome, the chromosomes still appear to be single threads. Another difference from mitosis seen at this stage is the failure of the chromosomes to shorten by coiling.

In complete contrast to mitosis the homologous chromosomes now appear to *attract* each other and come to lie along-side, so that all parts of the two chromosomes correspond exactly. The pairs of chromosomes so formed are called *bivalents*, e.g. a cell with a normal complement of six chromosomes would have, at this stage, three bivalents.

In this paired state the chromosomes shorten and thicken by coiling, and now each chromosome is seen to consist of two chromatids. As soon as this occurs, however, the pairs of chromatids seem to repel each other and move apart, except at certain regions called *chiasmata*. In these regions the chromatids appear to have broken and joined again but to a different chromatid. The significance of this exchange of sections of chromosomes or 'crossing over', is discussed on p. 179. All these changes occur during prophase while the nuclear membrane is still intact.

2 **Metaphase.** The nuclear membrane disappears, a spindle is formed and the bivalents approach the equatorial region.

3 **Anaphase.** The paired chromatids of each bivalent now continue the separation that began in prophase and move to opposite ends of the spindle in a manner superficially similar to that of chromatids in mitosis. The outcome is that only half the total number of paired chromatids reaches either end of the spindle. Thus although there may originally have been six chromosomes in the nucleus, there are now only three paired chromatids at either end of the spindle.

4 **Second meiotic division.** A nuclear membrane does not usually form round the paired chromatids at this stage. Instead, two new spindles form at right angles to the first one and the chromatids of each pair separate and become chromosomes.

5 **Telophase.** The four groups of chromosomes are now enclosed in nuclear membranes so forming four nuclei, each containing half the diploid number of chromosomes (the *haploid* number). Finally, the cytoplasm divides to separate the nuclei, giving rise, in the case of males at least, to four gametes. In sperm formation (*spermatogenesis*) in most animals the four cells will develop 'tails' to become sperms (Fig. 20.20).

Since it gives rise to cells containing half the diploid number of chromosomes, meiosis is sometimes called the *reduction division*.

Formation of ova: oogenesis. During the formation of ova, the cytoplasm is not shared equally. After the first meiotic division,

171

one of the daughter nuclei receives the bulk of the cytoplasm and the other nucleus is separated off with only a vestige of cytoplasm to form the first *polar body*, which, although it may undergo the next stage of its meiotic division, cannot function as an ovum and subsequently degenerates (Fig. 20.20).

In a similar way, the next meiotic division of the remaining egg nucleus produces a second polar body and a mature ovum. In many vertebrates, the first polar body is not formed until after the potential ovum is released from the ovary, and the second polar body is not formed until after the penetration of the sperm in fertilization. In man, when a sperm bearing 23 chromosomes fuses with a 23-chromosome ovum, a 46-chromosome zygote is formed.

New combinations of genes in the gametes. In mitosis the full complement of chromosomes derived from both parents is first doubled and then shared equally between daughter cells. The result of this replication is that the daughter cells receive identical genetic information. In meiosis, on the other hand, the genetic information on the chromosomes is not shared in exactly the same way between all the gametes. If homologous chromosomes were identical in their gene content, this variability in chromosome distribution would have no effect. Since, however, an individual's parents are bound to be genetically dissimilar in many respects, there will be many gametes with combinations of genes quite different from either of the individual's parents (*see* p. 179).

Fertilization (Fig. 20.21)

The cytoplasm of the sperm fuses with that of the ovum and the male nucleus passes into the ovum, coming to lie alongside the egg nucleus: the zygote is formed, but in many cases there is no fusion of nuclear material at this stage. Each nucleus simultaneously undergoes a mitosis with the axes of the spindles parallel to each other, but at the telophase stage the adjacent chromatids, originally from different parents, become enclosed in the same nuclear membrane, thus restoring the diploid number of chromosomes. These events are followed by the first cleavage, the zygote dividing into two cells. Subsequent mitotic division produces a multicellular organism with the diploid number of chromosomes in all its cells.

Determination of sex. In humans, one pair of the smallest chromosomes is known to determine sex. In the female, these two chromosomes are entirely homologous and are called the *X chromosomes*, while in the male, one is smaller and is called the *Y chromosome* (Fig. 20.6b). Femaleness normally results from the possession of two X chromosomes and maleness from possession of an X and a Y chromosome. At meiosis, the sex chromosomes are separated in the same way as the others (Fig. 20.22), so that all the female gametes will contain an X chromosome, but half the male gametes will contain an X and half will contain a Y chromosome. If a Y-bearing sperm fertilizes an ovum, the zygote will be XY and give rise to a boy. Fertilization of an ovum by an X-bearing sperm gives an XX zygote which develops to a girl. There should be an equal chance of X or Y sperm meeting an ovum, and therefore equal numbers of boy and girl babies should be born. In fact, slightly more boys than girls are born in most parts of the world. The reason for this is not clear, but it also happens that the mortality rate for boy babies and men is slightly higher than for girl babies and women, which tends to restore the balance.

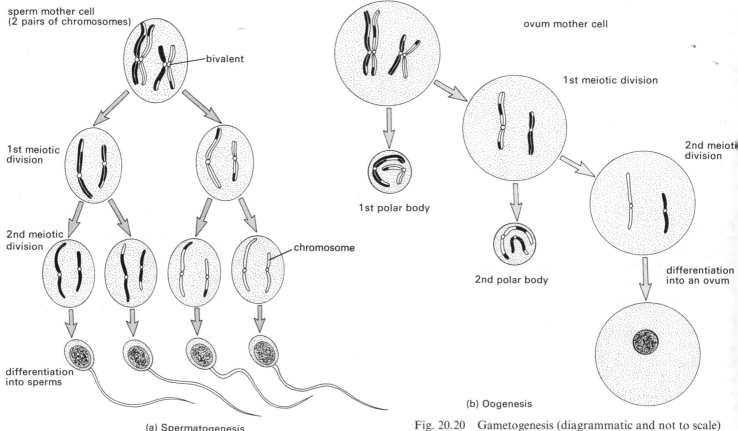

sperm mother cell
(2 pairs of chromosomes)

bivalent

1st meiotic division

2nd meiotic division

chromosome

differentiation into sperms

(a) Spermatogenesis

ovum mother cell

1st meiotic division

1st polar body

2nd meiotic division

2nd polar body

differentiation into an ovum

(b) Oogenesis

Fig. 20.20   Gametogenesis (diagrammatic and not to scale)

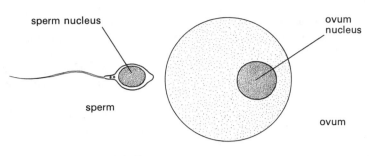

(a) Sperm meets ovum

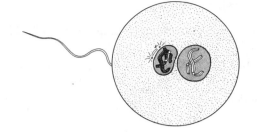

(b) Sperm nucleus enters ovum and both nuclei undergo mitosis

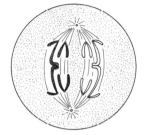

*'c) The spindles are parallel but sepa-
ate*

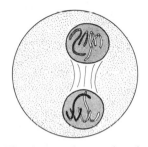

(d) The chromatids at each end of the spindle are enclosed in a common nuclear membrane

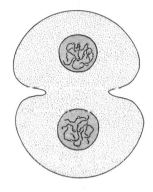

(e) The zygote divides to form two cells

Fig. 20.21 Fertilization (polar bodies not shown)

ovum
mother
cell

ova

all ova will contain
one X chromosome

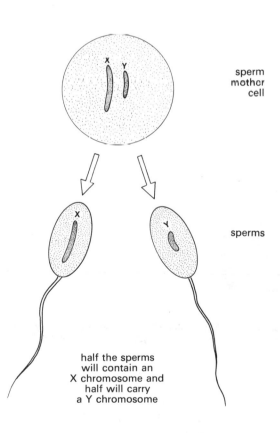

sperm
mother
cell

sperms

half the sperms
will contain an
X chromosome and
half will carry
a Y chromosome

Fig. 20.22   Determination of sex (diagrammatic only)

Although the X and Y chromosomes determine sex, it does not necessarily follow that male and female characteristics are determined by genes found only on the sex chromosomes. In man, genes for male and female characters may be scattered fairly evenly throughout all the chromosomes, but the presence of the Y chromosome in an XY zygote may tip the balance in favour of maleness. Femaleness results from the absence of the Y chromosome but this is not the case in all the animals studied; e.g. it is true for the mouse but not for *Drosophila*.

Practical Work

Experiment 1 **Squash preparation of chromosomes using acetic orcein**

Material. Allium cepa (onion) root tips. Support onions over beakers or jars of water. Keep the onions in darkness for several days until the roots growing into the water are 2–3 cm long. Cut off about 5 mm of the root tips, place them in a watch glass and

(a) cover them with 9 drops acetic orcein and 1 drop molar hydrochloric acid;

(b) heat the watch glass gently over a very small Bunsen flame till steam rises from the stain, but do not boil;

(c) leave the watch glass covered for at least five minutes;

(d) place one of the root tips on a clean slide, cover with 45 per cent acetic (ethanoic) acid and cut away all but the terminal 1 mm;

(e) cover this root tip with a clean cover-slip and make a squash preparation as described below.

Making the squash preparation. Squash the softened, stained root tips by lightly tapping on the cover-slip with a pencil: hold the pencil vertically and let it slip through the fingers to strike the cover-slip. The root tip will spread out as a pink mass on the slide; the cells will separate and the nuclei, many of them with chromosomes in various stages of mitosis (because the root tip is a region of rapid cell division) can be seen under the high power of the microscope (× 400).

Preparation of reagents

(i) **Clarke's fluid.** 25 cm^3 glacial acetic (ethanoic) acid 25 cm^3 ethanol.

(ii) **Acetic orcein.** 2 g orcein; 100 cm^3 glacial acetic (ethanoic) acid. Dilute a small portion with an equal volume distilled water just before use.

(iii) **Molar hydrochloric acid** (i.e. one gram molecule of HCl per litre). Make up 87.3 cm^3 of concentrated acid to 1 litre by adding distilled water.

Questions

1 Sometimes, at meiosis, the bivalent chromosomes fail to separate properly with the result that the gamete so formed contains the diploid number of chromosomes. If such a diploid sperm were to fertilize a normal, monoploid ovum, (a) what effect would you expect this to have on the zygote and offspring and (b) supposing the zygote grew into a normal individual, what might happen when the individual produced gametes by meiosis?

2 A horse and a donkey are related closely enough to be able to reproduce when mated together. The offspring from this mating is a mule and though healthy in all other respects is sterile. Suggest an explanation, to do with chromosomes and meiosis, for this phenomenon.

3 Revise the chemistry of proteins on pp. 17–18. Trace the steps involved in building up a tripeptide from alanine, glycine and serine starting from the appropriate segment of a DNA molecule. The DNA code for these amino acids is as follows: alanine, CGA; glycine, CCA; serine, TCA.

21
Heredity and Genetics

From its parents an individual inherits the characteristics of the species; e.g. man inherits highly developed cerebral hemispheres, vocal cords and the nervous co-ordination necessary for speech, a characteristic arrangement of the teeth and the ability to stand upright with all its attendant skeletal features. In addition, he inherits certain characteristics peculiar to his parents and not common to the species as a whole, e.g. hair and eye colour, blood group and facial appearance. The study of the method of inheritance of these 'characters' is called genetics.

In sexual reproduction a new individual is derived only from the gametes of its parents. The hereditary information must therefore be contained in the gametes. For many reasons, this information is thought to be present in the nucleus of the gamete and located on the chromosomes (*see* pp. 163–5).

Genes and inheritance

The term gene was originally applied to purely theoretical units or particles in the nucleus. These particles, in conjunction with the environment, were thought to determine the presence or absence of a particular characteristic. On p. 165 it was suggested that the genes may correspond to regions on the chromosomes and may consist of a large group of organic bases linked in a particular sequence in the chromosome.

In some cases, the presence of a single gene may determine the appearance of one characteristic, as in the eye colour of *Drosophila* (p. 164), but most human characteristics are controlled by more than one gene. This *multifactorial* inheritance, and the impossibility with humans of breeding experiments, make it difficult to collect and present simple, clear-cut genetical information about man. In addition, the readily observable human characteristics known to be under the control of single genes tend to be either severe abnormalities such as albinism or haemophilia, or they are rather trivial, e.g. the ability to roll the tongue or taste an obscure chemical. Consequently, in this chapter, the first example of certain types of heredity will be drawn from mice rather than men.

Single-factor inheritance. If a pure-breeding i.e. homozygous (*see* below) black mouse is mated with a pure-breeding brown mouse, the offspring will not be intermediate in colour, i.e. dark brown or some combination of brown and black, but will all be black. The gene for black fur is said to be *dominant* to that for brown fur, because although each of the baby mice, being the product of fusion of sperm and egg, must carry genes for both blackness and brownness, only that for blackness is expressed in the visible characteristics of the animal. The gene for brown fur is said to be *recessive*. The black babies are called the *first filial or F₁ generation*. If, when they are mature, these F₁ black mice are mated amongst themselves, their offspring, the *F₂ generation*, will include both black and brown mice, and if the total number for all the F₂ families are added up, the ratio of black to brown babies will be approximately 3 to 1. It must not be assumed, however, that if two black F₁ mice have four babies, three will be black and one brown. In a mating which produced, say, eight babies, it would not be at all unusual to find all black, or five black and three brown, etc. The ratio 3 : 1 appears only when large numbers of individuals are considered.

The appearance of brown fur in the second generation is proof of the fact that the F₁ black mice carried the recessive gene for brown fur, even though it did not find expression in their observable features.

In explanation, it will be assumed that a pure-breeding black mouse carries, on homologous chromosomes (*see* p. 163), a pair of genes controlling the production of black pigment. The genes are represented in subsequent diagrams (Figs. 21.1 and 21.2) by the letters BB, the capital letters signifying dominance. In the same position on the corresponding chromosomes in brown mice are carried the genes bb for brownness. The genes B and b are called *allelomorphic genes* or *alleles*.

The allelomorphic genes B and b influence the same characteristic, namely coat colour, but in different ways. *Two genes*, BB, Bb or bb, must be present, because the individual receives one chromosome from each parent. During the formation of gametes the process of meiosis (p. 171) will separate the homologous chromosomes, so that the gametes will contain only one gene from each pair. All the sperms from the pure-breeding black parent will carry the factor B and all the eggs from the brown parent will carry the factor b. When the gametes fuse, the zygotes will contain both factors B and b, but since B is dominant to b, only the former gene is expressed, i.e. the offspring will all be black.

When, later on, these black F₁ mice produce gametes, the process of meiosis will separate the chromosomes carrying the B and b factors (*see* Fig. 21.2) so that half the sperms of the male parent will carry B and half will carry b. Similarly, half the ova from the female will contain B and half b. At fertilization there are equal chances that a B-carrying sperm will fuse with either an egg carrying the B gene or an egg with the b gene, so producing either a BB or a Bb zygote. Similarly there are equal chances of a b-carrying sperm fusing with either a B- or a b-carrying ovum to give bB or bb zygotes.

This results in the theoretical expectation of finding, in every four F₂ offspring, one pure-breeding black mouse BB, one pure-breeding brown mouse bb, and two 'impure' black mice Bb.

The separation at meiosis of the alleles B and b into different gametes is called *segregation*. The pure-breeding black (BB) and brown (bb) mice are called *homozygous* for coat colour and the 'impure' black mice (Bb) are called *heterozygous*. The heterozygous mice will not breed true, i.e. if mated with each other their litters are likely to include some brown mice. The homozygous BB mice mated together can produce only black offspring and the bb homozygotes only brown offspring.

Genotype and phenotype. The BB mice and Bb mice will be indistinguishable in their appearance, i.e. they will both have black fur, and they are thus said to be the same *phenotypes*; in other words they are identical in appearance for a particular characteristic, in this case blackness. Their genetic constitutions, or *genotypes*, however, are different, namely BB and Bb. In short, the black phenotypes have different genotypes.

Single factor inheritance in man

The 'one gene–one character' effects described above illustrate very clearly the Mendelian* principles of inheritance, but they are the exceptions rather than the rule. Rarely do single genes control one trait. Colour in sweet peas, for example, is controlled by two pairs of genes, CC and RR. Gene C controls the production of the colour base and gene R the enzyme which acts on it to make a colour. The recessive cc will produce no colour base and rr will have no enzyme. CCrr and ccRR combinations will thus be unable to produce coloured flowers. At least six factors operate to produce coat colour in mice. In man, eight of the chemical changes involved in blood clotting are known to be under genetic control so that several genes are responsible for coagulation, and absence of any one of them may lead to a blood-clotting disease such as haemophilia (p. 180).

---

* The term is derived from an Austrian monk, Gregor Mendel, who in the 1850s first discovered the type of inheritance described here.

SINGLE-FACTOR INHERITANCE

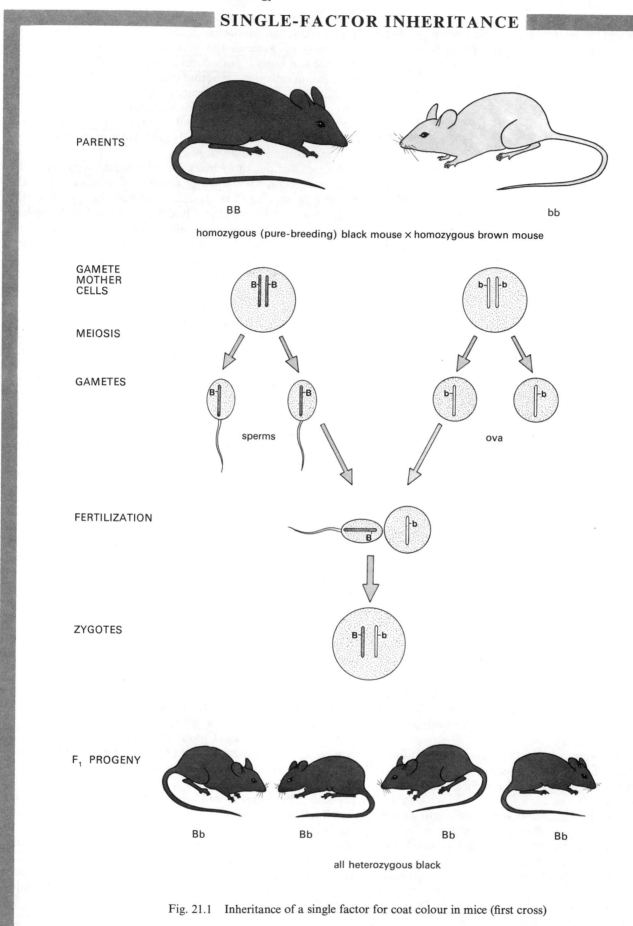

PARENTS

BB   bb

homozygous (pure-breeding) black mouse × homozygous brown mouse

GAMETE
MOTHER
CELLS

MEIOSIS

GAMETES

sperms   ova

FERTILIZATION

ZYGOTES

F₁ PROGENY

Bb   Bb   Bb   Bb

all heterozygous black

Fig. 21.1   Inheritance of a single factor for coat colour in mice (first cross)

SINGLE-FACTOR INHERITANCE

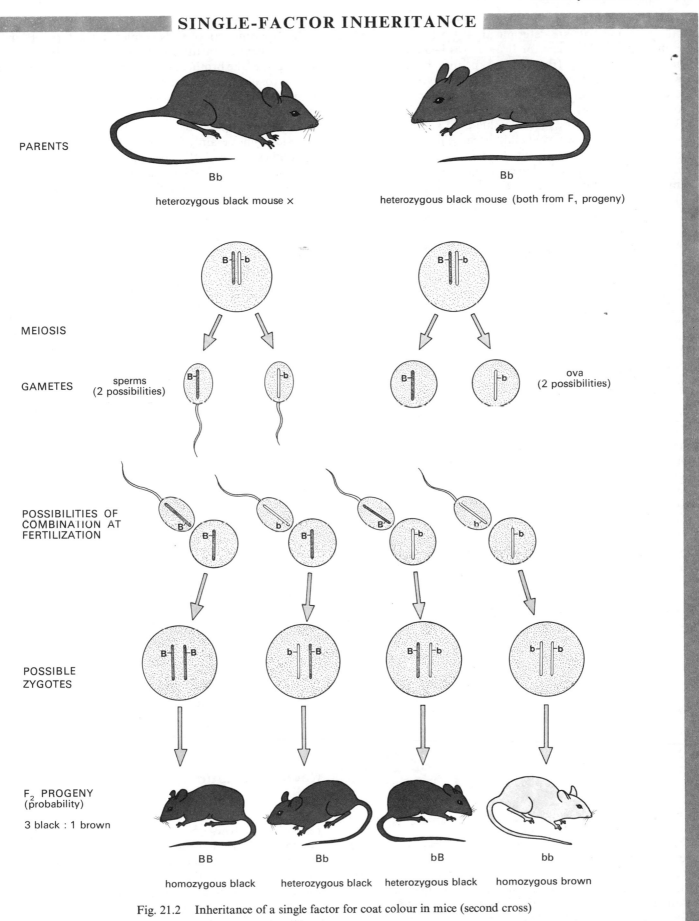

PARENTS

Bb

heterozygous black mouse ×

Bb

heterozygous black mouse (both from F₁ progeny)

MEIOSIS

GAMETES

sperms
(2 possibilities)

ova
(2 possibilities)

POSSIBILITIES OF
COMBINATION AT
FERTILIZATION

POSSIBLE
ZYGOTES

F₂ PROGENY
(probability)

3 black : 1 brown

BB

homozygous black

Bb

heterozygous black

bB

heterozygous black

bb

homozygous brown

Fig. 21.2   Inheritance of a single factor for coat colour in mice (second cross)

In the white-skinned races, characteristics such as the colour of the eyes and hair are determined, at least to some extent, by single genes. The gene for brown eyes is dominant to the gene for blue eyes. (Brown-eyed people have additional pigment in the irises of their eyes.) A blue-eyed person must therefore be homozygous recessive for the gene, i.e. his genotype is bb. A brown-eyed person's genotype could be Bb or BB. It follows therefore that two blue-eyed parents would not normally have a brown-eyed child because none of their gametes could carry the dominant B gene. On the other hand, if brown-eyed parents both have the genotype Bb, half their gametes will contain the factor b and there is a chance of one in four that they will produce a blue-eyed child (see Fig. 21.2). In fact, the inheritance of eye colour is probably controlled by more than one pair of alleles and some apparently blue-eyed people carry genes for eye pigment. Thus it is possible but unusual for a brown-eyed child to be born to blue-eyed parents.

Similarly in white-skinned races, red (ginger) hair is the result of a gene which is recessive to all other genes for hair colour. A red-haired person must be homozygous for the gene (nn) though both his parents could have black hair (Nn × Nn).

An example of single factor inheritance common to all races is the Rhesus factor in the red blood cells (see p. 76). In this case the Rh+ gene is dominant to the Rh− gene. The inheritance of the other blood groups is discussed below.

When one gene only is responsible for an important physiological change, its absence or modification will have serious consequences. Therefore most known instances of single-factor inheritance in man are associated with rather freakish abnormalities. These are usually rare conditions, e.g. occurring once in 10 000 to 100 000 individuals, but there are a great number of different kinds of genetic abnormality.

Examples of known single-factor inheritance involving a dominant gene in man are one form of night-blindness, one form of *brachydactyly* in which the fingers are abnormally short owing to the fusion of two phalanges, and achondroplastic dwarfism in which the limb bones fail to grow.

The achondroplastic dwarf will have the genotype Dd. This means that half his gametes will carry the dominant gene D for dwarfism, and if he marries a normal woman (dd) there is a chance of one in two that they will have an affected child.

	Affected man		Normal woman	
Genotype	Dd	×	dd	
Possible gametes	D	d	d	d
Possible zygotes	Dd	Dd	dd	dd
	affected		normal	

Similarly, there is a chance of one in four that two achondroplastic dwarfs Dd will have a normal child.

Some of the genetic disorders resulting from recessive genes are albinism, phenylketonuria, alcaptonuria, sickle cell anaemia, red-green colour blindness and haemophilia. The last two are inherited as sex-linked genes and discussed under this heading on p. 180. Phenylketonuria and alcaptonuria are described on p. 169. Albinism is a condition which results from the absence of pigment from the skin, hair and iris. The affected person has white skin, very blond hair and pink

irises to the eyes.

In experimental animals or plants, the type of inheritance and the genetic constitution can often be established by breeding together the brothers and sisters of the F_1 generation, or by back-crossing one of the F_1 individuals with the mother or father and producing numbers of offspring large enough to give results that have statistical significance. These methods are obviously not applicable to man and our knowledge of human genetics comes mainly from detailed analyses of the pedigrees of families, particularly those showing abnormal traits such as albinism, from statistical analysis of large numbers of individuals from different families for characteristics such as sex ratio, intelligence, susceptibility to disease, etc., and from individual studies of identical twins (see p. 181).

Incomplete dominance (co-dominance). Sickle cell anaemia results from the inheritance of a recessive gene (h) which affects the haemoglobin (p. 71). A child inheriting two recessive genes (hh) from both parents will produce red cells of which one third are likely to collapse in low oxygen concentrations and so lead to serious anaemia. The heterozygotes (Hh) can be normal healthy individuals but, even so, one per cent of their red cells are liable to distortion at low oxygen concentrations. The gene H for normal haemoglobin is thus not completely dominant over the recessive h gene.

The inheritance of the ABO blood groups in man is an instance of incomplete dominance. According to whether their blood will mix without clotting during a transfusion, people are classified into four major blood groups A, B, AB and O (see p. 75). The blood group is controlled by three genes, A, B and O, acting at the corresponding site on homologous chromosomes. A person will inherit two of these genes, one from each parent. Gene O is recessive to both A and B, but A and B are co-dominant, i.e. if a person inherits gene A from one parent and gene B from the other, he will be group AB, neither gene being dominant to the other. It follows that group O people must have the genotype OO while group A persons could be AA or AO and group B individuals BB or BO. The following example shows the possible blood groups of children born to a group A man and a group B woman both of whom are heterozygous for these genes.

Phenotype	group A		group B	
Genotype	AO		BO	
Gametes	A and O		B and O	
F_1 *Genotype*	AB	AO	OB	OO
Phenotype	group AB	group A	group B	group O

New combinations of genes

It was stressed in Chapter 20 that at mitosis the genetic information is passed on complete and intact to both cells. At gamete formation, however, meiosis gives rise to variations. It is evident that although offspring resemble their parents, they are not identical to them or to their brothers and sisters. This variability is largely the result of new combinations of genes which were present in the two parents. For example, a recessive gene may be present in the genotype of both parents but not be expressed until it appears in one of the offspring. Parents with the genotype Bb for hair colour may both have black hair and yet any one of their children could have red hair (bb).

On p. 171 it was explained that as a result of meiosis, only one of each pair of chromosomes could be present in the gamete. Since the genes are on the chromosomes it follows that only one of each pair of alleles can be present in a gamete. Which one of the pair appears in any one gamete is a matter of chance, and there are 2^{23} possible different combinations of chromosomes in the human gamete. The separation of alleles at gamete formation is called *segregation* of genes.

A European family might have a mother with red curly hair, bbCc, and a father with straight black hair, Bbcc (the gene for curliness, C, is dominant over straight, c). Each parent would produce two types of gamete with respect to these genes, bC or bc from the mother and Bc or bc from the father. Thus they could have children with curly red hair or straight black hair, like one or other of the parents, but there is an equal chance of their children having straight red hair or curly black hair, combinations which are not present in either parent (*see* Fig. 21.3).

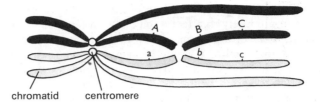

(a) Prophase; homologous chromosomes have paired up (the diagram shows the chromatids breaking at the chiasma but it is not known if this is actually what happens)

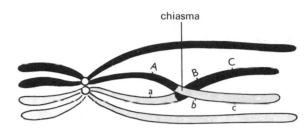

(b) Prophase (the terminal portions of the adjacent chromatids have become attached to the opposite chromatid)

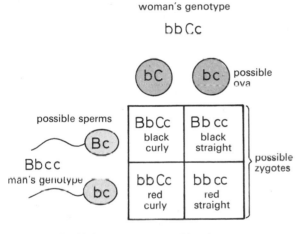

woman's genotype

bbCc

Fig. 21.3   New gene combinations

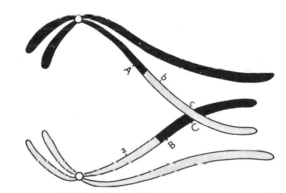

(c) Metaphase; the homologous chromosomes seem to repel each other except at the chiasma

Linkage and crossing over. During that early stage of meiosis when homologous chromosomes pair up, the maternal and paternal chromosomes exchange portions as mentioned on p. 171 and shown in Fig. 21.4. This leads to an even greater variability in the gene combinations of the gametes. In the absence of crossing over, the maternal genes A-B-C on the same chromosome would always appear together no matter how the chromosomes were assorted in meiosis. Similarly the paternal genes a-b-c would always remain together. For example, in *Drosophila*, since the genes for black body, purple eyes and vestigial wings occur on the same chromosome, one might expect that a black-bodied *Drosophila* would always have purple eyes and vestigial wings. Crossing over between chromatids, however, gives the possibility of breaking these *linkage groups* as they are called, so that new combinations, ABc, Abc, aBC, abC, aBc, AbC, could arise in the gametes, two of them being black body with red eyes and normal wings, or black body with purple eyes and normal wings.

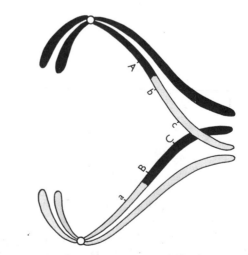

(d) Anaphase; the chromosomes separate, but as a result of crossing over, the genes A, B, C and a, b, c on the 'inner' chromatids are rearranged

Fig. 21.4   Crossing over

Sex linkage. Certain genes that occur on the X chromosome are more likely to affect a male than a female. The gene or genes for a certain form of colour blindness in man are carried on the X chromosome. Normal vision is dominant to colour blindness so that if a colour-blind woman, who must be homozygous for the character, marries a normal man, all their sons but none of their daughters will be colour blind. This can be explained by the fact that the Y chromosome is homologous with only a small section of the X chromosome and the non-homologous part of the X chromosome carries genes which are not represented on Y. It is assumed that the Y chromosome plays no part in the determination of colour vision. Fig. 21.5 shows how this type of sex linkage produces its effect.

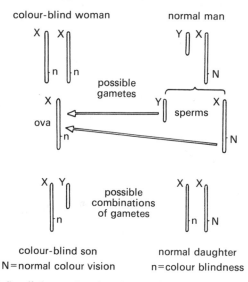

Fig. 21.5 Sex linkage, showing the possible distribution of X and Y chromosomes between the gametes and the chances of combination in the zygotes

The normal daughter is heterozygous for colour blindness and is therefore a 'carrier' for the recessive gene. If she marries a normal man the possible combinations of genes in the children are shown by:

Parents:	XN Xn		XN Y	
	carrier woman		normal man	
Gametes:	XN	Xn	XN	Y
Possible combinations of gametes:	XN XN	Xn XN	XN Y	Xn Y
	normal girl	girl carrier	normal boy	colour-blind boy

The theoretical expectations are that all the girls will be normal but half of them will be carriers, half the boys will be normal and half of them colour blind. The types of children expected from the marriage between a woman carrier and a colour-blind man, or a normal woman and a colour-blind man can be worked out in a similar way.

Other X-linked factors are *haemophilia* and brown enamel on the teeth. Haemophilia causes a delay in the clotting time of the blood. Although there are two kinds of sex-linked haemophilia, at least three other clotting disorders are known which are controlled by genes not on the sex chromosomes.

Sexual characteristics such as bass voice, beard and muscular physique in males, mammary glands and wide pelvis in females are not the result of sex-linked genes but the different expressions of the same genes present in both sexes. Both sexes carry genes controlling the growth of hair, mammary glands and penis, but in the physiological environment of maleness or femaleness they have different effects, with the result that, for example, the mammary glands in males are small and functionless; the penis in females is represented by only a small organ, the *clitoris*.

Only a few rare abnormalities are thought to be linked to the Y chromosome and even these are now open to doubt.

Discontinuous and continuous variation

The individuals within a species of plants or animals are alike in all major respects; indeed, it is these likenesses that determine that they belong to the same species. Nevertheless, even though an organism recognizably belongs to a particular species, it may differ in many minor respects from another individual of the same species. A mouse may be black, brown, white or other colours, the size of its ears and tail may vary; but despite these variations, it is still recognizably a mouse.

Discontinuous variation. The variations in coat colour are examples of discontinuous variation because there are no intermediates. If black and brown mice are bred together they will produce black or brown offspring. There are no intermediate colours and no problems arise in deciding in which colour category to place the individuals. It is not possible to arrange the mice in a continuous series of colours ranging from brown to black with almost imperceptible differences of colour between adjacent members of the series. The way sex is inherited is another example of discontinuous variation. With the exception of a small number of abnormalities, one is either male or female and there are no intermediates.

Discontinuous variation in humans is rather more difficult to illustrate. There are, for example, four major blood groups designated A, B, AB and O. Blood from different groups cannot be mixed without causing a clumping of the red cells. A person must be one or other of these four groups; he cannot, for example, be intermediate between group O and group A. In general terms, eye colour in white races appears to be inherited in a discontinuous manner; one has blue eyes or pigmented eyes, but there are some individuals who would be difficult to classify. Clear-cut examples of discontinuous variation occur among the more serious variants e.g. one is either an achondroplastic dwarf or one is not; intermediates do not occur.

The features of discontinuous variation are clearly genetically determined; they cannot be altered during the lifetime of the individual. You cannot alter your eye colour by changing your diet. An achondroplastic dwarf cannot grow to full height by eating more food. An albino cannot acquire a darker skin colour by sunbathing. Moreover, the variations are likely to be under the control of a small number of genes. One dominant gene makes you an achondroplastic dwarf; the absence of one gene for making pigment causes albinism.

Continuous variation. When one tries to classify individuals according to height or weight rather than eye colour, the decisions become more difficult and the classes more arbitrary. There are not merely two classes of people, tall and short, but a whole range of intermediate sizes differing from each other by barely measurable distances. Categories can be invented for convenience, e.g. people from 1.4 to 1.6 m, 1.6 to 1.8 m, 1.8 to 2.0 m, but they do not represent discontinuous variations of 0.2 m between individuals.

There is no reason why continuous variations should not be genetically controlled but they are likely to be under the influence of several genes. For example, height might be influenced by twenty genes, each gene contributing a few centimetres to the stature. A person who inherited all twenty would be tall whereas a person with only five would be short. Although this example is purely hypothetical, it is known that height is at least partially genetically determined because tall parents have, on average, tall children and vice versa, but how many genes are involved is not known.

Continuous variations are also those most likely to be influenced by the environment. A person may inherit genes for tallness but if he is undernourished in his years of growth he will not grow as tall as he might if he had received adequate food. In fact, most continous variations result from the interaction of the genotype with the environment. A person will grow fat if he eats too much food; he will lose weight if he goes on a diet. This seems to be an entirely environmental effect until one realizes that another person may eat just as much food and yet remain slim because of his different, inherited constitution. Whether one catches a disease or not would appear to be dependent on exposure to the disease germs, an exclusively environmental effect, and yet it is apparent that one may inherit susceptibility or resistance to a disease. If a person with inherited susceptibility to an infectious disease is never exposed to the infection, he will not develop the disease.

Heredity or environment?

It is possible to experiment with plants and animals to discover whether an observed variation is due primarily to the genetic constitution or to environmental differences. A species of plant growing in a valley may have larger leaves and taller stems than individuals of the same species growing on a mountain side. If the two varieties are collected, planted in the same situation and grown through one or two generations and still show the differences of leaves and stem size, one may assume that the differences are genetically controlled. If, however, the two varieties, after growing in the same environment, produce offspring which are indistinguishable, the original variations must have been due solely to the environmental differences.

Similar experiments with man are not possible or desirable. Even when situations occur which resemble the experiment, such as the 'uniformity' of an institutional environment for orphaned children, the observations are always susceptible to more than one interpretation. Thus, there is usually a great deal of argument about very little evidence when people discuss whether our intelligence, for example, is predominantly due to the genes we inherit or the conditions of home and school in which we were brought up. One source of evidence in the 'nature v nurture' controversy is the study of identical twins.

Identical twins

Twins may be either identical or fraternal. If they are fraternal, they are the result of the simultaneous fertilization of two separate ova by two separate sperms. The resulting zygotes will thus contain sets of chromosomes very different from each other, as explained on p. 172, and the twins, although they develop simultaneously in the uterus, will not necessarily be any more alike than if they were brothers or sisters born at different times, e.g. they can differ in sex. Identical twins, on the other hand, result when a single fertilized ovum, usually after a period of cell division, separates into two distinct embryos. The two embryos will thus have in their cells identical sets of chromosomes, since they are derived by mitosis (p. 161) from a single zygote. The twins often share a placenta, although they may be enclosed in separate amnions. Such twins, having the same genotypes, usually resemble each other very closely and are invariably of the same sex, though variations in their position and blood supply while in the uterus may produce differences at birth.

Since the one-egg twins carry identical sets of genetic 'instructions', it can be argued that any differences between them are due, not to their genes, but to the effects of their environment. Identical twins, therefore, are a valuable source of evidence for assessing the relative importance of heredity and environment. For example, the average difference in height of fifty pairs of identical twins reared together was only 1.7 cm while the average difference for the same number of non-identical twins was 4.4 cm. These and other points of comparison are given in the table below.

Average differences in selected physical characteristics between pairs of twins

Difference in :	50 pairs of identical twins reared together	50 pairs non-identical twins reared together	19 pairs of identical twins reared apart
Height (cm)	1.7	4.4	1.8
Weight (lb)	4.1	10.0	9.9
Head length (mm)	2.9	6.2	2.2
Head width (mm)	2.8	4.2	2.85

(From Freeman, Newman and Holzinger, *Twins: A study of heredity and environment*, Univ. Chicago Press, 1937)

The scores of identical twins in intelligence tests (*see* table below) show a greater correlation than those of non-identical twins even when the former have been brought up in different environments, but the results show that educational background can make a considerable difference.

Corrected average differences in IQ tests for 50 pairs of identical twins

Identical, reared together (50 pairs)	Non-identical (52 pairs)	Identical, reared apart (19 pairs)
3.1	8.5	6.0

(From Curt Stern, *Principles of Human Genetics*, 2nd edn., W. H. Freeman & Company, 1960)

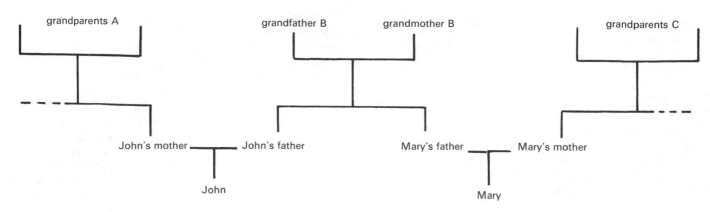

Fig. 21.6 Lineage of first cousins

Detailed histories of identical twins give even more impressive results. There is the case of girl twins, separated soon after birth; one was brought up on a farm and the other in a city, and both became affected with TB at the same age. Identical twin sisters were separated and adopted shortly after birth but both became schizophrenic within two months of each other in their sixteenth year. Such individual examples are of interest but cannot lead to any far-reaching conclusions about inheritance of human characteristics in general.

Applications of genetics to human problems

(a) **Eugenics** is the study of human genetics from the point of view (i) of encouraging breeding for good characteristics to improve human stock and (ii) of eliminating or reducing harmful characteristics. The simplest notions of eugenics as appreciated by the layman have tended to fall into some disrepute since they are based on naïve assumptions and insufficient evidence. It would seem obvious at first sight that if all the congenitally* insane were sterilized or prevented from breeding in some way, the numbers of congenital idiots in the world would be greatly reduced or the condition completely eliminated. That this is not the case is shown by considering the condition of recessive albinism. Only people with the two recessive genes, aa, will show the characteristics. These number about one in 20 000 of the population. The marriage of two albinos would give rise to all albino children but such a marriage is unlikely. Calculations show that 1 in 70 of the general population must be a carrier for albinism, i.e. have the genetic constitution Aa. Such persons are indistinguishable, at the moment, from normal AA individuals but a marriage between two such people could produce some albino children aa. Of all albinos, 99 per cent arise from such marriages between unwitting carriers and clearly there could be no question of sterilization or voluntary birth control at least until after the first albino child was born and the genetic constitution of the parents so revealed. If no homozygous recessive persons, aa, were to breed, it would take 22 generations to reduce the frequency of a harmful gene from 1 per cent to 0.1 per cent.

Similarly, if every congenitally mental defective were sterilized, the incidence of the disease would fall by only 8 per cent. This fall, however, represents the elimination of

* In this context the term *congenital* means a hereditary condition rather than an effect resulting from environmental causes during gestation or birth.

suffering for a large number of people; mentally defective people can hardly provide a suitable home even if they have normal children.

The elimination of a harmful dominant trait, Dd or DD, can theoretically be accomplished in one generation provided that the condition appears before the reproductive age.

(b) **Genetic advice.** Even if the more drastic measures of sterilization, etc. are not adopted, advice based on sound knowledge of genetics can sometimes avoid unsatisfactory breeding and several countries have 'heredity clinics' to give information about inborn defects.

For example, a person suffering from congenital juvenile cataract (a defect of the eye), caused by a dominant gene would be told that, if he married a normal person, half their children might inherit the disease; this can be seen by considering the possible F_1 offspring from the mating of Dd (affected) and dd (normal). An albino (aa) marrying a normal person who might be either AA or Aa would find that the chance of any one of his children being an albino is 1 in 140, while the normal brother of an albino, who might be a carrier, Aa, has a chance of 1 in 420 begetting an albino child if he marries a normal person. The chances for other relations, such as aunts and uncles, can also be calculated.

Genetic advice could be far more accurate if heterozygous affected people could be distinguished from homozygous normal. In some hereditary diseases such a distinction is becoming possible. Heterozygotes for the disease *phenylketonuria* can be detected with reasonable certainty by a test for the level of *phenylalanine* in their blood as the condition shows incomplete dominance (*see* p. 178).

(c) **Consanguinity.** The study of human genetics enables predictions to be made on the chances of the recombination of two harmful recessive genes in the children of marriages between first cousins.

Fig. 21.6 shows diagrammatically the theoretical pedigree of two cousins, John and Mary. Cousin John is assumed to be heterozygous for a comparatively rare recessive gene, Nn. (He would be known to be Nn for certain, only if one of his parents was nn.) John could have inherited this gene from his grandparents, A or B. There is a 1 in 2 chance that the gene came from grandparents B and in this case there is also a 1 in 4 chance that Mary has inherited the gene. There is thus a chance of 1 in 8 ($\frac{1}{2} \times \frac{1}{4}$) that cousin Mary is also Nn, in which case the chance of an affected child from their marriage is 1 in 4. The overall chances of an affected child if John is Nn and marries Mary, are thus 1 in 32 ($\frac{1}{8} \times \frac{1}{4}$).

If the gene is fairly rare in the general population, e.g. occurs once in 100 individuals, the chances of John marrying an Nn person from the general population are 1 in 100. The overall chances of an affected child then are $1/100 \times 1/4$, i.e. 1 in 400.

Although these considerations would apply equally well to beneficial genes, cousin marriages are not usually encouraged and brother-sister marriages forbidden by law. This does not reduce the total number of homozygous recessives which occur in a population but does reduce the chances of their occurring in a particular family. Consanguinity is bound to occur sooner or later, otherwise we should need to have had an impossibly large number of ancestors.

Intelligence

Intelligence is a product of a person's genetic constitution and the effect of his environment; i.e. he may inherit from his

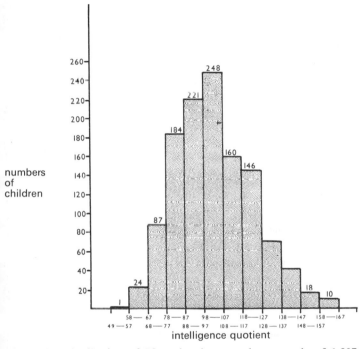

Fig. 21.7 Distribution of IQ rating in a random sample of 1 207 Scottish 11-year-old children

(From C. O. Carter, *Human Heredity*, Penguin Books, 1962)

parents the mental equipment for intelligent thought, but this will not produce his full potential of intelligent behaviour unless he is educated.

That part of intelligence which is genetically controlled, i.e. over half, is almost certainly influenced by a large number of genes and is not susceptible to simple analysis. When a graph or histogram is plotted to show the different numbers of individuals possessing a particular IQ value, the type of picture obtained is that shown in Fig. 21.7, often called a 'normality' curve or *curve of normal distribution*. Similar curves are also obtained for factors such as height and skin colour and can be explained on the basis of several genes influencing the characteristic. Instead of the straightforward presence or absence of a condition, such as albinism, there is a continuous variation with every grade of intermediate.

Practical Work

Breeding experiments with Drosophila

Drosophila is a small fly which is easy to breed in large numbers in the laboratory. By carrying out controlled cross-breeding experiments with mutant forms and wild types, it is possible to illustrate and investigate some of the principles of heredity.

Sources. Wild types and several mutant strains can be obtained from the usual biological supply firms.

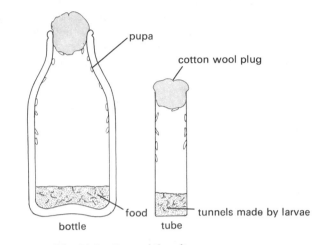

Fig. 21.8 *Drosophila* cultures

Culture medium. Mix together 50 g maize meal, 15 g agar, 13 g dried yeast, 25 g brown sugar and 800 cm^3 water and boil gently for several minutes. Dissolve 2 g 'Moldex' (or other mould-inhibitor) in 40 cm^3 boiling water and add it to the mixture. Pour the mixture into 100 mm × 25 mm specimen tubes to a depth of 20 mm, plug the tubes with cotton wool wrapped in butter muslin and sterilize in an autoclave at 10^5 N/m^2 (15 lb/in^2) for 15 min. On the day before introducing the flies, add 3 drops of a suspension of fresh yeast to each tube.

The tubes will hold about one hundred flies for experiments but for maintaining stocks of *Drosophila*, wide-mouthed bottles such as half-pint milk or cream bottles should be used and new cultures started every five or six weeks (Fig. 21.8).

Setting up experiments. It is essential that the females used for the breeding experiments have not already mated with the males in the culture bottle. From a flourishing culture with many unhatched pupae, all the flies are shaken into a clean, dry bottle and the culture bottle re-plugged. The flies that emerge from the pupae in the culture bottle during the day will be virgins and can be easily recognized by the unexpanded wings. These flies are etherized, and males and females sorted into separate dry tubes where they can recover from the ether. About three virgin females of a given strain, e.g. wild type, are transferred to a fresh culture tube and six males of a different strain, e.g. vestigial wings, are introduced. The males need not be virgins and can be taken directly from stock cultures.

The flies will mate and lay eggs in the culture medium. Larvae hatch from the eggs, burrow through the food, grow, and in about 10–14 days from laying, pupate on the sides of the tube. The parent flies should be removed after one week. When the F_1 progeny have been emerging from the pupal cases for about 10 days they should be etherized, the different sexes and strains counted and recorded, and the flies killed in alcohol or retained for F_2 experiments. From the results, the ratios of the different strains can be calculated, and interpretations attempted on the lines of the principles of Mendelian inheritance.

Etherizing (ether is very inflammable; no naked flame should be allowed while it is in use). The technique is depicted in Fig. 21.10a. The flies should not be exposed to ether for more than one minute. If they begin to recover while being counted, etc. they can be covered for a few seconds by a Petri dish lid carrying a small pad of ether-soaked cotton wool (Fig. 21.10b). If etherized flies are placed directly into a culture tube, the latter should have dry sides and be placed horizontally, otherwise the anaesthetized flies will stick to the food or the glass.

Sexing (see Fig. 21.9a and b). The presence or absence of sex combs on the fore-legs is the surest guide. A hand lens or binocular microscope is essential.

Suitable crosses. Wild type × vestigial wing; wild type × ebony body; wild type × white eye. Each cross should be made in two ways, reversing the sexes, e.g.

              vestigial winged male × wild type female

and   wild type male × vestigial winged female.

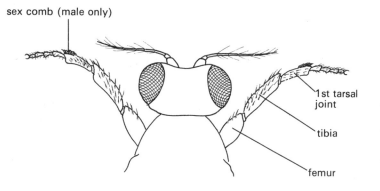

(a) Sex-combs on male Drosophila

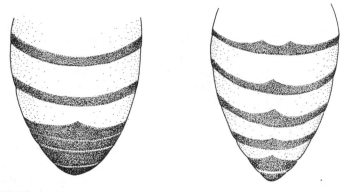

MALE more rounded, last 4   FEMALE more pointed, bands
segments fully pigmented   of pigment separated

(b) Drosophila *abdomen: dorsal aspect (these differences are not easy to see on newly hatched flies or ebony-body mutants)*

Fig. 21.9   Distinguishing the sexes

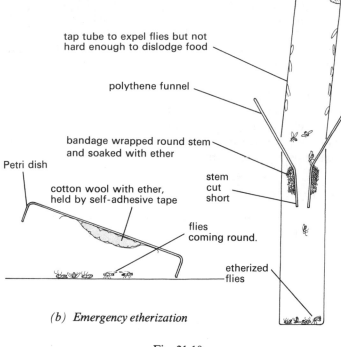

(a) Etherizing (the same method, without ether, is used to transfer flies from one container to another)

tap tube to expel flies but not hard enough to dislodge food

polythene funnel

bandage wrapped round stem and soaked with ether

Petri dish

cotton wool with ether, held by self-adhesive tape

stem cut short

flies coming round.

etherized flies

(b) Emergency etherization

Fig. 21.10

Further information

More detailed instructions can be obtained from the following books.

Practical Heredity with Drosophila, by G. Haskell (Oliver & Boyd, 1961).

Genetics for Schools (Modern Science Memoir No. 31), by Professor K. Mather (John Murray, 1953).

Cytology, Genetics and Evolution (Association for Science Education, John Murray, 1973).

Questions

1 Two black guinea pigs are mated together on several occasions and their offspring are invariably black. However, when their black offspring are mated with white guinea pigs, half of the matings result in all black litters and the other half produce litters containing equal numbers of black and white babies.

From these results, deduce the genotypes of the parents and explain the results of the various matings, assuming that colour in this case is determined by a single pair of genes (alleles).

2 (a) What are the possible blood groups likely to be inherited by children born to a group A mother and group B father? Explain your reasoning.

(b) A woman of blood group A claims that a man of blood group AB is the father of her child. A blood test reveals that the child's blood group is O. Is it possible that the woman's claim is correct? Could the father have been a group B man? Explain your reasoning.

3 The first child born to a married couple with normal phenotypes is an albino. What are the chances that their second child will also be an albino? Explain your reasoning.

4 A woman whose blood group is O, Rh− marries a group AB, Rh + man. What are the possible blood groups of their children? Explain your reasoning.

5 Individuals of a pure-breeding line of *Drosophila* are exposed to X-rays to induce mutations in their gametes. Most mutated genes are recessive to normal genes. How could one find out if mutations had occurred?

6 Two black rabbits thought to be homozygous for coat colour were mated and produced a litter which contained all black babies. The F_2, however, resulted in some white babies which meant that one of the grandparents was heterozygous for coat colour. How could you find out, by breeding experiments, which parent was heterozygous?

22
Population Statistics

Censuses

Population means the number of people living in an area. The area may be a town or a district, a country or the whole world. To discover the number of people in a selected area it is necessary to take a census, and the practice of recording the numbers of people in a country was probably started by the Romans. A census was being taken throughout the Roman Empire at the time when Christ was born, and the records of populations have been taken for particular reasons ever since that time. 'Bills of Mortality' were required by law in Britain after the outbreaks of bubonic plague in the sixteenth century and these originally gave information about the numbers of people who had died each week from the disease. In the following century more detailed information was called for which included reference to the trade or profession of the person who had died, together with a note of their sex and age.

By 1758 the Swedish government had instituted a regular census and in 1839 the General Register Office was established in London to collect information about births, marriages and deaths throughout Britain. This information, although useful, as we shall see, did not disclose the size of population and it was only the institution of a national census taken every ten years that revealed not only the size of the population of Britain but the way in which it changed with the passage of time.

The scientific study of population changes is termed demography, and the information or data on which the study is based is obtained by a census, and by the registration of vital statistics (literally, the statistics of life). A modern census involves a counting of people either where they are on the day appointed for the census—a *de facto* census—or else according to where they usually live—a *de jure* census. The information is obtained either by sending people (called enumerators or canvassers) into the community to do the counting and write down the statistics of sex, age, occupation and so on, or else by the householder method, in which the head of a house is provided with a form on which he or she has to fill in all the statistics on the appointed day. In Britain the householder method is used at ten-year intervals. By 1961 it was realized that the rate of change of the population was such that ten years was too long to wait to bring certain pieces of information up-to-date, and in 1966 for the first time a subsidiary census was taken in which statistics were collected from 10 per cent of the population.

Vital statistics

The registration of births, marriages and deaths provides a continuous flow of information. Birth statistics provide at least information about the numbers of live births and stillborn infants (babies born dead) and the sex of each baby. This information may be related to the health and marital status (that is, married or unmarried) of the mother. Marriage records indicate the age and sex of the persons married and whether they have been married before or not. Death certificates carry not only the name of the dead person and details of where he died but the cause of death and, if this was due to a disease, how long the deceased had suffered from it. Where there is doubt about the cause of death, a post-mortem ('after death') examination is required to be carried out in most countries of the world and this examination must be done by qualified medical men. The World Health Organization has drawn up a classification of diseases, injuries and other causes of death with a view to standardizing the recording of death statistics throughout the world, but the classification suggested is not very detailed.

The information gained by the census and registration enables the *vital rates* to be calculated. These express the frequency of events such as birth or death in proportion to the total population.

The *crude birth rate* is the number of live births per 1 000 of the population per year. This is calculated from the total number of live births per year and the mid-year population, as follows:

$$\frac{\text{number of live births in a year}}{\text{population at the middle of that year}} \times 1\ 000$$

e.g. 900 live births in a population of 30 000 gives a crude birth rate of

$$\frac{900 \times 1\ 000}{30\ 000} = 30.$$

This information is essential if a country is to prepare for the education of its children and provide the right number of school places. If long-term planning is to be effective, it is necessary also to know the *fertility rate*. This is calculated as follows:

$$\frac{\text{number of live births in a given year}}{\text{number of women aged 15 to 45 in that year}} \times 1\ 000.$$

A population with a large proportion of young women in this

age group will have a higher fertility rate than one with a large number of elderly women, incapable of child-bearing.

The *specific fertility rate* gives a more detailed picture by showing the numbers of babies born to each 1 000 women in five-year age bands. Women in the 20- to 25-year-old age band are likely to have a higher fertility rate than those in the 40- to 45-year-old age band.

Fertility varies from one social group to another. Generally the better-educated members of a population have a lower fertility rate. This does not mean that they are biologically less able to produce children but that they feel there are reasons for limiting the size of the family. If the data obtained in a census include details of education, age and family size, then instead of talking of a 'general trend' it is possible to calculate a precise fertility rate for that group.

The *infant mortality rate* is a useful guide to the standards of hygiene and sanitation in a community. When the standard is poor, many young babies die, chiefly from intestinal diseases and respiratory infections. The infant mortality rate is calculated as follows:

$$\frac{\text{number of deaths in a given year of babies under 1 year old}}{\text{number of babies born in that year}} \times 1\ 000.$$

The infant mortality rate in Norway in 1970 was 12.8, in Britain 18.8; in Jamaica the rate was 30 and in Pakistan, 142. Merely to quote the rate can be misleading and does not indicate the fact that hurricanes and famine had very seriously disturbed life in Pakistan, resulting in outbreaks of diseases to which young babies are particularly vulnerable.

The information from death certificates is used firstly to calculate the *crude death rate*, which is:

$$\frac{\text{total number of deaths in a population}}{\text{total population at the middle of the year}} \times 1\ 000.$$

When compared with the crude birth rate, this figure shows whether a population is growing, stable or declining. Comparison of birth and death rates over a number of years gives the *rate of population change.*

The crude death rate is indeed crude in the sense that it gives no indication of whether people are dying in old age or in infancy, from disease or starvation or as the result of war. To study the first two of these factors, *age-specific mortality rates* have to be worked out. The method is similar to that used in calculating infant mortality, that is the number of deaths in a particular age group is related to the total number of persons in that age group.

When age-specific mortality rates are known, it is possible to construct life expectancy tables. Such tables were first used by people whose business was to sell life insurance. To do this it is necessary to calculate the customer's probability of dying before his next birthday and, from this, his *expectation of life.*

A *life table* starts with a population of 1 000 at birth. Knowing the age-specific mortality rate for the population concerned it is then possible to work out the numbers of people who are likely to survive at the end of each year of age, and therefore their expectation of life. The figures given below are part of a life table for males and females in Britain in the years 1866 and 1966, and represents how many more years the various age groups can expect to live.

Expectation of life at age	*1866*		*1966*	
	Males	*Females*	*Males*	*Females*
0	40.2	42.5	68.4	74.7
15	43.8	44.3	55.4	61.3
25	36.5	37.4	46.0	57.5
45	22.8	24.1	27.1	32.5
65	10.7	11.5	12.0	15.7

From this table it can be seen that over 100 years the expectation of life at the time of birth has risen dramatically whereas in middle age the increase in life expectancy is very much smaller. However, many more people are now surviving to middle and old age than in 1866.

The *increase* in the expectation of life at age 15 over the expectation at age 0 in both sexes in 1866 deserves comment. This reflects the high infant and child mortality rates of the time. Children who survived into adolescence, having avoided or recovered from such diseases as typhoid fever, tuberculosis, malaria and diphtheria, could indeed look forward to a better chance of surviving to middle age.

This change in life expectation is seen more clearly in the two graphs in Fig. 22.1. The graph or *population pyramid* for 1866 has a shape characteristic of a population with a high birth rate and a high infant mortality rate. Improvements in the standard of hygiene and sanitation in the intervening hundred years have reduced the infant and childhood mortality rates. The pyramid for 1966 shows a population that is ageing, with the death rate increasing rapidly above the age of 45. The reasons for this are discussed in Chapter 23. By superimposing the two pyramids, drawn to the same scale (Fig. 22.2), it can be seen that not only have the numbers of people in different age groups changed, but the total population, represented by the *area* of each pyramid, has increased. The population of every country in the world is believed to have increased in the last

Deaths in the United Kingdom: analysis by age and sex

	All ages	Under 1 year	1–4	5–9	10–14	15–19	20–24	25–34	35–44	45–54	55–64	65–74	75–84	85 and over
Males														
1902	340 664	87 242	37 834	8 429	4 696	7 047	8 766	19 154	24 749	30 488	37 610	39 765	28 320	6 563
1972	342 605	8 393	1 460	1 024	801	1 779	2 092	3 661	7 629	25 184	64 379	109 448	85 535	21 220
Females														
1902	322 058	68 770	36 164	8 757	5 034	6 818	8 264	18 702	21 887	25 679	34 821	42 456	34 907	10 099
1972	331 333	6 198	1 238	665	416	770	878	2 107	5 267	15 897	36 260	77 261	113 076	71 300

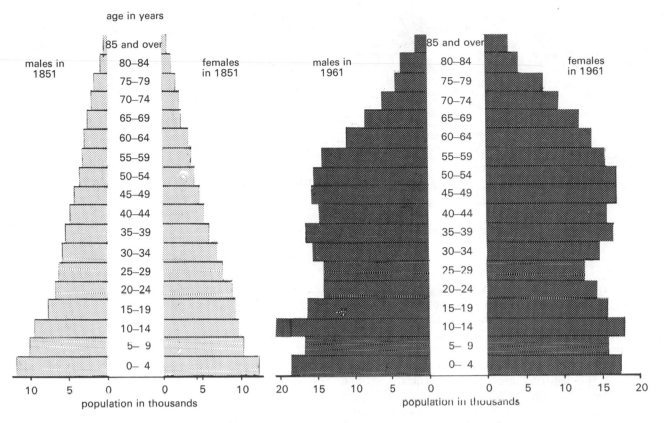

Fig. 22.1 Population pyramids showing the structure by age and sex of the population of England and Wales in 1851 and 1961

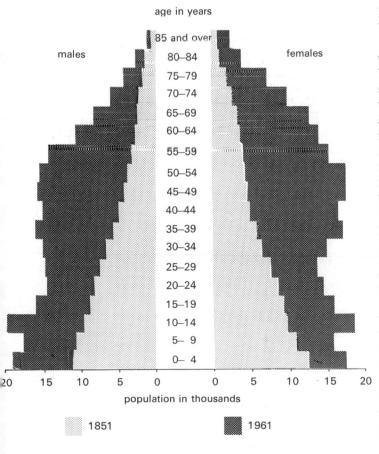

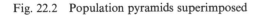

Fig. 22.2 Population pyramids superimposed

hundred years and in some countries the *rate* of increase has been much greater than in Britain.

When the population of a country increases, more food has to be produced to keep the people nourished. More houses also have to be built, with increased water supply and facilities for sewage disposal. More schools and hospitals are required. If the increase in food production and in the provision of housing and other facilities does not take place at the same rate as the increase in population then the *standard of living* falls. The information about population change and about the composition by age of the population enables a thoughtful government to plan ahead and try to provide facilities at the time when they will be needed. Thus if an increase in the birth rate is recorded, not only will there be more mouths to feed but more primary school places will be needed in five to seven years' time. On the other hand, resources of all kinds are limited. Farming methods have become more productive in many parts of the world but there seems to be no reason to believe that productivity will increase indefinitely.

In 1798 an English priest, the Reverend Thomas Malthus, wrote his *Essay on the Principle of Population*. His main theme was that a population would reproduce and increase in numbers by geometric progression, unless checked. Food supply for that population would only increase by arithmetic progression.

Geometric progression (or increase) is illustrated by the series 1, 2, 4, 8, 16, in which the numbers are *multiplied* by two at each step, and by the series 1, 4, 16, 64, 256, where each successive number is multiplied by four. *Arithmetic progression* is illustrated by the series 1, 2, 3, 4, 5, where one unit is *added* to each number, and by the series 1, 4, 7, 10, 13, where three units are added at each step (*see* Fig. 22.3).

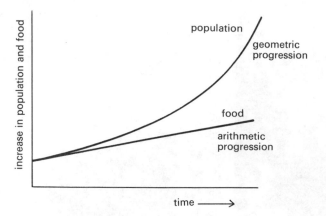

Fig. 22.3   A graphic comparison of geometric and arithmetic increase

In simple terms, Malthus said that food supply does not increase as rapidly as population. In fact, improvements in the methods of raising crops and rearing animals for food have increased productivity much more dramatically than Malthus would have predicted, but the population of many countries of the world continues to increase at rates that outstrip food production and this leads to undernourishment at least and often to death by starvation.

Charles Darwin was made aware of the Malthusian principle before he started to formulate his theory of evolution. He was impressed by the fertility rate (which he called reproductive capacity) of all species of animal and plant and said in his book *The Origin of Species*, 'There is no exception to the rule that every organic being naturally increases at so high a rate that if not destroyed, the earth would soon be covered by the progeny of a single pair'. He also recognized that there are many 'checks to increase' which limit the size of populations.

For human populations the checks have included disease and famine over which, until recent times, man had very little control. Even now his control is far from complete, but the degree to which the incidence of fatal diseases such as smallpox, cholera and malaria has been reduced since 1955 has resulted in an enormous increase in population throughout the tropics. With more mouths to be fed, the threat of starvation has increased. Starving people are not as well able to work and increase food production as healthy, well-fed people. While food shortage is indeed a check to population increase in animal communities, it is not a pleasant check to contemplate in human communities. The alternative is to restrict the number of births, either by refraining from sexual intercourse or by contraception (*see* Chapter 15, p. 109).

In an industrialized country such as Belgium the birth rate is controlled to such an extent that the population increases at the rate of 0.4 per cent per year. It would take 175 years for the population of Belgium to double at this rate of increase. The average population growth rate for tropical South America is 3 per cent, and at this rate the population will double in only 24 years, thus doubling the demand for food and other resources.

The effect on world population of the removal of some of the checks to increase of population, principally epidemic diseases, is shown in Fig. 22.4.

From about A.D. 1500, when awareness of the importance of pure water and the need to remove sewage, as well as a spread of knowledge of the technology of food production began to influence societies, the growth of world population has become very clearly geometric or exponential. One wonders what the next check to increase will be. Already shortage of food is checking population growth in many parts of the world. A check on the birth rate would enable the increase in food production to 'catch up' and improve the standard of living of those surviving in the world.

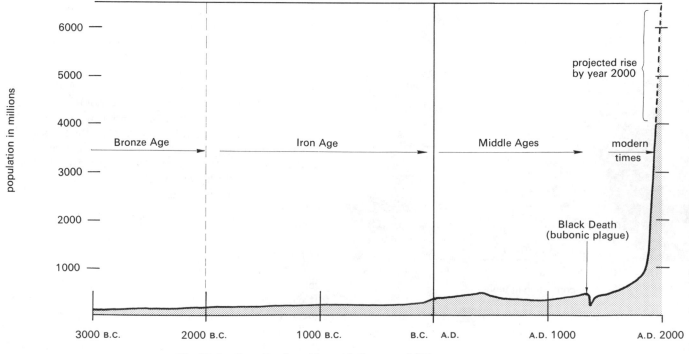

Fig. 22.4   Growth of world population over 5 000 years

Practical Work

Experiment 1   Censuses

Carry out a census among the pupils in your class. Start out with a census of family size, that is the number of children in each family. Plot the results in the form of a histogram or bar graph (*see* Fig. 22.5).

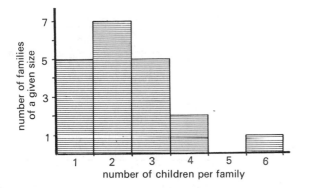

Fig. 22.5   Distribution of family size in class of twenty-four London schoolboys

Experiment 2

The mean family size can be calculated by multiplying the numbers of families in each group by the number of children in that group, adding the scores together and dividing by the total number of families. Thus:

No. of families		No. of children		
5	×	1	=	5
7	×	2	=	14
5	×	3	=	15
2	×	4	=	8
0	×	5	=	0
1	×	6	=	6

Total   48 ÷ 20 families = 2·4

The mean family size is 2·4 children for this group.

Experiment 3

Collect information about the age structure of the population in your road or village. Don't be too ambitious and attempt to collect information about too large a group. Find out how many people there are in five-year age groups, 0–5, 6–10, 11–15, and so on, and construct either a histogram or a population pyramid. Compare your results with the surveys carried out by other children in your class. Are there more children, or more people aged 60 or over in some streets than in others?

Questions

1 Why is the infant mortality rate usually considered separately from the general death rate of a population? Outline the factors that influence infant mortality in your country.

2 The population in the United Kingdom was 38 327 000 in 1902 and had increased to 55 798 000 by 1972. Use the table on page 186 and suggest why the total number of deaths in both years is almost the same. In which age group has the reduction in death rate between 1902 and 1972 been greatest?

23

Keeping Health Records

Notifiable diseases

Health authorities in most countries require doctors and other medical workers to send in reports of certain illnesses. Consequently these illnesses, which represent serious dangers to the community, have come to be known as *notifiable diseases*. Examples of these include

cholera	scarlet fever	diphtheria
smallpox	plague	typhoid fever
relapsing fever	typhus	yellow fever.

Of these diseases, outbreaks of cholera, plague, relapsing fever, smallpox, typhus and yellow fever must be reported to the World Health Organization. It is recognized that they can very easily be transmitted from one country to another and only by international co-operation can their spread be checked.

Epidemiology

Disease records are of limited use if they tell no more than the number of cases occurring in a given year. Information is needed about where the case occurred and at what time of year. The age, sex and occupation of the patient also enable a more detailed picture to be drawn up. *Epidemiology* is the study of such disease statistics and it can provide enormous support in planning preventive measures. Originally epidemiology was concerned with the study of those communicable diseases that give rise to epidemics. An *epidemic* is the occurrence of a number of cases of a disease very much in excess of what would normally be expected.

Bacillary dysentery is said to be an *endemic* disease in Britain because it is always present at least at a low level among the population. Each summer the number of reported cases increases, usually to *epidemic* proportions. Cholera, on the other hand, was once endemic in Britain but is now exceedingly rare. However, in Asia generally and in India in particular cholera is *endemic* and frequently *epidemic*. Occasionally the disease spreads from one country to another until one continent or more is affected. The disease outbreak is then said to be *pandemic*. Influenza provides an even more striking example of a disease that reaches pandemic proportions (*see* p. 222).

An early example of the value of the epidemiological approach is seen in the work of Dr. Snow on cholera in London in the 1840s and 50s. From observations, he felt convinced that cholera was spread by contaminated drinking water (*see* p. 205). The provision of water supply was in the hands of private companies such as the Southwark & Vauxhall Co. and the Lambeth Water Co. which drew water from the river Thames to supply south London. Much of London's sewage ran into the Thames which was, in consequence, heavily polluted. During the years 1849–1852 the Lambeth Water Co. moved its works upstream to Thames Ditton where the river water was uncontaminated. The Southwark & Vauxhall Co. continued to draw water from the Thames at Battersea where the level of pollution was high (Fig. 23.1).

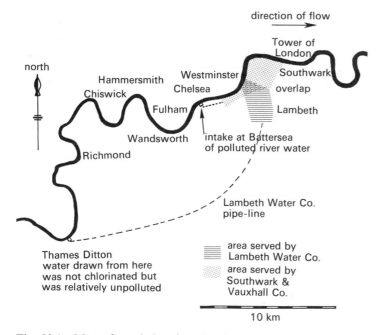

Fig. 23.1 Map of south London showing the areas served by the Lambeth Water Co. and the Southwark & Vauxhall Water Co. and their water intakes

During the summer of 1853 there was a cholera epidemic in south London and Snow observed that the districts served by the Lambeth Water Co. were almost entirely free of the disease, whereas the districts taking water from the Southwark & Vauxhall Co. had a death rate from cholera of 114 per 100 000. Some areas were supplied with water by both companies and in these the death rate was 60 per 100 000. While giving a lead, this evidence was not conclusive.

The area served by the Southwark & Vauxhall Co. was a more crowded, working-class area than the well-to-do areas of Lambeth, and Snow realized that overcrowding might itself be a factor in the spread of the disease. Besides, the 60 per 100 000 death rate in the areas with two water suppliers was puzzling. Snow discovered that, since a charge was made for piped water, there was competition for custom between the two companies in the marginal areas between the two boards. When a further cholera outbreak occurred in 1854 he discovered the address of each person who died of the disease and visited their houses to find out from which company they took their water. He then found out the total number of houses served by each company and calculated the death rate from cholera per 10 000 houses.

Water company	Number of houses supplied	Number of deaths from cholera July–August 1854	Death rate per 10 000 houses
Southwark & Vauxhall	40 046	286	71
Lambeth	26 107	14	5
All other water companies in London	287 345	277	9

This showed a death rate from cholera in homes supplied by the Southwark & Vauxhall Co. which was fourteen times greater than that in homes served by the Lambeth Co., although in earlier years, before the company moved its works, the cholera deaths in Lambeth had been at as high a rate as anywhere in London. Snow deduced that a micro-organism breeding in the gut and spread in faeces to drinking water was responsible for the disease. This deduction was made thirty years before Robert Koch identified the cholera vibrio (p. 196).

The marking on a map of the location of cases of a disease is now a standard method of studying the pattern of spread of epidemic diseases, whether within a town or a state or across a continent. Such maps are called *spot maps* or *dot maps* (Fig. 23.2). These often enable the source of a disease to be traced.

The incidence of a particular disease may be studied in relation to social class. In Britain the Registrar-General's

Fig. 23.2 World Health officials map the distribution of an insect vector of disease before planning a campaign to control its spread
(WHO

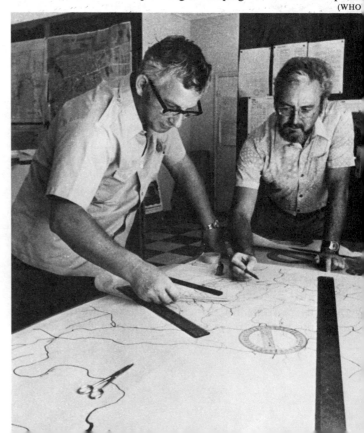

Occupation Classification gives a useful reference base (*see* table below).

Class	Description	Percentage of male employed population
I	Higher professional; doctors, lawyers, managers of large organizations	3.6
II	Minor professions; businessmen, school-teachers, farmers	14.5
III	Skilled occupations; clerical and manual, requiring training	48.6
IV	Semi-skilled; factory and agricultural workers	19.8
V	Unskilled workers; labourers	8.7

The histogram in Fig. 23.3 shows clearly that unskilled labourers have a five times greater death rate from bronchitis than top professional and administrative men, and one may well wonder whether they take less care over their health, are less well nourished or are more exposed to factors influencing

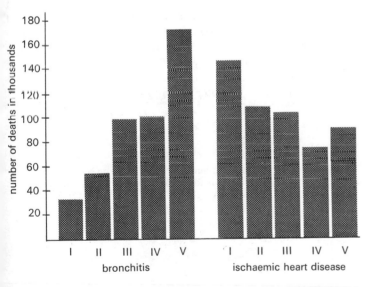

Fig. 23.3   Social class and the occurrence of death from bronchitis and ischaemic heart disease in men aged 20–64 years, England and Wales, 1951

the development of bronchitis. Ischaemic heart disease means disease involving a reduction in the blood supply to the heart muscle. It may result from thrombosis in the coronary artery (p. 79) or from a thickening of the wall of the coronary artery, reducing the size of the passage through it. Here, top executives are nearly twice as much at risk as men in social classes IV and V. Factors believed to influence ischaemic heart disease include mental stress, obesity (overweight), cigarette smoking and lack of exercise. It seems likely that men in social class V will take more exercise in their daily routine than businessmen sitting at

their desks, and they may well have less to worry them and cause mental stress than top executives. Cigarette smoking habits offer a conflicting picture and provide an opportunity to study yet another kind of health record.

In 1950 Prof. Doll and Dr Hill published the result of a survey designed to test the hypothesis that cigarette smoking and lung cancer were associated. They looked at the case histories of patients suffering from lung cancer and found out about their smoking habits. The figures for this group were compared with those for a control group of otherwise similar men, not suffering from lung cancer.

	Lung-cancer patients	Control group
Cigarette smokers	99.7%	95.8%
Non-smokers	0.3%	4.2%

This table suggests some connection, but the fact that the control group contained 95.8 per cent of cigarette smokers who were *not* suffering from lung cancer was confusing. A further investigation into the number of cigarettes smoked per day by men in each group produced the following results.

	Lung-cancer patients	Control group
Non-smokers	0.3%	4.2%
Smokers		
1– 4 cigarettes per day	5.1%	8.5%
5–14 ,, ,,	38.5%	45.1%
15–24 ,, ,,	30.2%	29.3%
More than 24	25.9%	12.9%

This shows that among the patients suffering from lung cancer a high proportion are heavy smokers. These figures do not prove that smoking causes lung cancer, since heavy smokers in the control group clearly did not suffer from the disease. However, it provided the sort of evidence that encouraged a different kind of survey. The previous investigations depended on information gained retrospectively, that is, from the past. Doll and Hill now chose to study the smoking habits of doctors whose names they took from the Medical Register. Having recorded their smoking habits at the time (1951) they proceeded to make continuous records of the pulmonary health of the group over the next few years, relying on the fact that doctors usually consult another doctor when they are ill. The death rate from lung cancer in this group or *cohort* over a five-year period is shown in the table below.

	Deaths from lung cancer per year per 100 000 doctors
Non-smokers	7
Light smokers	47
Moderate smokers	86
Heavy smokers	166

These figures, based on the doctors' assessment of their smoking habits *before* lung cancer was diagnosed, suggest a strong association between lung cancer and the amount a man smokes. The heavy smokers were 23 times more at risk than the non-smoking doctors.

Records of behaviour of vectors

Finally, records of climate and the breeding habits of a disease vector (Chapter 31) may lead to the development of methods of controlling a disease. Romans have known for centuries that the incidence of malaria in their city was high during the hot summer months. Wealthy Romans left the city to spend that period in villas high up in the nearby hills where malaria was, if not unknown, never spread from one person to another. We now know that the particular species of anopheline mosquito that transmits malarial parasites in central Italy will only complete its breeding cycle to produce new, adult mosquitoes when the temperature of the water in which the larvae develop is at least 15 °C. A combination of too low a water temperature for larval development and a night temperature too low for the adult mosquitos to fly in search of blood meals keeps the vector away from the hill villages.

Sometimes man is himself the carrier of disease from place to place. This is true for cholera epidemics (Chapter 29), and for smallpox. In Africa, smallpox is endemic only in the Sudan and Ethiopia. Records show that the greatest frequency of new cases occurs between January and March. The rainy season extends from September to early December as a rule and during this time the incidence of smallpox is known to be lowest. During the rains many roads are impassable and the movement of population is low. After the rains people start to move from one area to another again and the rise in the figures for smallpox infection coincides with this renewed travelling. If smallpox cases could be identified, treated and cured during the rainy season when the incidence is lower then it should be possible to wipe out smallpox as an endemic disease in Africa.

Practical Work

Experiment 1

In most countries people 'catch cold' at any time of year. Keep a record of the people in your class who catch cold, noting the month (or the week) in which they develop a cold. You might be able to obtain records for people catching colds in more than one class, perhaps in the whole school, if you make it a team effort.

Having collected your records for a year construct a histogram or bar graph to show the incidence of colds over the year. You will have to be persistent to collect records for the holiday period. Fig. 23.4 shows a histogram for a group of fifty boys over one year in a London school.

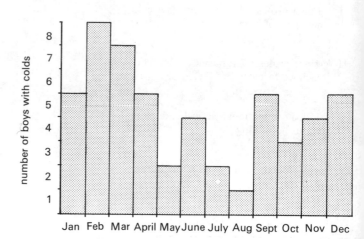

Fig. 23.4   Number of boys in a group of fifty suffering from colds each month over a period of a year

Experiment 2

You can carry out such a survey for any other illness that affects your group. You can also compare the incidence of illness in the first three weeks and the last three weeks of any term. Very often the 'score' for the first three weeks is the higher, at a time when everyone should be fresh and fit from the holidays. If this is so in your class can you suggest why this should be? Perhaps Chapter 32 will give you some ideas.

Question

Not all the people who die from lung cancer are cigarette smokers and this is sometimes used as an argument in favour of encouraging smoking. What facts justify a campaign against smoking?

24

Health and Disease

Good health is something that many of us take for granted. It is much more than an absence of disease; it involves a state of physical well-being in which all the organs of the body function efficiently. It also involves *feeling* well, both in body and in mind. We may become too concerned about small ailments and develop a feeling of being unwell. Worry about school, work or friendships or indeed worry about anything is likely to affect health, and such a state of ill-health requires medical attention as much as an illness such as tuberculosis.

For our physical well-being we require a balanced diet (*see* p. 37) in adequate quantity, safe drinking water and living conditions that are clean and not overcrowded.

Disease is not easy to define. If a person suffers from influenza then his body temperature will be above the normal 37 °C (the average daily temperature of people living in most countries) and he will probably have a headache as well as aches in his back and limbs. He will *feel* ill. A person suffering from tuberculosis, on the other hand, may have a persistent cough or may not feel very strong, but he is able to do work that does not require physical effort and he probably will not complain of feeling ill. Both influenza and tuberculosis are diseases in which parts of the body do not function normally or efficiently and both are the result of the invasion of the body by micro-organisms which, since they cause signs and symptoms of disease to develop, are called *pathogens*. Signs of disease can be seen by a doctor or a trained observer and may include such features as a skin rash, profuse sweating or diarrhoea. Symptoms are felt by the patient suffering from the disease and have to be described by him. A doctor cannot see or measure a pain and he relies on the patient to tell him where it is and whether it is acute or not. Influenza and tuberculosis are caused by pathogenic organisms which can be transmitted to other people. Because of this they are both described as infectious diseases.

In contrast to the large group of diseases caused by transmissible pathogens there are many others that cannot be transferred or caught.

Type of disease	Examples
Transmissible	
1 Diseases caused by micro-organisms	influenza; cholera
Non-transmissible	
2 Metabolic disorders	diabetes; phenylketonuria
3 Nutritional deficiency diseases	kwashiorkor; beriberi
4 Degenerative disease	arthritis; coronary heart disease
5 Cancer	breast cancer; leukaemia
6 Mental illness	depression; schizophrenia

Metabolic disorders

The disease phenylketonuria has already been discussed in Chapter 20 as due to the inheritance of defective genes. Haemophilia is another disease condition resulting from a defective gene. In this case the gene controlling the production of one of the factors enabling blood to clot fails to act and, as a result, an affected person may lose a great deal of blood from quite a small cut. This gene is carried on the X chromosome, one of the chromosomes determining the sex of an individual, and the disease is said to be sex-linked.

Diabetes is the name given to a condition in which the body is unable to regulate the concentration of glucose in the blood plasma. It results from a failure of the islet cells in the pancreas to produce the hormone insulin. Secretion of the hormone in a healthy person normally follows an increase in the concentration of blood glucose and it stimulates cells in the liver to convert excessive glucose to an insoluble compound called glycogen. If excessive sugar cannot be stored it is excreted by the kidneys. The name *diabetes mellitus* reflects the fact that urine of a diabetic is sweet, due to the presence of sugar. Diabetes can be serious in itself but it also increase the patient's

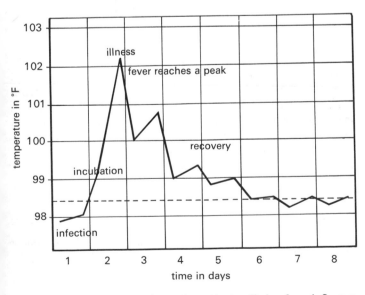

Fig. 24.1   Temperature chart of a patient suffering from influenza

susceptibility to tuberculosis and to disorders of the retina of the eye, leading to blindness.

Diabetes is certainly a disorder of the metabolism. It is not clear whether it is an inherited condition. At the present time it is believed that the tendency to develop diabetes is inherited, though some other factor is probably necessary to 'trigger off' the condition.

Nutritional deficiency diseases have been described in Chapter 6 and it is only necessary to add that an inadequate or unbalanced diet may result in a person being more susceptible to other kinds of disease. Thus the skin eruptions and slow healing that result from a shortage of ascorbic acid, vitamin C, in the diet may lead to infection by bacteria that would not cause harm to a healthy skin.

Better feeding and improved medical services reduce the likelihood of death from transmissible disease but, by enabling people to live longer, create situations in which the tissues of the body have time to degenerate. Thus in European communities the incidence of coronary thrombosis has increased during this century and it is most prevalent among the age group 45–65. A century ago the number of people living through this age range was little more than half what it is today.

Understanding of the nature and cause of cancer is increasing as more is discovered about the way in which cell division is controlled. Epidemiological studies (*see* p. 189) suggest that there is a relationship between the incidence of certain forms of cancer and chemicals which are thought to induce abnormal cell division. These chemicals that induce cancer are called *carcinogens*. Thus the tars that are distilled out of burning tobacco and inhaled during smoking are associated with a higher incidence of lung cancer in heavy smokers than in non-smokers, and also with cancer of the digestive tract and bladder. This is not to say that non-smokers are immune to such cancers, but that they appear to be significantly less likely to develop them. The cancer-producing (carcinogenic) effect of such tars has long since been demonstrated on laboratory animals.

Cancer occurs most commonly in those tissues in which cell division is a normal activity. Such tissues include the skin, where cell division ensures the replacement of cells that are worn away by physical contact; the liver, in which cells damaged during the detoxication of poisonous substances are replaced; and all kinds of epithelium or lining cells, such as those lining the stomach and bladder, which are also worn away during normal activity.

Mental health is quite as important as physical health though it is not as easy to define. Just as our bodies grow and develop through childhood and adolescence to maturity, so our minds and emotions develop. As babies and small children we are very dependent on our parents and other adults to provide not only food and physical protection but also emotional protection and affection. As we grow older and particularly when we enter the period of development called adolescence we feel increasingly independent of adults and often resent having our behaviour controlled by them. Most of us, however, would like to feel that somebody cares about our welfare. If we are fortunate, the concern expressed by our parents, which includes training and disciplining us during childhood, changes as we become more responsible for our own actions. They are still responsible, legally as well as emotionally, for our well-being and development but allow us increasing freedom. Views and ideas and behaviour patterns are challenged and if we ourselves are wise we do not assume that ours is the only possible 'right' view or behaviour. We should not be forced into complete submission to the authority of parents or of school. Ideally we should accept limits on our freedom to do absolutely what we want, when we want. Excessive restraint or repression generates emotional tension and mental stress and prevents full development. We are quite ready to believe this but are usually less willing to believe that life without any restraints can also result in emotional immaturity.

Always we have to adjust to living with other people, at any age. Failure or inability to do so leads to reactions in our minds. Mental illness is no more easy to define than mental health. Certainly it does *not* as a rule mean madness. We are *all* as likely to suffer from some form or other of mental illness as from the common cold, and just as likely to recover. In much the same way that mild colds pass unnoticed by most other people, so most mental illness such as slight depression or unreasonable behaviour is noticed only by people who observe us closely. On the other hand a person who is so depressed that he is unable to perform his daily work adequately is seen to be ill. If he is given appropriate medical treatment he is likely to recover his former good spirits, and acquaintances will say that he is normal again.

The many forms of mental disorder can be classified as follows.

1 **Disorders due to a failure in normal development** arising from genetic factors; virus infections affecting the mother during pregnancy and affecting the foetus; severe deficiencies in diet; or hormonal abnormalities, e.g. cretinism. Each of these may result in subnormal emotional and intellectual development.

2 **Disorders following a reaction to internal or external stress.** These include depressive illness, hysteria, drug addiction and alcoholism, but a detailed consideration of these is beyond the scope of this book.

The precise way in which stress, such as overcrowding, worry about financial or domestic matters or about status, can cause the disorders listed under (2) is not clear but they may result from overactivity of the pituitary and adrenal glands in response to particular patterns of activity in brain cells.

Practical Work

Follow up the survey suggested on page 192 by making a list of the members of your class at school and the illnesses from which they have suffered. Draw a histogram to show which diseases occur most frequently. Which diseases may affect a person more than once?

Question

Suggest reasons why the *number* of people suffering from most forms of cancer is increasing throughout the world whereas the number suffering from tuberculosis is falling steadily.

25

Organisms that Cause Disease

The possible connection between living organisms and the incidence of disease has been a matter of speculation for a long time. Fracastorius in 1546 suggested that syphilis was caused by a *contagium vivam*—a live contact.

It is likely that the first person to observe micro-organisms was the Dutchman, Van Leeuwenhoek, who first described 'little animals' (animalcules) in the scrapings from his teeth, about 1676, and noted that these organisms did not move if the scrapings were taken just after drinking hot coffee.

Both before and after Leeuwenhoek's time, theories were advanced to account for the appearance of maggots in rotting flesh and, indeed, to account for decomposition itself. Spallanzani is credited with having established that the breakdown of organic liquids depends on the introduction of live organisms from the air. Both he and Louis Pasteur, nearly a century later, conducted experiments to test the hypothesis that decay was brought about by micro-organisms. If these organisms were prevented from reaching the organic material then decay would not take place. At this time such a theory was revolutionary and met considerable opposition, particularly when extended to suggest that similar minute organisms were the cause of many diseases.

The connection between disease and micro-organisms did emerge, slowly. Robert Koch carried out investigations of the diseases anthrax and tuberculosis and showed that each disease was caused by a particular organism. In 1884 he summarized his findings in a series of statements known now as *Koch's postulates*.

1 The organism must be observed in *every* case of the disease.

2 The organism must be capable of isolation in a pure culture (*see* below).

3 The disease can be produced in a suitable experimental animal by injecting it with the pure culture.

4 The organism can be recovered in pure culture from the diseased experimental animal.

Koch devised methods for the culturing of bacteria including the use of gelatin with suitable nutrients to form a solid, easily handled material. One of his assistants, Petri, produced the glass vessel known as the Petri dish, which is still widely used.

Koch introduced the idea of a *pure culture*, that is a dish with a colony of a single kind of organism, uncontaminated by any other organism.

Within the last hundred years knowledge of the range of organisms that cause disease has increased enormously. Pasteur could speak of microbes, but we must distinguish between bacteria, spirochaetes, rickettsiae, viruses, fungi and protozoans, all of which are very small.

Bacteria

Structure. Bacteria are very small organisms, each being a living cell. Most bacteria are between 0.0005 mm and 0.002 mm long and they rarely exceed 0.01 mm in length. They are therefore visible only under a high-power microscope. A cell wall is present, made of protein and fatty substances. It encloses the cytoplasm and the nuclear or genetic material. Since the latter is not enclosed in a membrane, we cannot call it a nucleus (*see* Fig. 25.1).

Different kinds of bacteria show a range of shapes (*see* Fig. 25.2). Certain kinds possess long thread-like structures called flagella which produce movement, though many other kinds of bacteria, especially vibrios, can move about. Whether they move or not, all bacteria must respire; most use oxygen, respiring aerobically, while others, including several of the *pathogenic* or disease-causing bacteria, respire anaerobically.

All bacteria reproduce by fission, dividing into two. While this may not seem a spectacular rate of increase it is as well to remember that, in ideal conditions of warmth, food supply and disposal of waste products, certain bacteria may reproduce at intervals of only twenty minutes. Calculate the number of bacteria derived from one as a result of dividing three times each hour for twenty-four hours; is it so surprising that symptoms of bacterial disease, such as a sore throat, can

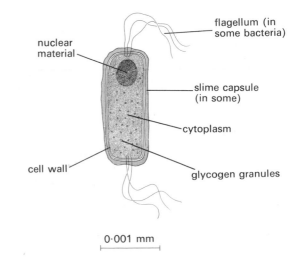

Fig. 25.1 Generalized diagram of a bacterium

literally develop overnight? In fact we usually develop symptoms of disease after being infected by millions of bacteria at one time.

The simpler bacteria may be classified as cocci when they are spherical, bacilli when cylindrical, vibrios when comma-shaped and spirilla when they are spirals that do not move (*see* Fig. 25.2*a*).

Activities. Most bacteria live in water, soil and in decaying matter. In these situations they feed on dead organic material and are called *saprophytes*. They secrete enzymes that digest the food material, which is then absorbed through the cell wall to be used inside the bacterial cell. We may find such activity a nuisance when it results in the decomposition of stored food, but in nature it is the means of bringing about the breakdown and recycling of dead material (*see* Chapter 8).

Certain kinds of bacteria are found in the intestines of animals, including man, where they may be beneficial in producing vitamins B_{12} and K. Other gut bacteria may cause diseases such as *cholera*. Still other bacteria are exploited in the making of cheese and yoghurt, while the oxidation of ethanol to ethanoic (acetic) acid, as in the souring of wine, was one of the bacterial activities investigated by Pasteur. An understanding of the role of bacteria in spoiling food is essential if food is to be preserved in a state fit for eating (p. 243).

Spirochaetes

Although spiral in shape, like spirilla, these organisms differ from most other bacteria by being motile (capable of moving of their own accord) and able to bend their shape. They are all pathogenic and include *Treponema* (Fig. 27.5), which cause syphilis.

Rickettsiae

These are smaller than most bacteria and vary in shape from spheres to thin rods, up to 0.002 mm in length. They are bacteria like in that they are visible under the light microscope, and are similar in structure to the bacteria shown in Fig. 25.2, having similar genetic material. However, like viruses, they are capable of growing only within living cells, and are therefore total parasites. Different species of *Rickettsia* cause the various forms of typhus.

Viruses

Viruses are even smaller than bacteria and rickettsiae, and most of our knowledge of their structure has been gained by studying them under the electron microscope (Fig. 25.2*b*). They differ from bacteria also in having only one nucleic acid in their genetic material, either DNA or RNA, but not both.

Viruses can only reproduce inside living cells. After the virus has entered a suitable cell, the nucleic acid of the virus takes over from the cell nucleus and acts on the cytoplasm, causing it to make new virus material instead of the substances that would normally be produced.

Once established in the body the virus is likely to be dispersed in the blood and transported to so-called *target cells*. In the case of the common cold, these include the epithelium of the nasal cavity, where the cells respond by producing a watery mucus and breaking down the cell membrane, resulting in a 'running' nose. Viruses are very specific, that is they usually affect only one host and, often, only certain tissues. Thus the virus of myxomatosis that is fatal to rabbits has no effect on man, and rabbits do not catch colds!

Fungi

Most of the fungi are saprophytes and these include several useful moulds, such as *Penicillium*, from which antibiotics are extracted. Pathogenic fungi are not numerous and we shall only consider one group causing infection of the skin, and another infecting the mouth, throat and vagina (Fig. 25.3).

Ringworm or tinea appears as athlete's foot between the

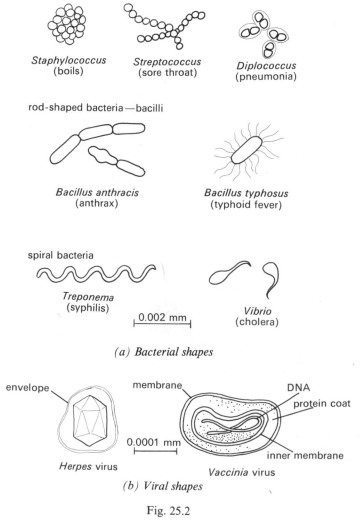

spherical bacteria—cocci

Staphylococcus
(boils)

Streptococcus
(sore throat)

Diplococcus
(pneumonia)

rod-shaped bacteria—bacilli

Bacillus anthracis
(anthrax)

Bacillus typhosus
(typhoid fever)

spiral bacteria

Treponema
(syphilis)

0.002 mm

Vibrio
(cholera)

(a) Bacterial shapes

envelope

membrane

DNA

protein coat

0.0001 mm

inner membrane

Herpes virus

Vaccinia virus

(b) Viral shapes

Fig. 25.2

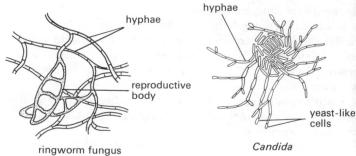

hyphae

hyphae

reproductive body

yeast-like cells

ringworm fungus

Candida

Fig. 25.3 Pathogenic fungi

toes, as dhobie itch in the groin, and is usually referred to simply as ringworm elsewhere on the body. Branched threads or *hyphae* of the fungus are found in the epidermis where their secretions produce dermatitis, an inflammation and irritation of the skin. Such infections are not dangerous in themselves, but by damaging the skin may open the way for other infections.

A group of yeast-like fungi called *Candida* are often present in the mouth and vagina where, like many other kinds of organisms, they only produce disease symptoms when the patient has a lowered resistance. Both groups of fungi form spores by which the organism can be dispersed to new hosts.

Protozoans

These are very small single-celled animals which abound in fresh water and moist soil, and were certainly seen by the early microscopists, Leeuwenhoek and Hooke. Most protozoa ingest small particles of solid food, much as *Amoeba* does, while others, like the malarial parasite, absorb nutrients through the cell membrane. They reproduce asexually by dividing into two, though some also have more complex patterns of sexual reproduction. Here we are concerned only with those protozoa that are pathogenic and parasitic in man (Fig. 25.4).

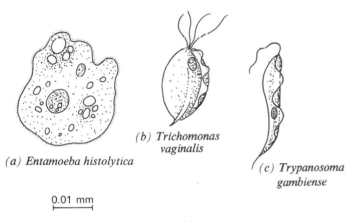

(a) *Entamoeba histolytica*

(b) *Trichomonas vaginalis*

(c) *Trypanosoma gambiense*

0.01 mm

Fig. 25.4 Parasitic protozoa

Entamoeba histolytica is smaller than most free-living amoebae and is visible only under a high-power microscope. It is usually taken into the body in contaminated drinking water and once in the large intestine begins to feed on the bacteria which are normally found there. It may remain feeding harmlessly in this way, or it may invade the epithelium lining the intestine and cause ulceration. This leads to bleeding and the parasites then feed on the red cells. Pain and acute diarrhoea result, the chief symptoms of amoebic dysentery, and in chronic cases, anaemia may follow. Those entamoebae that remain feeding among the bacteria inside the gut may encyst by secreting a material which 'sets' to produce a wall that, when the cyst is shed with the faeces of the host, protects the animal inside against drying up. Such cysts may remain viable (capable of becoming active again) for several weeks. No further activity takes place until the cyst is swallowed by a suitable host, when the wall is dissolved away in the small intestine and the parasite resumes activity.

Trichomonas vaginalis is a smaller protozoan (0.015 mm) that may be found in the vagina, where it causes an inflammation and irritation termed vaginitis. In human males it may cause urethritis when living in the urethra. Like *Entamoeba*,

it reproduces by fission, but does not form cysts. It is usually spread during sexual intercourse and vaginitis (and urethritis) is thus termed a venereal disease. Unlike the organisms causing two other, serious, venereal diseases, gonorrhoea and syphilis, *Trichomonas* may remain active in mucus or water on lavatory seats and towels for several days.

Trypanosoma is a protozoan with one flagellum. It is found in the blood stream and is transmitted from one host to another by the bite of a blood-sucking insect. The tsetse fly spreads the trypanosome of African sleeping sickness. After being sucked in with a meal of blood the protozoan works its way from the stomach of the fly to its salivary glands. Parasites are then injected with saliva through the skin of a new host as the fly prepares to suck blood again. Occasionally parasites are transmitted on the outside of the mouthparts of biting insects after feeding on the blood of an infected person.

Chagas' disease, from which Charles Darwin suffered, occurs in Central and South America and is caused by a trypanosome transmitted by blood-sucking bugs. This species of *Trypanosoma* leaves the blood stream to settle and develop in muscle tissue, frequently in heart muscle.

Plasmodium, the malarial parasite, is another protozoan living in the blood stream and liver cells in infected humans. It has a much more complex life cycle than any of the pathogens so far discussed. Like *Trypanosoma*, it is transmitted by a biting insect, in this case an adult female mosquito, but unlike *Trypanosoma*, it is obliged to undergo parts of its life cycle in the body of the mosquito. This aspect is discussed in Chapter 29, but at this stage it is sufficient to say that after injection of infected mosquito saliva into the human blood stream, the parasite is carried to the liver where it multiplies without producing any malarial symptoms. If released from liver cells into the blood stream the parasites penetrate red cells in which they multiply further by repeated division. This stage in red cells may take 48 or 72 hours to complete, depending on the species of *Plasmodium*. Accordingly, since the cycles of fever are spread over three or four days, the disease conditions are called tertian and quartan malaria. The patient reacts to the poisonous waste products (toxins) that are released with the parasites when the red cells containing them burst (*see* Fig. 29.3).

Roundworms or nematodes

Most roundworms are free-living in soil and water. Quite a number are responsible for diseases of plants and animals. The rather small number of species that cause disease in humans do, however, affect large populations in many countries.

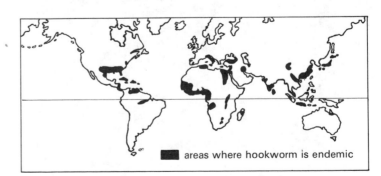

■ areas where hookworm is endemic

Fig. 25.5 World-wide distribution of hookworm

Pathogenic roundworms vary in size from *Ascaris* (Fig. 25.8), a parasite of the small intestine that may attain a length of 30 cm or more, to the microfilariae, larval stages of such animals as *Wucheria* that are only 0.25 mm long. Members of different species are very similar in structure.

The sites of attack vary; in the gut, *Ascaris* and particularly the hookworms *Ancylostoma* (Figs. 25.6 and 25.7) and *Necator* cause serious harm.

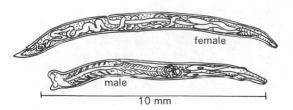

Fig. 25.6   *Ancylostoma duodenale*, hookworm

Filarial worms invade the lymphatic vessels and cause elephantiasis, while Guinea worms penetrate the skin and connective tissues. These differences in choice of site for invasion may reflect diversity in the physiology of these parasites.

Roundworms have a life cycle in six stages: egg, four larval stages, and an adult stage which is often referred to as the fifth stage. The end of each larval stage is marked by the moulting of the cuticle or outer covering. Hookworms, which are notorious, widespread parasites, are free-living in water as first and second stage larvae and only in the third stage are they infective. They are then able to enter the human host, by boring their way through the skin of feet and ankles of people wading in infected water or walking through vegetation or on damp soil. Once inside the skin they enter the blood and lymphatic systems and are swept along to the lungs. Leaving the capillaries, they enter the alveoli and are carried in the mucus stream and by coughing to the oesophagus and, if swallowed,

Fig. 25.7   Head of *Ancyclostoma duodenale*, showing hooks

(Wellcome Museum of Medical Science)

develop to become active egg-laying adults in the gut. They pierce the lining of the gut and suck blood, causing anaemia if they are numerous and the infection is unchecked. Carelessness over defaecation in fields, gardens and waterways enables the eggs to be dispersed and the life cycle to be continued.

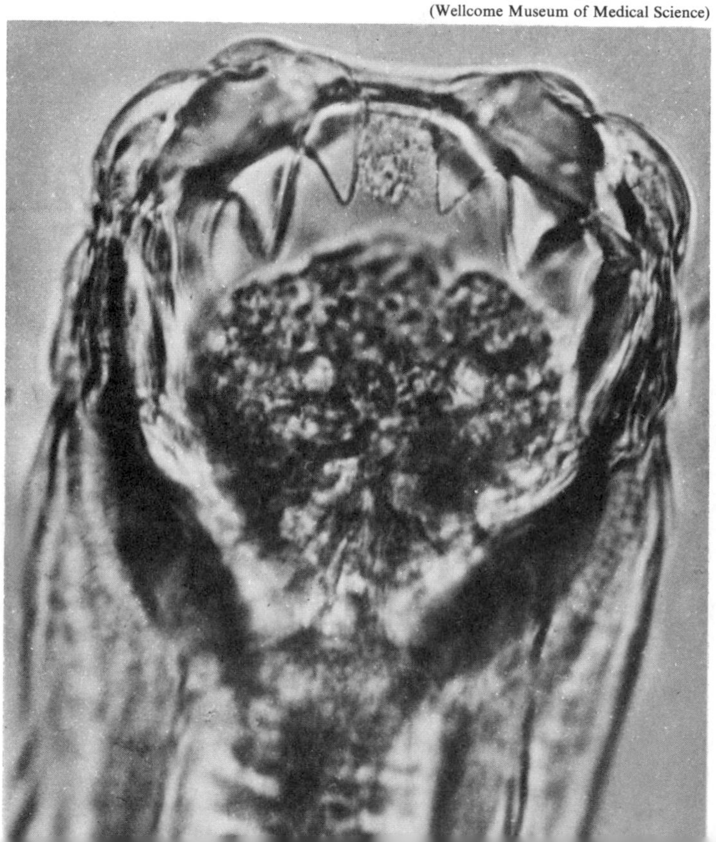

Ascaris eggs are shed in human faeces and the first larval stage is completed before the egg hatches. If an egg is swallowed with contaminated food then the 'shell' is dissolved and the stage two larva enters the blood stream through the mucous membrane. As with hookworm, the larva is carried to the lungs to emerge into an alveolus and be carried in the mucus to be swallowed again.

Heavy infections result in damage to the lungs, causing haemorrhage, and in the intestine may cause obstruction as well as producing toxic wastes to which the host reacts.

Adult filarial worms are found chiefly in the lymphatic system, though the larvae (referred to as microfilariae) may live for long periods in the blood stream where they seem to be relatively harmless. Worms in the lymphatic system cause damage in two chief ways.

Firstly they produce antigens (*see* p. 74) that produce an immunological response by the body's white cells with accompanying pains in the tissues. At a later stage, as a result of destruction of tissue in the lymph nodes, obstruction of the lymphatic system occurs and, since lymph continues to be formed by drainage of fluid from the tissues, either this lymph must be re-routed in its journey to the thoracic duct and back to the blood stream or oedema results. Oedema is the distension of tissues with fluid that is not being removed at an adequate rate. It is the obvious feature of elephantiasis, when blockage of the lymphatic drainage from the legs has taken place, but oedema may occur in the scrotum or indeed in any other tissue dependent on efficient lymph drainage. The growth of connective tissue in the affected parts is not reversible after treatment. Not surprisingly it is most frequently noted in the lower part of the body where gravity is an already existing factor to be overcome in removing lymph (Fig. 25.9).

Loa-loa is a filarial infection found in West Africa in which the worm, though present throughout the body, makes its appearance particularly in the conjunctiva of the eye. Here it gives rise to swelling and irritation and may cause blindness.

Fig. 25.8   *Ascaris* male and female (the male is smaller)

(Wellcome Museum of Medical Science)

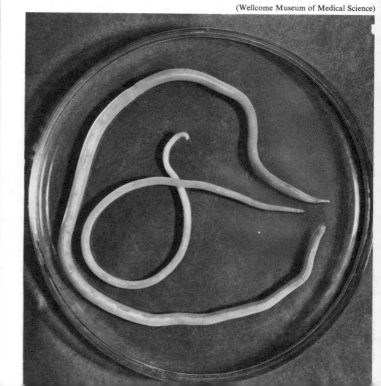

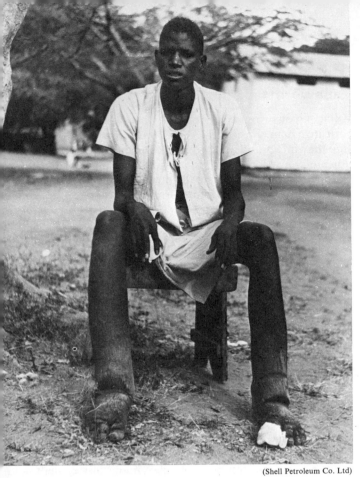

(Shell Petroleum Co. Ltd)

Fig. 25.9   Young man suffering from elephantiasis

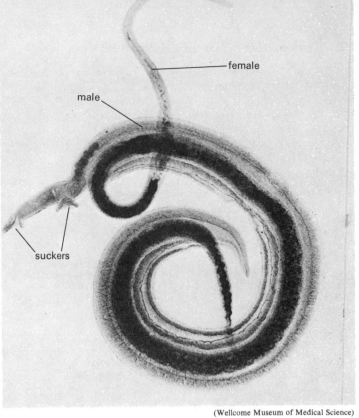

(Wellcome Museum of Medical Science)

Fig. 25.10   Male and female *Schistosoma*

Flatworms or *Platyhelminthes*

Although some of the parasitic flatworms are of spectacular size (e.g. tapeworms) the group generally is of less importance as a cause of disease than the parasitic roundworms; but there are exceptions, and the three species of *Schistosoma*, the human blood fluke, are widespread and important. *Schistosoma mansoni* is found in its adult stage in the hepatic portal vein and the small vessels of the gut; *S. haematobium* invades chiefly the blood vessels of the urinary bladder and associated organs; while *S. japonicum* causes extensive and sometimes fatal damage to the liver and spleen as well as the gut.

All three species are similar in appearance. Male worms are larger than the females and both are between 1 cm and 2 cm long. After pairing has occurred a female is usually held by the male in a groove that runs the length of its body, thus facilitating repeated fertilization (Fig. 25.10). Eggs are released into the host's blood stream, and if this occurs in a blood vessel close to the intestine or bladder surface then, by the use of a short spine (*see* Fig. 29.16) and the action of digestive enzymes, the egg may enter the intestine or the bladder. Eggs later leave the body in either faeces or urine and, if elimination of waste takes place in water or where the eggs can be carried into water, they hatch (Fig. 25.11). The ciliated larva that emerges must enter the body of a particular freshwater snail if further development is to occur. Secretions from the appropriate snail attract larvae which may penetrate the snail's skin partly as a result of enzyme action and partly by mechanical effort. Inside the blood space of the snail each larva is bathed in soluble food; it grows

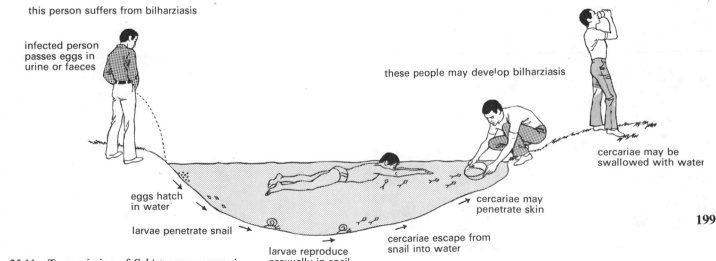

Fig. 25.11   Transmission of *Schistosoma mansoni*

199

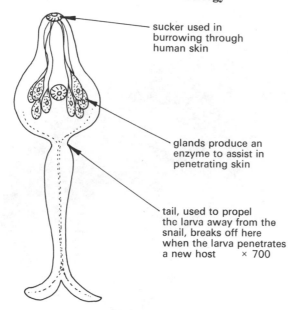

Fig. 25.12   Cercaria larva of *Schistosoma*

and eventually reproduces asexually. Since reproduction may take place two or three times a considerable increase in numbers of potentially infective parasites occurs.

Eventually thousands of larvae called cercariae emerge from the snail into the surrounding water (Fig. 25.12). If this water is then drunk by man, the larvae may burrow through the gut wall. They can also penetrate the skin, usually of the ankles and legs of people bathing or simply walking in infected water. Either way the larvae gain access to the blood stream and settle in the regions mentioned earlier, mature, pair and begin producing more eggs.

Since the parasites become sexually mature in humans, man is said to be the *primary host* while the snail, though essential for the completion of the life cycle, is called the *secondary host*.

Tapeworms

Adult tapeworms are probably the largest organisms to parasitize man (Fig. 25.13). Along with the nematode *Trichinella*, they infect humans by being consumed in the flesh of another animal. Man is the primary host since tapeworms become sexually mature in his small intestine. The secondary host varies from one kind of tapeworm to another: *Taenia solium* undergoes larval development in the pig, *T. saginatum* in cattle and *Diphyllobothrium* in freshwater fish; any of these are infective if the flesh is eaten raw or only lightly cooked.

Larvae taken in with the flesh of the secondary host are activated by human digestive juices. They resist digestion, though the reason for this is not clear. The presence of a resistant cuticle is a possible reason. A head or, more accurately, a *scolex* is already present, and this carries suckers and, in some species, hooks with which the young tapeworm attaches itself to the wall of the small intestine between the villi (Fig. 25.14). The scolex carries no mouth but the worm is bathed in digested food which is absorbed actively over the body surface.

Growth follows an interesting pattern. The region behind the scolex 'buds off' segments. These start as short units of tissue which subsequently develop as they increase in size, to form male and female reproductive organs. Each segment is therefore hermaphrodite and fertilization is made easy.

The adult worm comprises a scolex, immature segments and, at the end furthest down the intestine (towards the rectum), sexually mature segments and ripe or gravid segments packed with fertilized eggs (Fig. 25.15). These segments may break off spontaneously or be detached by the movements of the host's

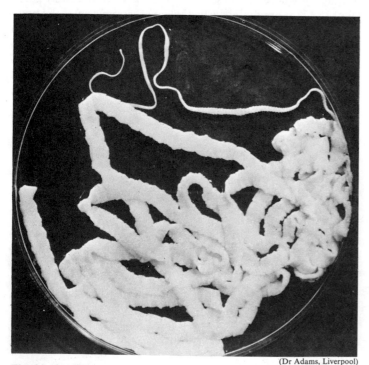

(Dr Adams, Liverpool)

Fig. 25.13   *Taenia saginata* expelled intact after patient was treated with mepacrine

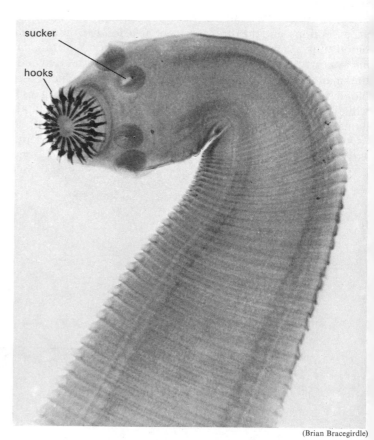

(Brian Bracegirdle)

Fig. 25.14   Hooks and suckers of *Taenia*

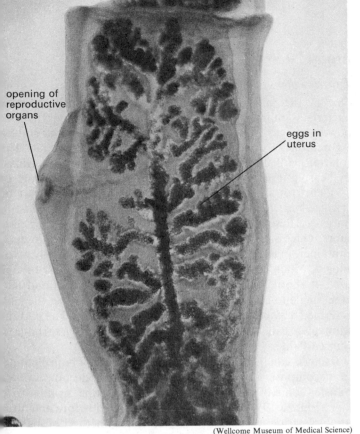

opening of reproductive organs

eggs in uterus

(Wellcome Museum of Medical Science)

Fig. 25.15   Ripe segment of *Taenia*, containing eggs

If the eggs are taken in at all by the secondary host then they are usually consumed in large numbers. In the case of cattle or the pig, the digestive juices liberate the embryos, which have already developed hooks. These are used to tear a passage through the delicate lining of the gut, allowing the embryos to pass into the blood stream or a lymph vessel and so to be carried around the body. Larvae usually settle in muscle where they develop into a fluid-filled bladder surrounding the scolex, like the pushed-in finger of a glove. In beef the bladder-worms are most common in the muscles of the heart and the jaws, though they can be found elsewhere. In pork the larvae are present in the muscle of the neck and shoulder, though again they may be found elsewhere.

Heavy infestation causes the meat to look spotty when cut, hence the phrase 'measly pork'. If this meat is eaten raw or undercooked then the larvae will infect man, as described.

Man may swallow eggs of either of the two species of *Taenia* if hygienic precautions are not observed. The eggs can, rarely, be regurgitated from the intestine to his own stomach. When the egg case has been digested the larvae are quite capable of boring through the gut wall and forming cysts in the tissues.

Most carnivorous vertebrates are subject to tapeworm infections and while the larvae will only become sexually mature in the appropriate host, the eggs of many tapeworms will hatch and develop in the bodies of unusual hosts. Thus children playing with dogs infected with *Echinococcus* may swallow eggs transferred to the mouth by fingers soiled from the body of the dog or from contaminated bedding. Dogs and other pets also nose around faeces and may be passive agents transferring eggs on their snouts to people stroking, handling or being licked by them. Such eggs hatch and release larvae that may settle in the liver, lungs or brain, for example. Subsequent development is often abnormal in that a large cyst develops. If the site of development is the brain, then pressure

gut and are carried out with the faeces. Further development depends on where defaecation takes place or whether faeces will be carried to a point where the secondary host has access to them. Thus for the two species of *Taenia*, infected faeces must be shed where pigs or cattle graze, while *Diphyllobothrium* eggs must be released into fresh water (*see* Figs. 25.16 and 25.17).

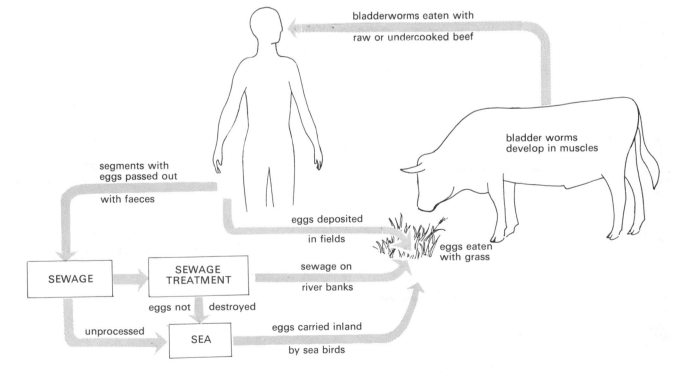

bladderworms eaten with raw or undercooked beef

bladder worms develop in muscles

segments with eggs passed out

with faeces

eggs deposited in fields

eggs eaten with grass

SEWAGE

SEWAGE TREATMENT

sewage on river banks

eggs not | destroyed

unprocessed

SEA

eggs carried inland by sea birds

Fig. 25.16   Life cycle of *Taenia saginata*, the beef tapeworm

of the cyst causes damage and behavioural changes. In the liver or lungs such a cyst may press on vessels and interfere with circulation.

The fish tapeworm, *Diphyllobothrium*, differs from the pork and beef tapeworms in that its life cycle requires two intermediate hosts for its completion (Fig. 25.17). It also differs in that it may become adult in a variety of fish-eating mammals. Thus the fact that man disposes of his faeces hygienically does not mean that there is then no chance of infection, since other mammals may contaminate the water in which the second and third hosts live.

All the organisms described in this chapter are parasitic in man and cause disease. To be a successful parasite, whether it be a bacterium or a tapeworm, the organism must have some means of being transferred from one host to another, and in the next chapter we shall review the methods adopted. Success depends also on its ability to obtain food from the host. However, it must not take so much food or produce such damaging effects that the host dies or, if this should happen, the parasite must have some means of protection or transfer ready. The likelihood of encountering a new host is often slender, and most parasites have spectacular rates of reproduction. One bacterium may give rise to several million within twenty-four hours, and one tapeworm may release many millions of eggs during its adult life, so that while there is undoubted wastage, there is a high probability of the life cycle being repeated.

The control methods are dealt with in detail in Chapter 30.

Practical Work

Experiment 1 Culturing bacteria

One of the most convenient materials on which to grow bacteria is nutrient agar. This is made by stirring 1.5 g of powdered agar into 100 cm^3 of hot distilled water and adding 1 g peptone, 1 g meat extract and 0.5 g sodium chloride. The solution, called the culture medium, must now be sterilized by heating in a pressure cooker (Fig. 34.12) at a pressure of 1 kg/cm^2 for 15 minutes. The containers to be used must be sterilized in the same way to destroy any bacteria that are present. These containers may be glass Petri dishes or test-tubes. Once sterilized, 5 cm^3 of medium is poured into each container. In a Petri dish this provides a thin layer of jelly when cooled, which covers the bottom of the dish. If a test-tube is used, it should be plugged with sterile cotton wool and laid at an angle to cool, as shown in Fig. 25.18. When set the jelly is termed a *slope*. It can be handled at any angle. The cotton-wool plug can be sterilized by passing it swiftly through a Bunsen flame.

Bacteria can be obtained by allowing a piece of boiled potato to decompose in water. After two days' decomposition transfer some of the water to a plate or a slope, using a wire loop (Fig. 25.19). The loop must be sterilized before and after use by heating to red heat in a flame. The method of making the culture is shown in Fig. 25.18. As bacterial colonies grow they show up as glistening blobs on the jelly.

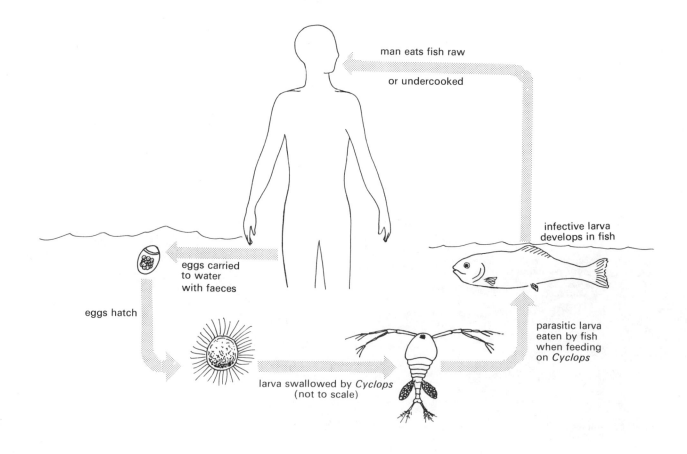

Fig. 25.17   Life cycle of *Diphyllobothrium*, the fish tapeworm

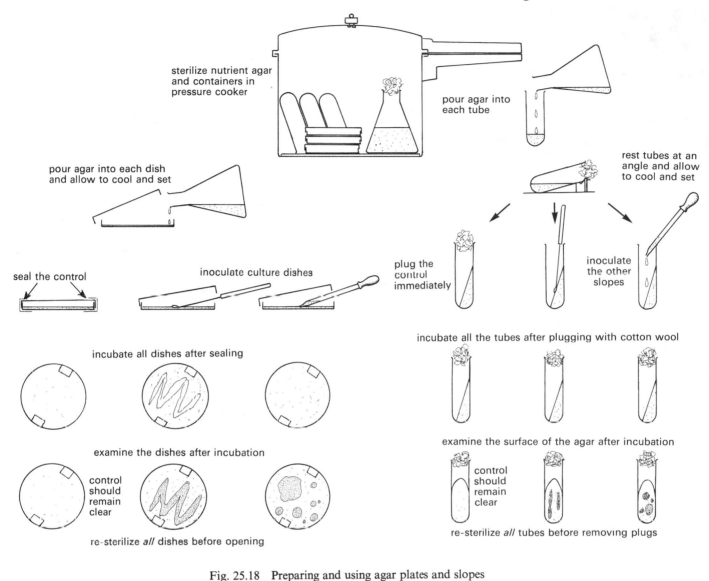

Fig. 25.18   Preparing and using agar plates and slopes

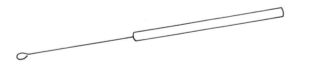

Fig. 25.19   Wire loop used for subculturing bacteria

Experiment 2   Sources of bacteria

Collect samples of river water, pond and tap water in separate, sterile vessels and make a fourth sample by placing soil in a vessel with just sufficient water to cover it. Transfer water from each sample to each of four plates or slopes using a wire loop. Keep a fifth plate or slope, sterilized like the others, as a *control*. This provides a check that sterilization has been effective, since no bacterial colonies should appear on it. The cultures are all compared with the control after they have been sealed and incubated at 37 °C for two days. They should not be opened, since pathogenic organisms may be present. All plates

and slopes should be re-sterilized in the pressure cooker before the containers are opened or re-used.

Experiment 3   Nematodes or thread worms

A nematode called *Rhabditis* is usually obtained if an earthworm, killed swiftly by dropping into boiling water, is cut open lengthwise, laid on a dish of fresh garden soil, and covered with polythene or other waterproof material for two days. The nematodes can be seen moving on the surface of the worm and may be transferred to a drop of water on a slide for examination under a hand lens or a microscope.

Questions

1   Draw up two tables, one showing the ways in which bacteria, viruses, protozoa and fungi resemble each other and one showing the ways in which they are different from each other, e.g. in methods of feeding and reproduction.
2   What evidence is there for the statement that it is not in the interest of a pathogenic organism to kill its host? For what organisms might this statement appear at first sight to be untrue?

26

How Disease-causing Organisms Enter the Body

Commensal bacteria which normally live harmlessly within the body may become pathogens with a change of circumstances. Here we are concerned with the ways and means by which they and other more obvious pathogens gain access to human tissues (Fig. 26.1).

Natural openings

Many micro-organisms can enter the body through the natural openings. The nasal passages, mouth, urinary passage, anus and, in females, the vagina all present pathways for the entry of pathogens. Each of these openings leads to a tube lined with a soft, moist mucous membrane. The mucus itself often contains enough food material to sustain microbial life such as the bacterium *Staphylococcus aureus*. Fortunately, if a person is in a state of good health, the cellular membranes seem able to resist penetration by most kinds of micro-organism, but the extent of this resistance varies from one individual to another and also within one individual from

time to time. In any case, these tubes lead on to other organs which may possess less resistance.

The different openings are often associated with particular methods of spread (*see* Chapter 27). Thus the nose and mouth are the principal means of entry for airborne infections. The mouth provides access for organisms present in drinking water and food, as well as for organisms transferred to the lips by contaminated fingers or cups and cutlery. Entry of organisms to the urethra or vagina is often associated with venereal diseases though many other disorders of these passages arise from organisms that are spread other than by sexual intercourse.

Wounds and breaks in the skin

Human skin provides a remarkable degree of protection against micro-organisms. The kinds that can penetrate the skin of their own accord are, fortunately, few, but include the larvae of *Schistosoma* and hookworm (p. 199) which enter through a combination of enzymic and mechanical action. The staphylo-

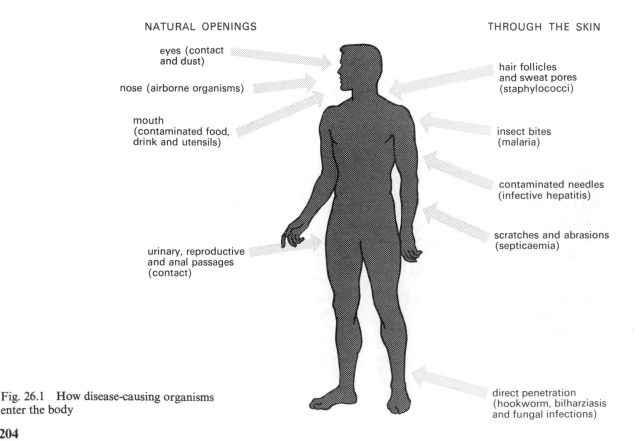

NATURAL OPENINGS

eyes (contact and dust)

nose (airborne organisms)

mouth (contaminated food, drink and utensils)

urinary, reproductive and anal passages (contact)

THROUGH THE SKIN

hair follicles and sweat pores (staphylococci)

insect bites (malaria)

contaminated needles (infective hepatitis)

scratches and abrasions (septicaemia)

direct penetration (hookworm, bilharziasis and fungal infections)

Fig. 26.1 How disease-causing organisms enter the body

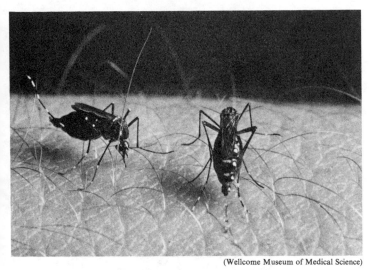

(Wellcome Museum of Medical Science)

Fig. 26.2   Yellow fever mosquitoes piercing human skin

cocci that cause boils and pimples invade hair follicles and set up local infections. Abrasion or damage to the skin provides an entry for bacteria such as those causing wounds to become septic, usually with the formation of pus, and for the fungi causing ringworm and athlete's foot.

Deep wounds provide access to muscle and other tissues such as bone which are normally sterile and disease symptoms may develop rapidly when the skin barrier is broken.

Bites, mostly by insects and other arthropods, are a particularly important source of infection. Thus certain species of blood-sucking mosquitoes may inject malarial parasites through the skin, directly into the blood stream (p. 197). No one ever suffered malaria as a result of parasites being rubbed on to his skin. Horseflies and similar biting flies may introduce micro-organisms through the skin on the outside of their biting mouthparts. The bite of a dog infected with rabies virus usually results in infection of the wound with the virus from the saliva on its teeth.

27

How Disease-causing Organisms are Spread

Very few of the organisms causing disease are able to spread by their own power of movement. We may consider that larvae of *Schistosoma* and hookworm (*see* p. 199) are mobile, but dispersal owes much to the movement of the water in which they often live.

Waterborne infection

Water is a splendid medium for the dispersal of the organisms causing gastro-intestinal infections such as amoebic dysentery, cholera and typhoid fever. When such organisms reproduce in the gut, eggs, spores or active organisms are carried out with the faeces and the sanitary habits of the infected person will determine the chances of the disease being spread (Fig. 27.1).

If faeces or urine carrying disease organisms are deposited directly in water that is used for drinking, the organisms may thus infect large numbers of people. If infected faeces are left on the ground or even buried within a few metres of a stream or lake, the disease organisms may be washed by rain into the water supply and contaminate it. One person suffering from an intestinal disease such as typhoid or cholera may thus infect hundreds of others. It is important for individuals to see that their faeces are buried as far as possible from streams,

Fig. 27.1   Water being carried away from a river in which people bathe and cattle are washed, to be drunk without any treatment

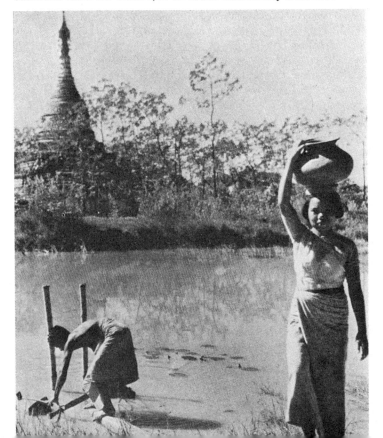

(WHO)

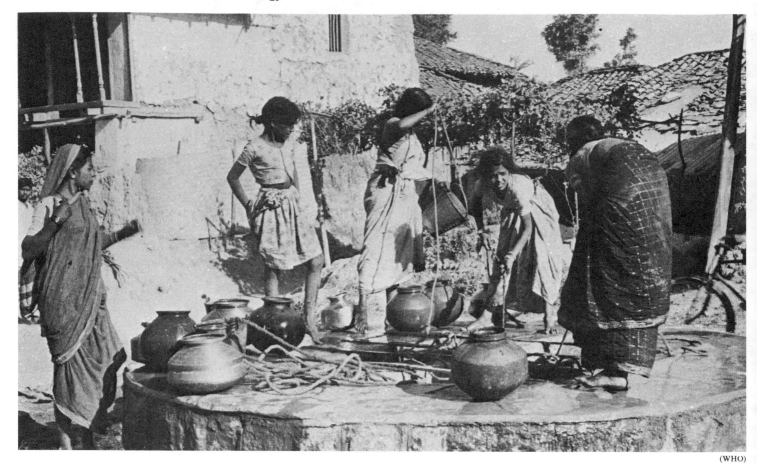

(WHO)

Fig 27.2 Contamination of drinking-water is not always obvious; this well is protected by a raised stone surround, but the feet of the villagers carry dirt and germs on to the surround and the ropes then contaminate the well

rivers and lakes, and even more vital for the sewage from towns to be disposed of in such a way that water supplies cannot be contaminated (*see* pp. 251–3).

After defaecation and urination, the hands are likely to carry minute amounts of faeces and urine. If such unwashed hands touch food, utensils for handling food or even door handles and other objects, the faecal matter with any germs it contains may be transferred to the object and later picked up by another person who eats the food or opens the door. For this reason it is essential to wash hands after each visit to the lavatory and before handling food. People handling and preparing food for others must be particularly careful in this respect.

Moving water can quickly spread micro-organisms over large distances. The sweet-water canals of Egypt have in the past been the means of spreading cholera from a point of contamination to people using the water for drinking many miles away. One of the unforeseen results of the irrigation of land by water from new dams such as those on the Nile has been the spread of the watersnail that is the host of *Schistosoma* larvae. Rivers similarly carry pathogens downstream. Even sterilized drinking water has been known to become re-contaminated through defects in pipe systems or by pollution of reservoirs for the storage of sterilized water. Severe flooding often means that sewage channels overflow, carrying raw sewage and therefore germs to places where one would not normally expect contamination to occur. In this way outbreaks

of gastro-intestinal diseases may occur in cities that normally take a pride in their record of good health (Fig. 27.2).

Foodborne infection (Fig. 27.3)

Many of the organisms transmitted in water are also carried on or in food. Washing food in contaminated water, or leaving food unprotected from the visits of flies that feed on faeces, may lead to infection (*see* p. 208) and food can also be contaminated when handled by people with unwashed hands and with unprotected septic wounds. In this section we are more concerned with bacterial food poisoning and fluke and worm infections. Some bacteria such as *Salmonella*, causing typhoid and paratyphoid, or *Clostridium*, causing botulism, an often fatal food poisoning, are able to multiply in proteinaceous food such as cooked meats, raw meat and milk, as well as in raw egg products. Bottle-fed babies in hospitals are sometimes at risk from such infection which spreads very quickly. We have referred already to tapeworms (p. 201), with the consumption of raw or undercooked meat as the source of new infection.

Bacillary dysentery, caused by several species of *Shigella*, occurs frequently among children in Britain and, as with waterborne organisms, the human hand is often an essential link in transferring the bacilli from faeces or anus to food. The commonest form is mild and characterized by an inconvenient diarrhoea.

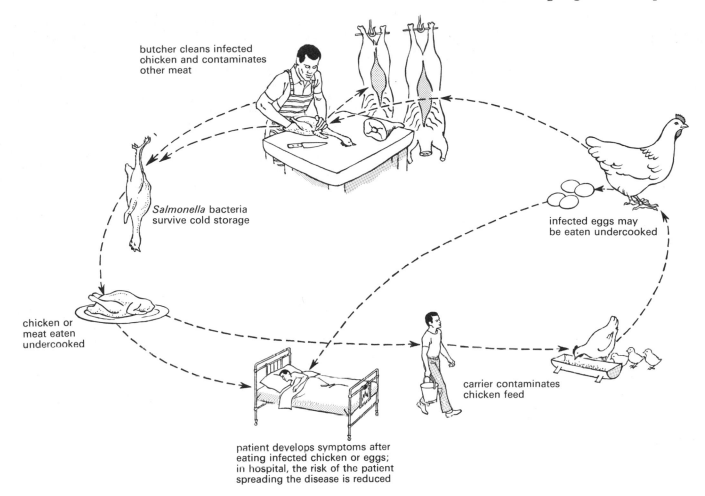

butcher cleans infected
chicken and contaminates
other meat

Salmonella bacteria
survive cold storage

infected eggs may
be eaten undercooked

chicken or
meat eaten
undercooked

carrier contaminates
chicken feed

patient develops symptoms after
eating infected chicken or eggs;
in hospital, the risk of the patient
spreading the disease is reduced

Fig. 27.3   Transmission of *Salmonella* food poisoning

Droplet infection

Coughing and sneezing, and also talking and normal breathing,
result in the discharge into the air of tiny droplets of moisture.
The larger drops may settle on food or utensils but it is the tiny
droplets, between 1 and 10 μm in diameter, that concern us
here. These usually evaporate speedily, having a very large
surface-to-volume ratio, and any virus particles or other
germs in the droplet are then suspended in the air as very
small bodies indeed. These may be breathed into the respiratory
passages. Evaporation of the moisture surrounding them would
kill many bacteria breathed into the air in this way, but viruses
remain infective (Fig. 27.4).

In conditions of high humidity such as occur in crowded
rooms or buses and trains at rush hours, the droplets evaporate
more slowly and even bacteria such as those causing pneumonia can survive, to be breathed in by other people. The
spread of colds and influenza is rapid among people using
crowded transport and ill-ventilated rooms, especially in cold
weather when windows are kept closed and the free movement
of air is restricted. Children in temperate climates are more
subject to epidemics of mumps, measles and chickenpox when
ventilation is reduced in winter months, though there are other
factors that may influence such epidemics.

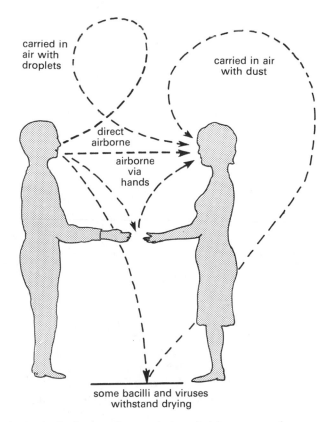

carried in
air with
droplets

carried in air
with dust

direct
airborne

airborne
via
hands

some bacilli and viruses
withstand drying

Fig. 27.4   Pathways of transmission of airborne organisms

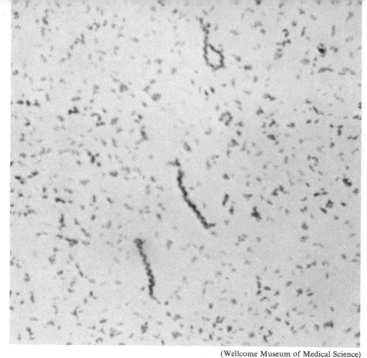

(Wellcome Museum of Medical Science)

Fig. 27.5 *Treponema*, causing syphilis (×2 000)

Contagious diseases

Certain diseases are normally spread *only* by direct contact. These include the venereal diseases, of which gonorrhoea and syphilis are the most serious. They are only spread by sexual contact, either during intercourse or during petting or touching of the genital organs. The bacteria of both these diseases are very susceptible to the effect of drying and die quickly outside the body.

Fungal diseases, such as ringworm and athlete's foot (Fig. 27.6) are spread by contact. Portions of the fungus may be rubbed from the skin of one person on to another, though a more likely path of infection is contact with skin fragments bearing the fungus that have been rubbed on to a towel or a floor surface from an infected person. Septicaemia is also transmitted mostly by contact, and the risk of infecting other people by touch when a person has, say, a septic finger should be clearly realized.

Leprosy is a disease with a long history, referred to in the Old Testament, and it has long been supposed that spread was by contact. It is caused by *Mycobacterium leprae* and while

Fig. 27.6 Athlete's foot; damaged skin between the toes is caused by a fungus transmitted by contact

(Blackwell Scientific Publications)

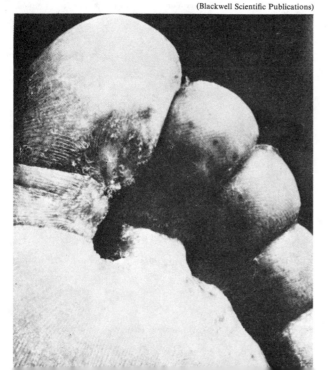

it is inappropriate here to discuss the various forms that the disease takes, it is clear that skin-to-skin contact, usually over a prolonged period of time, is the principal means of transmission. Invasion is through the skin, and it is in the skin that the first lesions (injuries) occur. Slow but devastating damage may be done to nerve tissue over a long period of time as the bacterium penetrates into these tissues. Infection is thought to occur frequently during childhood, particularly in communities in which the caressing of children is part of the family pattern, though signs of the disease may be slow in developing. Early diagnosis and control is therefore not easy but the organism, once seen to be present, can be destroyed by such drugs as dapsone and certain sulphonamides. The patient will retain the signs of any damage to tissues but he is then not infectious to other people.

Infection by insects

Insects transmit disease organisms (i) on the outside of their bodies and (ii) inside their guts or salivary glands. A remarkably wide variety of insects comes into the first group. The houseflies (*Musca* species) form the most notorious vectors or spreaders of many intestinal diseases. The adult insects are attracted by smell to faeces and also to food destined for humans. In feeding they place a proboscis or tube on the food and pump out saliva which, having dissolved part of the food, is then sucked up. The moist proboscis becomes well contaminated

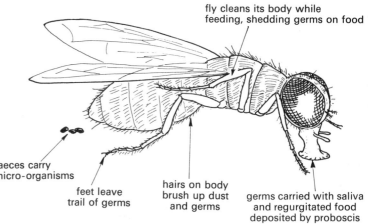

fly cleans its body while feeding, shedding germs on food

faeces carry micro-organisms

feet leave trail of germs

hairs on body brush up dust and germs

germs carried with saliva and regurgitated food deposited by proboscis

Fig. 27.7 Transmission of disease organisms by the housefly

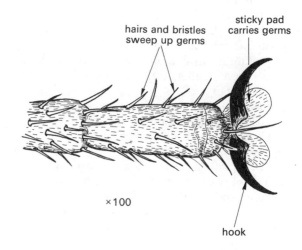

hairs and bristles sweep up germs

sticky pad carries germs

×100

hook

Fig. 27.8 Foot of housefly

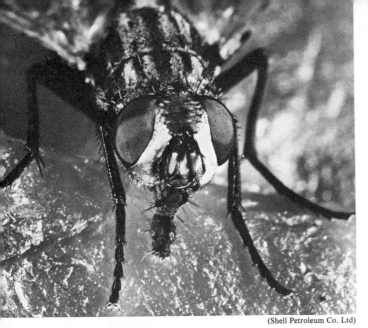

(Shell Petroleum Co. Ltd)

Fig. 27.9   Head of housefly

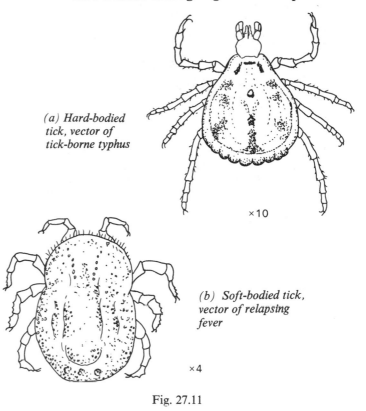

(a) Hard-bodied tick, vector of tick-borne typhus

×10

(b) Soft-bodied tick, vector of relapsing fever

×4

Fig. 27.11

with any micro-organisms present, and should these include pathogens such as the bacteria of cholera or bacillary dysentery then infection from eating food over which flies have subsequently walked is highly likely. Bacteria may also be left by the flies on utensils, cups and surfaces which are subsequently touched by human fingers. Organisms can also be carried on the hairy bodies, the feet and in the faeces of the flies (Figs. 27.7–9).

Cockroaches, though not specifically attracted to faeces (which are a source of pathogens), are vectors of many diseases, mostly intestinal, and at one time they were shown to be capable of carrying the virus of poliomyelitis. They hide under floorboards, in cracks in walls, under sacks and generally in places where dirt and germs accumulate. They are notorious for feeding on and contaminating human food on which they can lay a trail of micro-organisms (Fig. 27.10).

The insects of the second group are blood suckers with mouthparts modified for piercing human skin. Certain mosquitoes and ticks have such slender mouthparts that their bites are not noticed until later, while horseflies and other tabanid flies give painful bites, as do some of the midges.

However, whether the bite is noticed immediately or not, organisms may be introduced into the blood stream on the mouthparts or in the saliva during the act of biting. In this way malarial parasites, filarial worms and yellow fever virus are spread by mosquitoes, the trypanosomes of sleeping sickness by tsetse flies, and the bacteria of bubonic plague and rickettsiae of murine typhus are transmitted by fleas.

Infection by other animal vectors

Ticks and mites are often associated with fleas and lice in their role as vectors though the former are not in fact insects. The spirochaetes of relapsing fever are carried by soft-bodied ticks, while the hard-bodied or Ixodid ticks are responsible for the spread of many viruses and rickettsiae (see Fig. 27.11).

Blood-sucking mites carry the rickettsiae of murine typhus and scrub typhus. The itch mites, however, which are responsible for scabies, are not vectors but do direct damage to the skin in which they burrow and reproduce, causing intense irritation (Fig. 27.12). They themselves are spread from one host to another by direct contact.

Fig. 27.10   Cockroaches feeding on a tomato

(Rentokil Ltd)

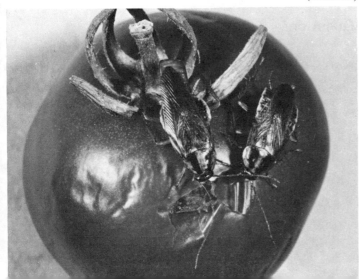

Fig. 27.12   Characteristic distribution of scabies on the body of a child

(Blackwell Scientific Publications)

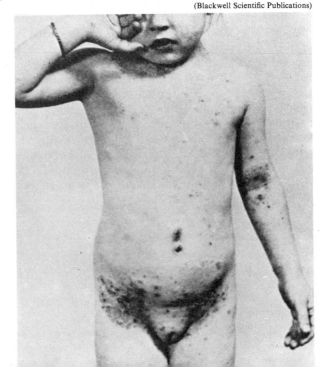

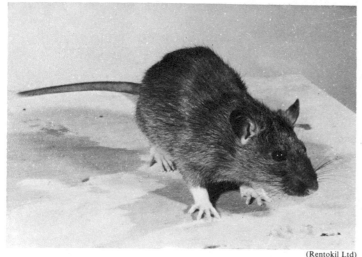

(Rentokil Ltd)

Fig. 27.13   The brown rat, *Rattus norvegicus*, is also known as the sewer rat; it is a good swimmer and emerges from sewers to contaminate food with its urine and faeces, transmitting *Salmonella*, causing food poisoning, and *Leptospira*, causing Weil's disease

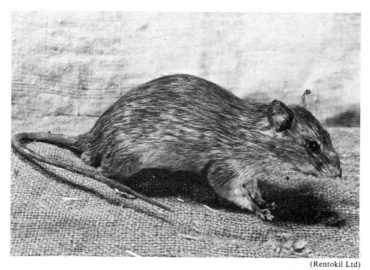

(Rentokil Ltd)

Fig. 27.14   The black rat, *Rattus rattus*, is also called the ship rat; it is commonest around seaports and is the reservoir of the bacterium causing bubonic plague. Like the brown rat, it also contaminates food

Rats, mice and other mammals form an interesting group of vectors. Since they frequent places where food is stored they often contaminate that food with pathogens carried on their fur and feet. They also carry *Salmonella*, causing food poisoning, in their urine and faeces. The spirochaete causing Weil's disease (infective jaundice), a severe and often fatal illness, is carried by rats and passed in their urine. Contact with rat urine may be made in sewage plant, rat-infested rivers and, in Australia, in sugar-cane fields. Apart from this, rats act as reservoirs for a remarkably wide range of pathogens including that of bubonic plague, the cause of the Black Death of Europe in the Middle Ages and the Great Plague of London in 1665 as well as innumerable other notorious outbreaks. We are wise to eliminate rats from human environments (*see* Chapter 37).

How disease organisms are spread

Method of spread		Examples of disease
contaminated water	drinking	intestinal diseases, e.g. dysentery, cholera, typhoid fever
	bathing, washing or paddling	bilharziasis, hookworm
contaminated food	eating	intestinal diseases, salmonella, tapeworm
airborne	droplet	diseases of respiratory tract, common cold, TB
		diseases entering by respiratory tract, measles, influenza, smallpox
	dust	diseases of respiratory tract (e.g. tuberculosis) and eyes (e.g. trachoma)
contact (contagion)	skin to skin, skin to clothing to skin	smallpox, ringworm, scabies, septicaemia
	sexually transmitted	gonorrhoea, syphilis, candidiasis
insect vector	carried externally, e.g. housefly, cockroach	dysentery, salmonella
	carried internally, e.g. mosquito	malaria, yellow fever
other animal vectors	rat (urine) dog (saliva)	Weil's disease rabies

Practical Work

Experiment 1

Prepare three agar plates or slopes (p. 202). Hold one of them before your mouth and cough hard on to it. Place a small quantity of saliva on the jelly in the second and keep the third as a control. Incubate for two days at 37 °C and compare the results. Destroy the cultures by re-sterilizing the plates or slopes.

Experiment 2

Prepare two agar plates. Catch a housefly and allow it to walk over the jelly of one of the plates and allow a cockroach to walk over the other. Remove the creatures and then incubate the plates. Discuss the results, and destroy the cultures by re-sterilizing.

Questions

1   In Europe in the sixteenth and seventeenth centuries it was believed that bubonic plague was spread by touch or contact. Plague is not a contagious disease but the belief is understandable if one knows how the disease organisms really are transmitted. Suggest reasons why the belief persisted.
2   Make a list of the transmissible diseases from which you and the other people in your class have suffered. How is each of these spread?

28

The Course of an Infectious Disease

We have discussed the means by which pathogenic organisms are transmitted and gain access to the body. Infection literally takes place when the organisms first penetrate tissue, whether this be the skin, the mucous membrane of the throat or the lining of the gut. However, germs of many kinds enter the bodies of each one of us every day and usually we experience no feelings of illness and show no sign of disease.

Before disease can result, a person must be *susceptible*, the organisms must be present in sufficient numbers and they must be virulent. The susceptibility of the host—the state of his defence mechanisms—is discussed in the section on immunity on page 238. At present it is sufficient to note that immunity to attack by pathogens takes various forms. There is genetic or innate immunity, and immunity acquired either as the result of a previous attack by a disease or through artificial immunization. Susceptibility to many diseases also varies with a person's general state of physical health.

The defence mechanisms of the body are substantial and include the action of phagocytes (p. 72) and of those white blood cells that produce antibodies (p. 74). A small number of invading pathogens, e.g. the few virus particles breathed in while talking in the open air to a friend with a cold, may be dealt with successfully. The same defences may be literally overwhelmed by the sheer quantity of virus breathed in during a train or bus journey sitting close to a fellow passenger who is breathing out virus-laden droplets into a humid atmosphere. The level of the infective dose required to produce disease varies also from one pathogen to another. Thus for *Salmonella* food poisoning it is high—the number of organisms swallowed at one time must be large—while only a small number of typhoid bacilli appear necessary to produce violent disease symptoms.

The *virulence* of an organism is a different matter. In the years 1905 to 1935 scarlet fever was regarded as a serious disease among children in western Europe. The streptococcus causing the disease is still found and recognized but it now produces only a mild reaction. Its virulence has diminished.

Virulence varies in the effect produced by pathogens in different hosts. Tuberculosis mycobacteria exist in three strains as reflected by the normal hosts. Thus one strain is normally associated with man, a second with cattle and a third with birds. While the second and third can parasitize man, neither produces the devastating effects in man that they do in the natural hosts. Their virulence towards man is diminishing.

Louis Pasteur discovered that it was possible to reduce the virulence of pathogenic bacteria by growing them in abnormal conditions such as at unusual temperatures or in unusual hosts. The use of such *attenuated* strains with reduced virulence is discussed on p. 239.

Incubation period

The period of time that elapses between the entry of pathogens into the tissues of a susceptible host and the onset of the first signs and symptoms of disease is termed the *incubation period*. The duration of this period varies greatly from one disease to another as may be seen from the table below.

Duration of incubation period	Disease
2– 4 days	bubonic plague
2– 6 days	cholera
3– 7 days	bacillary dysentery
5–10 days	gonorrhoea
10–14 days	smallpox
14–21 days	chickenpox
up to several years	leprosy

A knowledge of these incubation periods is helpful in the control of the spread of infectious diseases and particularly in deciding the period of quarantine or isolation of contacts. The term quarantine originates from the belief that isolation of travellers arriving from an infected area for a period of forty days would be sufficient time for disease symptoms to develop and be recognized.

Infective period

It is even more difficult to be precise about the duration of the period in which a patient is infective, that is, capable of releasing pathogens to infect another person. As soon as the parasites begin to multiply and leave the body of a patient in airborne droplets, sputum, faeces or urine, or in insect vectors, he is *infective*. He ceases from being infective only when his normal defences have destroyed all the pathogenic organisms or when these have been destroyed by antibiotics or other drugs. During the infective period the patient should be isolated from other people as far as possible, and those who must have contact in nursing him should observe strict hygiene of hands and, where possible, clothing. Occasionally a person harbours pathogens without showing symptoms of disease. If he is capable of transmitting those organisms he is said to be a *carrier*.

Signs and symptoms of disease

These are sometimes considered together as the *clinical features* of a disease. The signs can be seen sometimes by direct examination of the patient, sometimes by examining faeces, urine or a blood sample. Thus a rash, patches of yellow matter on the tonsils, diarrhoea, an enlarged spleen, or presence of the eggs of the parasite in faeces would be termed *signs of disease* (Fig. 28.1).

Complaints by the patient of a feeling of nausea, of pain, headache or loss of sensation (feeling) cannot be seen by the medical observer and are termed *symptoms*. They may be invaluable to the person who is trying to determine or *diagnose* the cause and nature of a disease in order to prescribe appropriate treatment.

One sign of reaction to disease organisms that is almost universal is a rise in body temperature. Man is homoiothermic (*see* p. 98). His body temperature is usually about 37 °C and it is reduced only by long exposure to cold and increased by vigorous physical activity. Most pathogens invading the tissues and those gut parasites that excrete toxic substances are associated with a temperature rise. This may be a small rise, from 37 °C to 38 or 39 °C if the patient is suffering from the common cold. Pneumonia or acute tonsillitis may result in temperatures of 40–41 °C.

The rise in temperature seems to result from an interaction between the pathogen or its toxins and certain white cells (Fig. 11.3). This causes the release of a substance that acts on the temperature regulatory centre in the brain. Temperature rise increases the metabolic rate within the tissues and the activity of the white cells in ingesting micro-organisms and producing antibodies is speeded up. The heartbeat similarly increases its rate.

While an increased temperature assists the body defence mechanisms, it is also the cause of some of the discomfort of disease—headache, profuse sweating and loss of appetite.

The rapid reaction of a malaria sufferer to the release of merozoites (p. 214) and their toxins as the invaded red cell burst involves a cold stage followed by a dramatic rise in temperature, accompanied by headache and vomiting.

Treatment of disease

An account of the treatment of disease in general terms would be inadequate and misleading but the treatment of a number of specific diseases is described in Chapter 29.

Secondary effects of disease

Disease organisms produce a variety of effects on the body and upset the feeling of well-being of the patient. Some such organisms cause changes in the body which result in further effects such as *anaemia* (p. 71).

Anaemia is the condition that occurs when the capacity of the blood to carry oxygen is reduced, either by a reduction in the numbers of red cells or in the amount of haemoglobin they contain, or by both factors. The signs of anaemia may include pallor (paleness) of the mucous membranes, shortness of breath during exertion and a low red cell count (assuming that a normal count is 4–6 million red cells per mm³). Symptoms may include general tiredness and giddiness during exertion, experienced by the patient but not measurable by an observer.

There are many causes of anaemia, but here we are only concerned with those that result from the activities of pathogens. The strictly infectious diseases rarely result in anaemia though it occasionally results from cholera. More frequently it is a secondary effect of attack of blood flukes, hookworms and malarial parasites. In each case heavy infestation with parasites results in destruction of large numbers of red cells; in the case of blood flukes or hookworms by the direct ingestion of blood. In chronic malaria the red cells are destroyed by the parasites living inside them.

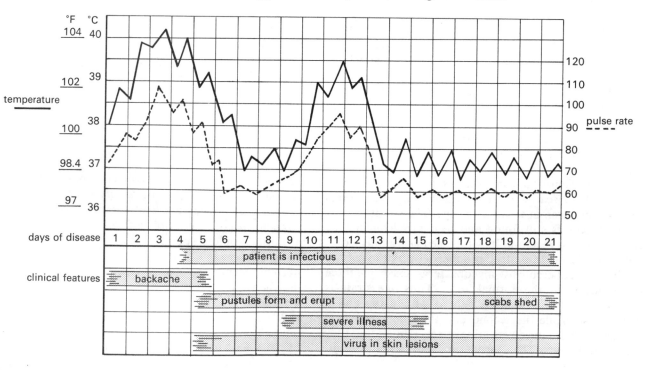

Fig. 28.1   Relationship between temperature, pulse rate and other clinical features in a smallpox patient

29

Some Diseases of World-Wide Importance

Malaria

Malaria is endemic in many tropical countries and until recent years it was widespread throughout many European countries. It occurred in Britain until the last years of the nineteenth century under the name of *fen ague*, because of its association with the fens, marshy breeding grounds of the mosquito vector, and ague, referring to the violent shaking or shivering that accompanies one stage of the disease.

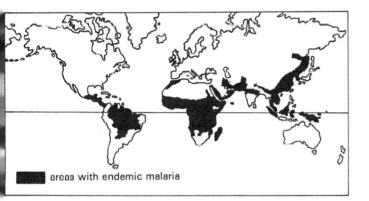

areas with endemic malaria

Fig. 29.1 World-wide distribution of malaria in 1974

Causative agent and vector. The parasite causing the disease is a microscopic single-celled animal (protozoan) belonging to the genus *Plasmodium*. It lives in the red blood cells and liver cells of man. There are several species of *Plasmodium* but only four affect humans and these are listed in the table below.

Four types of malaria

Type of malaria	Causative organism	Duration of cycle in blood stream	Geographical distribution
benign tertian	Plasmodium vivax	48 hours	Europe, N. America, Argentina, Australia
quartan	Plasmodium malariae	72 hours	commonest form throughout tropics
subtertian	Plasmodium falciparum	24 or 48 hours (irregular)	Central America, Brazil, Sri Lanka
ovale tertian	Plasmodium ovale	48 hours	mostly West Africa

Infection is normally the result of being bitten by a female anopheline mosquito that has already sucked blood from a malaria victim and is therefore carrying the parasites (*see* Fig. 29.2). A complex development, involving sexual fusion followed by rapid increase in numbers of the parasites, takes place in the mosquito and a stage known as a *sporozoite* develops in the salivary glands of the mosquito. The mosquito thrusts its feeding tube or *stylets* through the human skin, and injects saliva containing an *anticoagulant*, a chemical that prevents blood from clotting. Thus it can suck blood freely and also withdraw its stylets after feeding. When an infected mosquito injects saliva into its human host it introduces hundreds of malarial parasites into his blood stream.

The sporozoites are carried around the body in the blood stream but they can only develop further in cells in the liver, where they multiply over a period of about one week. Some remain multiplying in the liver while others are released in their thousands into the blood stream, where they invade red blood cells. Inside the red cells the parasites feed, grow and again reproduce asexually by dividing to form sixteen offspring as a rule. This reproduction is completed about 48 hours (72 hours for *P. malariae*) after the red cell was first invaded, and the cell now collapses. The sixteen merozoites together with their

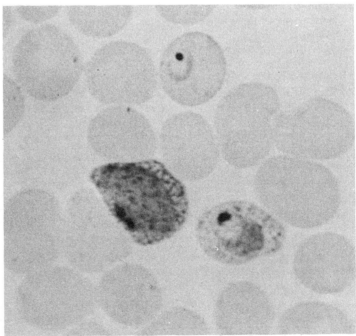

(Wellcome Museum of Medical Science)

Fig. 29.2 Three stages in the development of malarial parasites in red blood cells (×2 000)

213

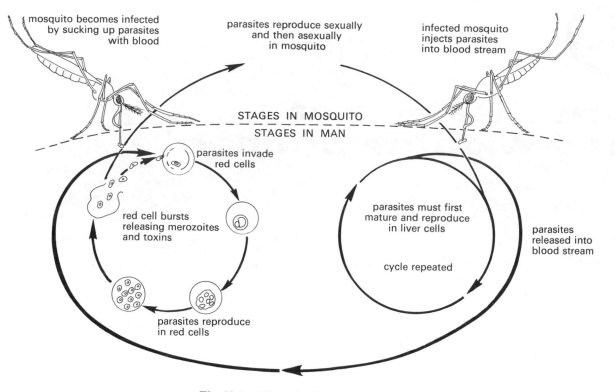

Fig. 29.3   Life cycle of the malarial parasite

waste products are released into the blood plasma, but by some curious mechanism not clearly understood, this release of parasites seems to occur almost simultaneously from all the affected red cells. The numbers of parasites released into the blood plasma may number many millions, and Sir Ronald Ross, a pioneer in research into malaria, reckoned that at least 150 million must be present before a patient would show signs of fever (Fig. 29.3).

Course of the disease (Fig. 29.4). The first attack usually takes place ten to fourteen days after infection and is often preceded by tiredness, aching and sometimes by vomiting.

Cold stage. This is the ague, characterized by shivering and chattering of the teeth, and it lasts for one to two hours. It

follows the release of the parasites from the red cells. The parasites quickly enter fresh red cells and the disease passes to the next stage.

Hot stage. The patient feels hot and his temperature may rise to 40 °C (104 °F) or higher. Rapid breathing and pulse rate are accompanied by headache and general discomfort for three to four hours.

Sweating stage. Sweating is profuse over a period of two to four hours, but the patient's temperature falls to below normal and eventually he experiences a feeling of relief. He is likely to feel exhausted, but is capable of rising from his bed and moving about until the onset of the next fever, two or three days later according to the type of malaria.

Principles of control. Malaria is a community disease, large numbers of people usually being affected. Application of a combination of the following principles is essential if the disease is to be controlled.

(i) Prevention of the mosquitoes from breeding.
(ii) Use of insecticides to prevent mosquitoes from becoming effective carriers (Fig. 29.5).
(iii) Prevention of mosquitoes from gaining access to both patients and uninfected individuals.
(iv) Use of drugs to kill malarial parasites in the blood and liver of infected persons.
(v) Use of drugs in a healthy person so that parasites are killed as soon as they are injected into the blood stream.

These preventative measures are called *prophylaxis*.

Mosquitoes lay their eggs in still water in lakes, ponds, swamps, roof gutters, drains and even in water-filled pots and tin cans. The eggs hatch into larvae which live and feed in the water for several days before turning into adults. Measures to prevent the adults from breeding include drainage of swamps and the spraying of lakes and ponds with oil and insecticide.

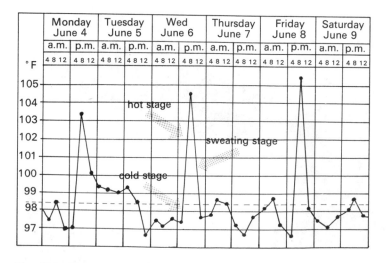

Fig. 29.4   Temperature chart of a patient suffering from benign tertian malaria

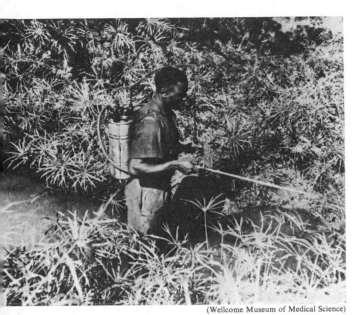

(Wellcome Museum of Medical Science)

Fig. 29.5 Spraying the breeding grounds of anopheline mosquitoes

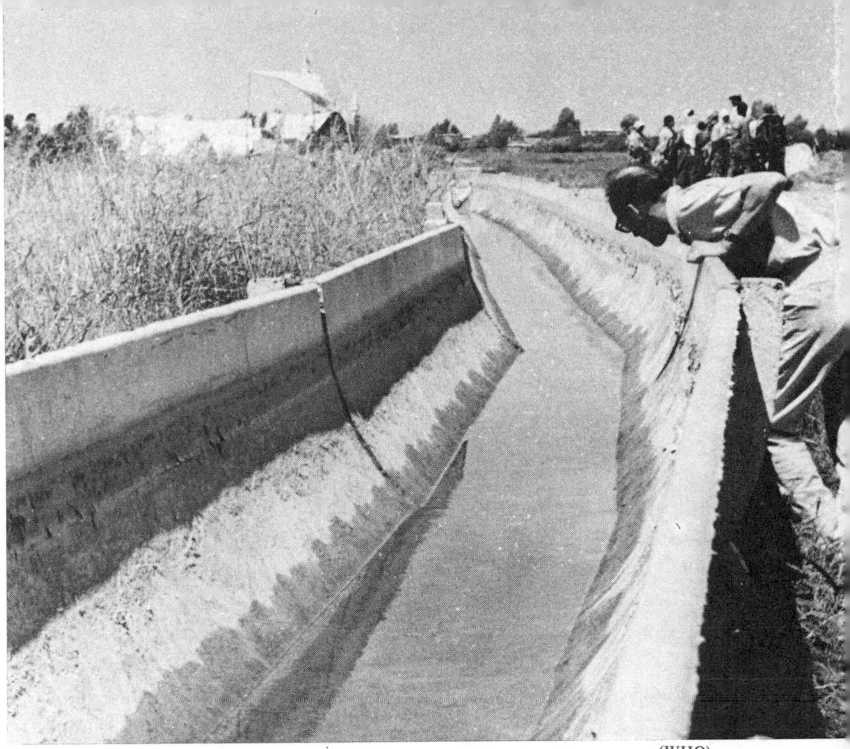

(WHO)

Fig. 29.6 Concrete-lined irrigation canal in Turkey boosts agriculture but does not provide breeding grounds for mosquitoes

il forms a thin film on the surface of water, clogging the breathing tubes with which the larvae take in air so the larvae suffocate. An insecticide in the oil provides a second line of attack in killing both larvae and egg-laying adults that settle on the water. Roof gutters and drains should be treated with insecticides, as should any other places containing still water. Old jars, pots and tins should be destroyed or buried so that they will not contain even the small amount of water needed for eggs to be laid.

Malaria had been endemic in much of Italy until measures were taken to drain breeding grounds such as the Pontine Marshes near Rome, thus reducing or eliminating the possibility of anopheline mosquitoes breeding. Drainage of areas of stagnant water has been effective in reducing malaria in Malaysia. The introduction of fish that feed on mosquito larvae, so reducing the numbers of vectors, is an interesting biological feature though it is doubtful whether it is of as much significance as either the drainage of breeding grounds or the use of insecticides.

The introduction and use of insecticides first began on a large scale in 1935 and the material used was pyrethrum. The newer synthetic insecticides such as DDT, gamma BHC and dieldrin have had an incomparably greater success and the massive reduction in the world-wide incidence of malaria in the 1960s owes more to the systematic use of insecticides than to all other methods. The aim is not to kill all mosquitoes at once but to prevent the adults from living for more than twelve or fourteen days, the time taken for the parasite to complete its sexual reproduction in the mosquito and migrate to the salivary glands.

To achieve this control, insecticides such as DDT are sprayed on the walls of buildings, particularly where the roof hangs over the wall, since mosquitoes often rest there. Such an insecticide remains effective for weeks or even months and the mosquito has only to land on or walk over the sprayed surface to be affected.

Mosquitoes sometimes become resistant to DDT and then the use of another insecticide is necessary.

It is not always feasible to prevent mosquitoes from breeding

or to kill all the adults, and it is thus wise to prevent them from reaching malaria patients, the only source of parasites, and healthy persons who could be infected. Here it is essential to know the habits of the female anopheline mosquito. It feeds on blood before producing eggs and does so almost entirely at night. If patients and healthy persons alike are protected by mosquito nets, or by fly gauze over doors and windows from dusk to dawn, then mosquitoes will not reach them. This fact was demonstrated in 1909 when a team of researchers, working in the Pontine Marshes in Italy, retired before dusk to a small hut and stayed inside until after dawn. They remained healthy in an area ravaged by malaria, though they took no other precautions (Fig. 29.7).

The use of drugs to cure malarial patients by killing the parasites in their blood and liver cells means that the patients are no longer a source of parasites. This approach to control is possible only where hospitals and medical supplies exist.

Drugs that will prevent the parasites from ever developing, even in a person bitten by an infected mosquito, have been in use for some time. These drugs are available under many

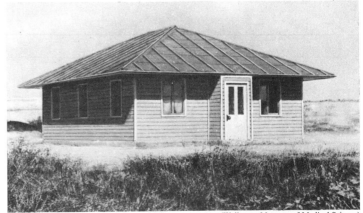

(Wellcome Museum of Medical Science)

Fig. 29.7 Hut in the Campagna, Italy, used in establishing the role of the mosquito as the vector of malaria

proprietory names which cover just four chemicals: chloroquine, amodioquine, pyrimethamine and proguanil. They have superseded quinine, an extract of the bark of the cinchona tree, which for three centuries or more was the only effective drug against malaria.

Use of any one of the four drugs listed gives a visitor travelling to a malarious area almost complete protection, if he is bitten by a malaria-carrying anopheline mosquito. As a means of providing protection to an entire population it could, theoretically, succeed but it depends on the reliability of each member of the population taking the drug at the right frequency. It is also costly and at the present time mosquito eradication is seen to give the most encouraging results.

In the early 1950s there were thought to be at least 250 million cases of malaria in the world each year, with 2.5 million deaths. A world-wide campaign mounted by WHO reduced that figure to 100 million cases, and many countries in which malaria was endemic are now free from it. Nevertheless, vigilance is essential and the small outbreak of malaria in Stockwell in south London in 1953 illustrates the point. Stagnant water in the basements of bomb-damaged buildings provided a breeding ground for anopheline mosquitoes. Soldiers returning from service in a malarious region overseas brought the parasites, and the mosquitoes were able to spread the disease to a small number of people before it was recognized and the cycle broken by draining the breeding grounds. The spread of malaria can be checked by eliminating the parasites or eliminating the vectors, or, of course, by combining both measures.

Cholera

Cholera is an acute infection of the intestines and is caused by invasion by a bacterium of the kind classed as a vibrio (p. 196). *Vibrio cholerae* and *V. el tor* are the species causing this disease in man.

Through historical time the disease has been endemic in Bangladesh and in Burma and central China. Epidemics have occurred in most parts of Asia from time to time, but it was only in the nineteenth century that the disease spread to Africa, Europe and America. In each of these continents sporadic outbreaks may assume epidemic proportions (*see* Fig. 29.8).

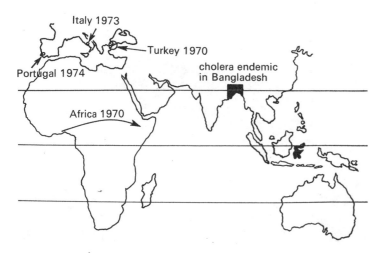

Fig. 29.8 Distribution of endemic cholera and cholera outbreaks 1970–1974

Method of spread. The spread of cholera within a population through contamination of the water supply (Fig. 29.9). The vibrios grow well at 25 to 30 °C. Where a population draw its water from a river or canal and consumes this water withou further treatment, then contamination with the faeces of cholera victim will make the water dangerous and put tha population at risk. Such was the case in the Suez Canal Zone o Egypt in the autumn of 1947. The canal, fed by water pumpe from the Nile, became infected by vibrios brought by a travelle from Bengal where an epidemic was raging. Within week thousands of Egyptians were stricken with the disease an many died. The direction and rate of spread coincided with th flow of water in the sweet-water canals from which the peopl drank.

In the summer of 1973 an outbreak at Bari on the Adriati coast of Italy was traced to the eating of contaminated shel fish. Untreated sewage, which included the faeces of a choler victim, had been passed into the sea where the shellfish, in th natural process of breathing and feeding, filtered out an retained the vibrios from the seawater. Presumably the shel fish were not adequately cooked to destroy the vibrios befor they were eaten.

Houseflies which as adults are attracted to and feed on huma faeces may also spread the vibrios when they subsequentl walk over food intended for human consumption.

Course of the disease. After an incubation period of two to si days diarrhoea begins as a result of the cholera toxin. Havin cleared out the bowel of faecal matter, the diarrhoea continue with the passage of colourless, watery material. The patient i likely to vomit violently. In these two ways the patient lose not only the fluid that he drinks but also the considerabl volume of digestive juices secreted by different parts of th digestive system such as the stomach and pancreas. Water i withdrawn from the tissues to maintain the secretion of juice and the body quickly becomes dehydrated. The patient' condition resembles that of medical shock. Death may resul though in mild cases recovery occurs within two to thre weeks.

Treatment. It is necessary to kill the vibrios but it is als important to replace the water and salts lost from the tissue as a result of the action of the toxin on the gut lining. This i done ideally by the careful injection of biologically balance salt solution into a vein or by the use of a saline drip transfusior Each of these methods requires medical supervision.

The swallowing of a sulphathiazole drug or tetracycline t kill the vibrios is necessary not only for obvious choler victims but also in the treatment of those people, terme carriers, in whose faeces vibrios are identified but who show no signs or symptoms of the disease.

Control. To control the spread of cholera, patients must b isolated in a place where neither vomit nor faeces will contam inate water supplies, food or even clothing, or be reached b flies. Both vomit and faeces carry large numbers of vibrios.

People who have been in close contact with patients may b given the drug tetracycline, and other people in an infecte area may be inoculated against the disease (p. 238). Inocula tion gives protection for a period of at least three months an possibly up to a year, in which time an epidemic is likely t have died down.

Thorough control of houseflies near hospitals, lavatories

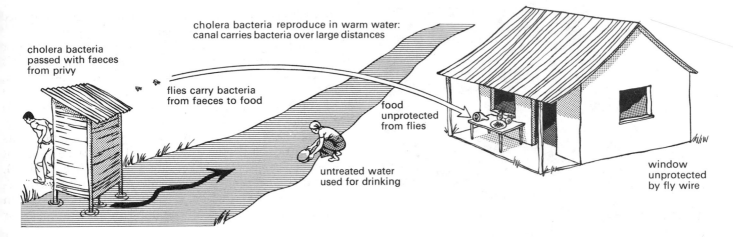

cholera bacteria reproduce in warm water:
canal carries bacteria over large distances

cholera bacteria
passed with faeces
from privy

flies carry bacteria
from faeces to food

food
unprotected
from flies

untreated water
used for drinking

window
unprotected
by fly wire

Fig. 29.9   How cholera is spread

kitchens and eating places must be maintained and it is usual to chlorinate drinking water supplies more heavily than normal.

Outbreaks of cholera should be notified to local health authorities, whose duty it is to inform the World Health Organization. Restrictions on travel from infected areas and strict quarantine of those travellers who do enter a country from an infected area help enormously in checking the spread of a cholera epidemic.

Prophylaxis. Effective prevention is achieved by ensuring that people drink only filtered and chlorinated water, free from vibrios, and by controlling houseflies.

The killed vibrio vaccine used to immunize people gives only short-term protection. Protection for the resident population of a country normally free from the disease when an epidemic breaks out elsewhere is best gained by very vigorous quarantine measures.

Tuberculosis or TB

Tuberculosis is caused by a very small bacillus, known as *Mycobacterium* (Fig. 29.10). The micro-organism, which varies from 1 µm to 5 µm in length and 0.2 µm to 0.6 µm in breadth, was first isolated by Robert Koch in 1882. There are several species of *Mycobacterium* and the one most commonly causing tuberculosis of the lung is *M. tuberculosis*. In countries where a great deal of unpasteurized milk is drunk (p. 245) *M. bovis* may be the commoner organism, and infection having started in the alimentary canal may spread to other parts of the body. Since children drink more milk than adults as a rule, the risk to them from infected, unpasteurized milk is greater.

Spread and course of the disease. *Mycobacterium tuberculosis* is spready chiefly by droplet infection (p. 207). The bacteria are inhaled and the first lesions or signs of damage to tissues develop in the lungs. The pathogen develops slowly and quite often is destroyed by the antibodies produced by the infected person. Small scars may be left in the lung and can be detected by careful X-ray examination.

However, if resistance to the pathogen is low then it may do extensive damage to lung tissue over many years. This damage includes the formation of masses of epithelial cells which, unlike the alveoli, offer no surface for gaseous exchange. Breathing efficiency is reduced and irritation set up by the

Mycobacterium results in violent coughing. Pathogens are blown out of the lung at each cough. If blood vessels are burst by the violence of the coughing then blood droplets may also be scattered with each cough. This stage of the disease is exhausting and the patient loses weight. In Victorian times the disease was known as consumption since it seemed to consume or burn away the patient's body.

The pathogen may invade lymphatic tissue and be spread to other parts of the body. This is more likely in the case of *Mycobacterium bovis*, present in milk from tubercular cows, which penetrates the body through the alimentary canal. In the 1930s children with tuberculosis of bone tissue and joints were commonly found in Britain, but pasteurization of milk together with improved standards of hygiene in dairies and amongst cow handlers have reduced this form of tuberculosis. The introduction of new and effective drugs has helped to cure those cases that have developed.

Treatment. Treatment for pulmonary tuberculosis involves complete rest, usually in hospital, together with a course of a drug such as streptomycin. This destroys the bacterium, but careful nursing is necessary to restore the patient to full physical vigour. Low resistance to the pathogen is often associated with inadequate diet, so good food with sufficient

Fig. 29.10   *Mycobacterium*, causing tuberculosis (× 2 000)
(Wellcome Museum of Medical Science)

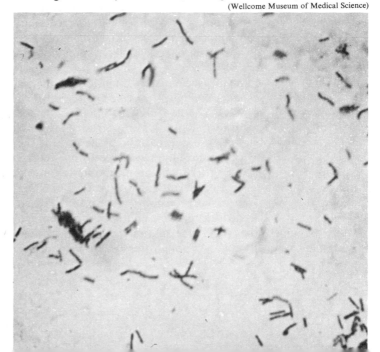

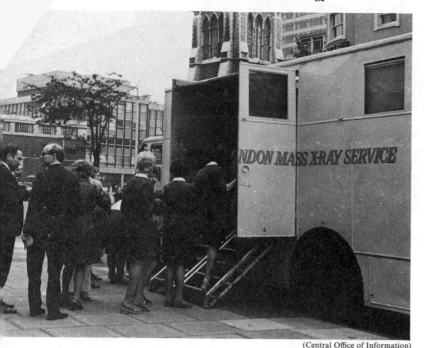
(Central Office of Information)

Fig. 29.11 Mass radiography is a means of discovering early signs of TB

protein is essential for recovery. Patients are kept in very well-ventilated wards, partly to reduce the risk of infecting patients suffering from other complaints and partly because fresh air and sense of space seem to improve the patients' morale, an important factor in recovery.

Prophylaxis. Since sufferers from tuberculosis may be infectious for years before signs and symptoms are noticed, it is important to apply hygienic principles in order to prevent the spread of the pathogens, particularly in those areas where the disease is known to exist. As with all diseases spread by droplet infection, living in overcrowded, humid conditions increases enormously the risk of infection. Conversely, good ventilation and space, in schools and factories as well as in the home, play a considerable part in reducing the spread of this disease.

The use of *mass radiography* (Fig. 29.11), in which mobile X-ray machines visit factories, schools and villages for chest X-rays to be taken, has made it possible to *screen* or check large numbers of people for early signs of tuberculosis. Tubercular lesions show up as shadows on the lung in an X-ray and, when noticed, can give an indication that further tests and investigations should be carried out. Early treatment not only gives a greater chance of a successful cure but enables measures to be taken to prevent that person from spreading the pathogens.

In 1920 two French medical scientists, Calmette and Guérin, used a strain of *Mycobacterium bovis* to make a vaccine which is still referred to as BCG (Bacille Calmette–Guérin). Before vaccinating, a skin test is carried out. Antigens from a preparation of dead mycobacteria are injected under the skin. If the person has previously contracted and recovered from TB (and many do without knowing it) then the antibodies resulting from this infection react with the antigen to give a red swelling in two to four days. If there has been no previous infection then there is no antibody–antigen reaction and such a person can usefully be given the BCG vaccination to encourage the development of antibodies. Although this is active immunity

it does not last very long and re-vaccination is recommended after three to five years, particularly for young people.

Both mass radiography and BCG vaccination tend to be abandoned when the incidence of TB falls to a low level. This is largely because both methods of protection cost money, and when only a very few people are shown by X-ray to have the disease or, by the skin test, to have had it, then health authorities tend to concentrate on keeping infection out of the community. A careful check on visitors to a country and on immigrants from countries where the disease is still widespread is one of the most effective ways of keeping a country free from TB. In countries where the disease is still common then the widespread use of BCG vaccine, as in the WHO programme in India and parts of Africa, certainly produces spectacular results.

Smallpox and variola

Smallpox has been described in the writings of mankind from earliest times. Evidence from the mummified body of Pharoah Rameses V suggests that he died of the disease about 1160 B.C. In Europe it has caused disfigurement, blindness and death until recent times. Epidemics commonly killed 20 to 40 per cent of the people afflicted and, when the disease was introduced to the Americas by invaders, the death rate was frequently much higher. However, from being endemic throughout Europe, Asia, Africa and, later, America, the endemic areas are now restricted to India, Pakistan and Bangladesh, and the Sudan and Ethiopia. From these centres there are still occasional transmissions to other parts of the world (*see* Fig. 29.12).

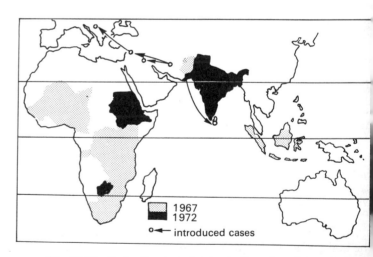

1967
1972

o← introduced cases

Fig. 29.12 Reduction in endemic smallpox over five years

Causative agent and means of spread. Smallpox is caused by the variola virus. This is a large virus that can, unlike most viruses, just be recognized under a high-power light microscope. Although spread is chiefly by the inhalation of droplets (*see* p. 207) carrying the virus, it can also be contracted by contact with a patient or with his clothing, since the virus is resistant to drying.

Course of the disease. The first symptoms are headache, fever and aching limbs and back, usually arising twelve days after infection. Three or four days later a rash develops, particularly

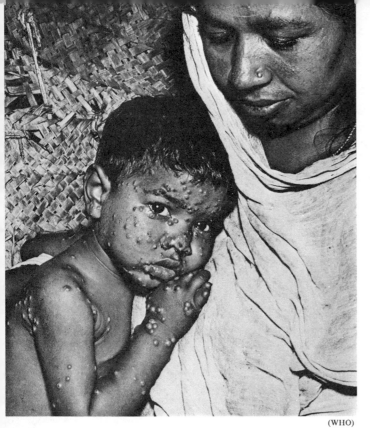

(WHO)

Fig. 29.13 Smallpox pustules. This child is at the 'severely ill' stage of the disease

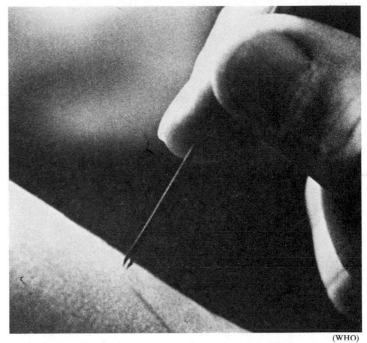

(WHO)

Fig. 29.14 A bifurcated needle is used to scratch anti-smallpox vaccine into the skin

on exposed parts of the body. The spots, red at first, develop into pustules filled with fluid (Fig. 29.13). These dry, if the patient survives, to form crusts or scabs filled with active virus particles which can be spread by contact. However it is the unseen pustules in the respiratory passages releasing virus into the droplets breathed out that provide the greatest danger.

Secondary infections may arise from staphylocci (*see* p. 196) invading the pustules, and these accentuate the scarring that frequently is a legacy of smallpox.

Treatment. Isolation in special hospitals is essential if this highly infectious disease is to be prevented from spreading. Sedatives ease the patient's discomfort, and the irritation associated with the rash can be reduced by frequent bathing.

Control and prophylaxis. Control involves the isolation of patients, already mentioned, coupled with a vigorous vaccination programme which also forms the basis of prophylaxis (prevention).

The principle of vaccination against smallpox was established in the eighteenth century by Edward Jenner, a young doctor in a village near Bristol in England. People noticed that milkmaids and cowmen who had contracted cowpox, a mild disease caught from the animals in their charge, were never stricken with smallpox. Jenner planned a bold experiment and on 14 May 1796 he made a scratch on the arm of a healthy eight-year-old boy and rubbed in pus from a pustule on the arm of a milkmaid suffering from cowpox. A small sore developed on the boy's arm after seven days and later disappeared. Two months later he inoculated the child with matter from pustules on a smallpox victim, but the infection did not take and the boy remained healthy (*see* p. 238).

Within ten years Jenner's technique of vaccination was being tried in Europe though there was still plenty of mistrust to be overcome at home! However, by 1840 a Vaccination Act had been passed in England making vaccination compulsory. New

and improved methods of producing vaccine were developed. At the present time it consists of lymph obtained from calves or sheep after inoculating the skin with *Vaccinia* virus.

A variety of methods of introducing it through the skin have been tried. The most effective method is little different from that used by Jenner. A sterile, double-pointed needle is dipped in vaccine and then used to scratch the skin of the person to be immunized (Fig. 29.14).

When outbreaks of smallpox do occur, then a person from the infected area wishing to enter a country free from the disease is required to produce a certificate of vaccination, usually on a form issued by WHO. Failing this, such a person may be placed in quarantine for sixteen days. In this period it is reckoned that signs and symptoms of the disease would develop if the traveller were infected.

Such precautions are particularly necessary when air travel makes it possible for the disease to be transmitted at high speed over great distances. In the winter of 1961–62, five people entered Britain from Pakistan without having been vaccinated. They developed smallpox shortly after arrival. The disease affected sixty-two other people before it was controlled and of these twenty-four died. In spite of setbacks such as this and the persistence of endemic smallpox in a few countries, there are clear indications that smallpox is being controlled.

Schistosomiasis or bilharziasis (human blood fluke)

Although this disease was recorded in drawings in Egyptian tombs over 3 000 years ago, it was only in 1851 that Theodor Bilharz, a German doctor working in the Medical School in Cairo, described the causative organism, the human blood fluke. The disease was known as bilharzia for many years, but it is also known as *schistosomiasis* since the animal causing the disease belongs to the genus *Schistosoma*, a group of tiny

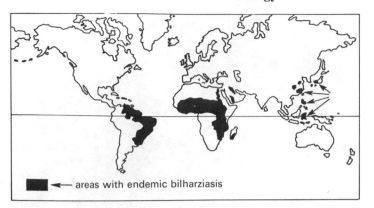

Fig. 29.15   Distribution of endemic bilharziasis

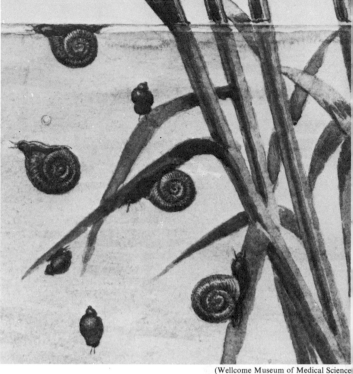

(Wellcome Museum of Medical Science)

Fig. 29.17   Water snails act as intermediate hosts for the larvae of *Schistosoma*

parasitic flatworms or flukes; the name bilharziasis is also sometimes used.

The disease is most widespread in countries where agricultural land is irrigated by canals (Fig. 29.15). Thus *Schistosoma haematobium* causes the disease in the Nile valley and areas of East and West Africa, in the valleys of the Tigris and Euphrates and in the Malagasy Republic (Madagascar). *Schistosoma mansoni* is found in the Nile delta, the Sudan and parts of East and West Africa, and also in Brazil, the Guianas and Venezuela. *Schistosoma japonicum* occurs in the Yangtze valley in China, in the Philippines and parts of Japan.

The causative agent and its life cycle. The adults of *S. haematobium* are found in the blood vessels of the bladder while *S. mansoni* and *S. japonicum* are present in branches of the portal vein. Male blood flukes are larger than the females which they carry in a groove in the body surface. Eggs (Fig. 29.16) are laid in the smaller blood vessels of the gut or bladder and can pass through the walls of the vessels and enter the intestine or the bladder, to be dispersed either in faeces or in urine. If released in fresh water, the eggs hatch and ciliated larvae emerge which must penetrate the bodies of freshwater snails (Fig. 29.17) within a day if they are to survive. Once inside a suitable species of snail the larvae feed on the tissues of the snail and reproduce asexually. Eventually, after four to eight

weeks, they change into cercariae (Fig. 29.18). These creatures, about 0.5 mm long, leave the snail and swim in the surrounding water for up to two days, after which they die unless they can penetrate the body of a human (*see also* pp. 199–200).

Penetration through human skin can occur when people bathe or wade through or simply get their feet wet with infected water. The larvae may also penetrate the body from the gut if they are swallowed in untreated drinking water. Partly by the secretion of enzymes and partly by a wriggling movement the cercariae make their way through, for example, the thin skin at the ankle, and shed their tails. Inside the body, the larvae enter lymph vessels and are then carried slowly to one of the large veins near the heart and so into the circulatory system (*see* p. 83). They appear in the liver after a few days and develop there into adult worms which then re-enter the blood stream. *S. mansoni* and *S. japonicum*, after a total of twenty-three days in the body, establish themselves in branches of the hepatic portal vein near the intestine; while *S. haematobium*,

Fig. 29.16   Egg of *Schistosoma*

(Wellcome Museum of Medical Science)

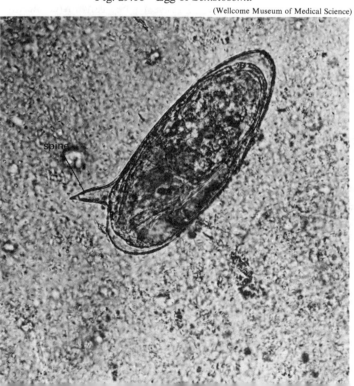

spine

Fig. 29.18   Cercaria larvae of *Schistosoma*

(Dr M. Blair)

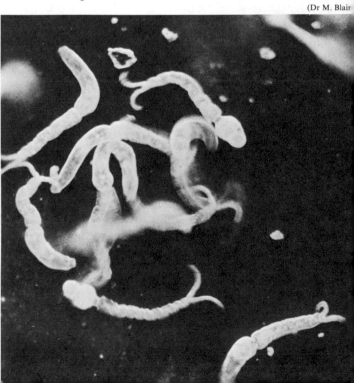

after a similar period, is found in the blood vessels of the bladder. Egg production soon begins and the cycle is resumed.

Course of the disease. Apart from some itching caused when large numbers of cercariae pierce the skin, little is felt until about a month after infection. Then, for five or six weeks the patient may feel ill and have a fever. Heavy infection with *S. mansoni* or *S. japonicum* is accompanied by diarrhoea with blood and mucus appearing in the faeces together with eggs, though these can only be found by examining faeces under a microscope. Over a period of time eggs may be carried in the blood stream to other parts of the body and although they do not develop into larvae, they may cause damage by obstructing small blood vessels, particularly in the brain and spinal cord.

S. haematobium by damaging blood vessels around the bladder causes blood to appear in the urine. Urination becomes uncomfortable and, over a period of years, the ureters are often scarred and obstructed with build-up of pressure in the urine back to the kidneys which may, in turn, be damaged.

Treatment. Diagnosis is usually made by the recognition of eggs in either faeces or urine. The usual treatment is to inject a compound containing antimony into a vein. Such a compound must, of course, be toxic to the blood flukes but there is a risk that the patient might react also. One new antimony compound can be injected into muscle, which is less uncomfortable for the patient but not as effective as those injected into a vein. Drugs known as Nilodin and Miracil D can be taken by mouth. One of the problems is that treatment and cure of individuals does not prevent re-infection.

Control and prophylaxis. If control of schistosomiasis is to be effective then it is necessary to know where infection is coming from. This means mapping an area carefully to show all canals, streams, ponds and other wet areas that may harbour the snails. Then the places where people bathe, wash clothes, obtain drinking water, plant rice, or come into contact with water used for irrigation must be noted on the map. Where the snails are found, they are examined for the presence of schistosome larvae, taking precautions against infection while handling them, for example by wearing rubber gloves.

When this preparatory work has been done, the following measures are put into operation.

(a) Treatment of drinking and washing water. Filtration of water followed by chlorination kills cercariae, but if treated water is to be stored then it is essential that the tanks and cisterns be snail-free, to prevent re-contamination. Boiling destroys these parasites as effectively as it destroys other micro-organisms.

(b) Preventing the eggs from reaching fresh water. It is not sufficient to provide latrines or an effective sewage disposal system if people suffering from schistosomiasis still urinate or defaecate in or near fresh water. People living in infected areas must be educated always to use latrines and this is not an easy or obviously practical goal to achieve. Children in particular should be told about the hazards of snail-infested water and taught the need for hygienic behaviour, since they often play near and splash in and out of water, exposing themselves to the risk of infection and of contaminating the water (Fig. 29.19).

(c) Cercariae can be prevented from reaching the skin either by keeping out of water or by wearing protective boots. Building bridges and culverts over streams and ditches is also helpful.

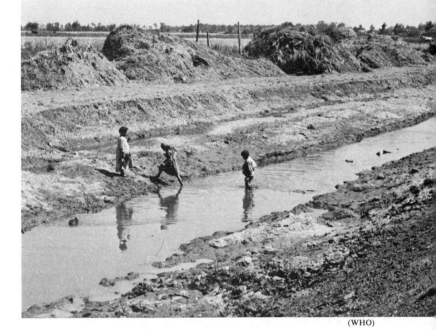

(WHO)

Fig. 29.19 Children paddling in this sweet-water canal in Egypt are exposed to infection with bilharziasis

(d) Control of the snails, the secondary hosts, can be achieved by regulating the flow of irrigation canals. A rapid flow with few obstructions discourages the growth of the water-weeds on which the snails feed. If the water can be cut off to allow ditches to dry out periodically then large numbers of the snails die. This has proved effective in Ghana where the periodic drying out of rice paddy fields has reduced the numbers of snails carrying larvae. Another method is to destroy the snails by the use of copper salts in the water. This requires careful control because copper molluscicides (snail killers) are expensive and can also be dangerous to humans, domestic animals and crops if used at too high a concentration.

In Sharkiah Province in Egypt a project was successfully launched following an investigation of the spread of schistosomiasis that accompanied a new irrigation scheme in the area. Irrigation of the land led to a rise in productivity and prosperity, and the money was used to provide piped, sterilized water and a simple but effective latrine system. Then the part of the canal where village children played was lined with stone and a control dam built at either end. In the hot season the water in this section is treated with a molluscicide to destroy snails and with bleaching powder to control bacteria and other micro-organisms. At the same time, to provide a check on the effectiveness of these measures and the accompanying health education programme, the children's faeces and urine were checked for schistosome eggs. The egg count is falling and the incidence of schistosomiasis in this community is being reduced.

In 1964 WHO estimated that 200 million people suffered from schistosomiasis and that the number was rising. This is particularly so where new irrigation schemes designed to make arid lands in the Philippines, Iraq, Egypt and West Africa more fertile also provided a habitat for snails whose previous absence meant freedom from blood flukes. Awareness of the biology of the schistosome life cycle and determination to break this cycle are leading now to a slow reduction in numbers of patients.

Influenza

Causative agent. Influenza is an illness affecting the breathing system. It varies in severity, and during the years 1933 to 1949 three distinct strains of causative virus were isolated.

Strain A is highly infective and causes epidemics at intervals of two years.

Strain B is irregular in its appearance and outbreaks are usually localized.

Strain C is very mild in its effect and the disease is often undiagnosed.

It is spread by inhaling the virus (Fig. 29.20) in droplets in the air breathed out by infected persons.

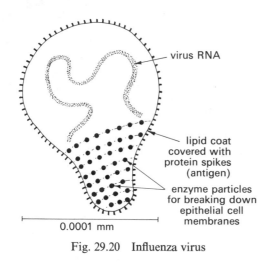

Fig. 29.20   Influenza virus

Course of the disease. Children aged 5 to 14 years are most susceptible, and young adults aged 25 to 35 are also likely to be affected. Of course people in other age groups can and do suffer from the virus, which first attacks the ciliated epithelium of the nasal cavity, pharynx and often the lungs. Symptoms include headaches and fever (Fig. 24.1) together with aches and pains and these all develop rapidly, usually within two days of infection. A person rarely remains infective for more than six days, though he may feel quite weak after an attack.

Treatment. There is no particular treatment other than allowing a person to rest, away from other people to reduce the chances of spreading the virus. However, since the virus damages the mucous membrane of the breathing passages, secondary infections may follow from bacteria which normally exist as harmless commensals (*see* p. 204) on these membranes. One of these, *Haemophilus influenzae*, is associated with bronchitis and inflammation of the nasal sinuses, while the pneumococci causing pneumonia often become active in elderly people following influenza. Pneumonia is often fatal and was probably the most frequent cause of death in the influenza pandemic of 1918–19 when between 15 and 20 million people died.

Prophylaxis. Vaccines containing inactivated strains of the A and B virus give some protection for a short time, but new substrains of these viruses appear as a result of changes in the RNA (the genetic material) of the virus, and there is rarely any immunity to a new strain. However, medical workers and others concerned with maintaining essential services are often vaccinated when it is known that an epidemic is likely to occur.

Influenza is one of the few diseases to show a truly pandemic spread during this century. The pandemic of 1918 has already been mentioned. In 1957 a virus known as A_2 caused a pandemic of 'Asian flu'. Its spread has been traced from China to Hong Kong and from there to most parts of the world. Hong Kong is a centre of world trade with an international sea- and airport from which infected persons may carry the virus to other countries.

It is still surprising that influenza, with its maximum of six days' infectivity in man and its rapid production of symptoms should be transmitted quite so widely and speedily. What happens to the virus between outbreaks is still uncertain. Possibly it is kept going by a chain of sporadic cases, though healthy carriers of the virus may exist. International co-operation through WHO enables outbreaks to be predicted, and some preparations to be made for dealing with a wave of infection by the preparation and administration of vaccines.

Rats, fleas and plague

Bubonic plague is a disease caused by bacteria. It appeared in epidemic proportions throughout most of Europe in the thirteenth to nineteenth centuries and was often referred to as the Black Death, because of the appearance of dark areas of diseased tissue on the bodies of victims, particularly after death. An epidemic in the fourteenth century killed about a quarter of the population of Europe.

The spread of plague throughout the tropics has been more recent and has followed the transport of rats, the principal reservoir of the causative agent, from one country to another with grain shipments, particularly as movements of grain food

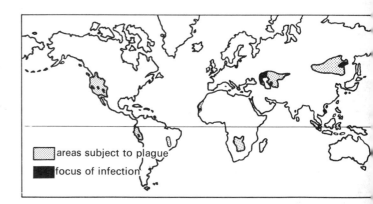

Fig. 29.21   Areas where plague was endemic in 1974

between countries have greatly increased. A major outbreak in India in 1896 lasted for fifteen years and killed over eight million people. The epidemic followed the extension of rail and sea transport facilities. It soon spread into East Africa but it was only in 1903 that it was first recorded on the west coast of South America where it is now endemic (Fig. 29.21).

Scientists believe that the disease was originally confined to wild animals which, being the hosts in which the pathogen normally lives, still form the reservoir of infection; from these animals it may be introduced or re-introduced to humans. An infection of this kind, originating in another vertebrate, is called a *zoonosis*. To understand its relationship to man one has first to know the ecology (life pattern in relation to its environment) of the reservoir animal and also of the vector, in this case the rat flea.

For plague to become endemic there must be a suitable host animal with a high resistance to disease. Rats such as the black rat, *Rattus rattus*, and the brown or sewer rat, *Rattus norvegicus*, certainly harbour the plague bacillus in such countries as India, Pakistan and Burma, though in other parts of the world to which plague has been introduced the rats have had a low resistance to the bacteria and have died. Marmots, mice, gerbils and other rodents are among the mammals that act as hosts in different parts of the world.

Causative agent and method of spread. The micro-organism causing plague is a bacillus with rounded ends called *Pasteurella pestis*, first identified in 1894. Experiments carried out in Hong Kong in 1898 showed that these bacilli were present in fleas that had fed on plague rats, and that these fleas could infect healthy rats. The details of transmission to humans were not discovered until 1914 when it was noted in India that only certain kinds of rat flea were capable of transmitting the bacilli. Fleas that digest the bacilli as well as the blood are not able to act as vectors. However, when the rat flea, *Xenopsylla cheopis* (Fig. 29.22), has fed on infected blood the bacillus

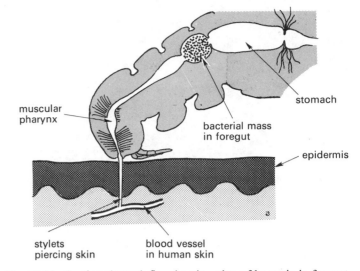

muscular pharynx · stomach · bacterial mass in foregut · epidermis · stylets piercing skin · blood vessel in human skin

Fig. 29.24   Section through flea showing plug of bacteria in foregut

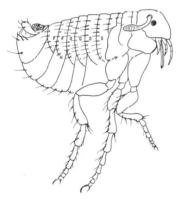

Fig. 29.22   Rat flea, *Xenopsylla* (× 15)

multiplies in the flea's foregut and forms a mass which blocks the gut and prevents further feeding until the flea, by now hungry, regurgitates the bacterial mass on to the host's skin (Fig. 29.24). As it pierces the skin to feed, some of the bacteria are introduced into the wound and, provided the numbers of bacteria are sufficient, a new case of plague results. When feeding, a flea can take about 0.5 mm³ of blood into its stomach. This volume of blood from an infected rat may contain large

numbers of bacilli, but 0.5 mm³ of human blood, unless the host is nearly dying of plague, will not contain sufficient numbers of bacilli to provide a minimum dose (*see* p. 211) so that no infection results. It was only in 1953 that the human flea, *Pulex irritans*, was finally shown to be capable of transmitting plague bacilli from one human host to another and then only when infection was very heavy and when the fleas are numerous. When many fleas feed together the numbers of bacilli entering the blood exceeds the minimum needed to produce an infection (Fig. 29.23).

Course of the disease. Plague bacilli produce a powerful antigen (*see* p. 74). In addition they inhibit the phagocytic activity of leucocytes. Symptoms develop after an incubation period of two to four days, occasionally longer, and include fever of 39–40 °C (103–104 °F) or higher, and the patient feels very ill and weak. The white cells of the blood stream combat the invasion of fast-breeding bacilli and the lymph nodes become choked with dead cells and bacteria. Lymph nodes in the groin and armpit in particular become swollen, sometimes to the size of a hen's egg, and the name 'bubonic plague' is a recognition of these buboes or swollen lymph nodes. Mortality from plague is high, particularly at the start of an epidemic, but the antibiotic drug streptomycin destroys the bacilli.

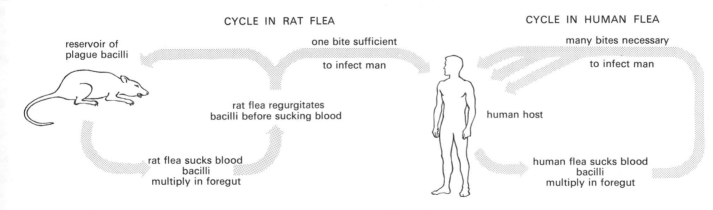

CYCLE IN RAT FLEA · CYCLE IN HUMAN FLEA

reservoir of plague bacilli · one bite sufficient to infect man · many bites necessary to infect man

rat flea regurgitates bacilli before sucking blood · human host

rat flea sucks blood bacilli multiply in foregut · human flea sucks blood bacilli multiply in foregut

Fig. 29.23   Transmission of bubonic plague

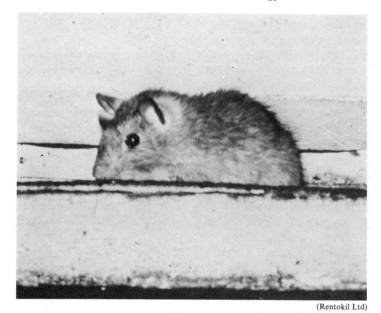

(Rentokil Ltd)

Fig. 29.25 The black rat, *Rattus rattus*, is the reservoir for *Pasteurella pestis*, the plague bacillus

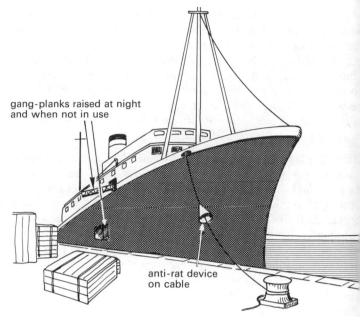

gang-planks raised at night and when not in use

anti-rat device on cable

Fig. 29.26 Precautions against the spread of rats by ship

Prophylaxis. The most effective way of preventing plague epidemics is to destroy both the reservoirs of the disease, usually rats, and the fleas that act as vectors. To destroy rats successfully one must know their habits and where they feed and breed (Fig. 29.25).

Stored food, particularly grain, is attractive to rats. Granaries and rice stores should be made rat-proof (*see* p. 261) and so should domestic food stores. Rats are good climbers, and rat-proofing a building at all levels is not easy and is often expensive. Rats also frequent rubbish tips, drains and sewers, each of which provide food for the animals. Methods of making these less accessible to rats are described in Chapter 37.

Where rats have already established themselves and are breeding they can be destroyed by poisons, laid in a bait, usually crushed grain. Warfarin is still widely used. It reduces the clotting properties of the blood, and rats that eat it die from internal haemorrhages. However strains of rats have evolved that are resistant to warfarin and the search for a new rodent destroyer is being intensified.

Attention to personal hygiene, particularly the wearing of clean underclothing (p. 226), eliminates or at least reduces the numbers of fleas on the body and therefore reduces the chances of a minimum infective dose of bacilli penetrating the skin. DDT powder on floors and DDT spray on walls of rooms where fleas may be present reduce the numbers of vectors.

Public health authorities must act quickly when plague outbreaks do occur but the fact that epidemics are now rare is a reflection of the attention given to control of rats. The introduction of plague to a healthy country is prevented by such measures as the use of anti-rat shields on the mooring ropes of ships and by drawing up gangways when these are not being used (Fig. 29.26).

Questions

1 Account for the enormous fall in the death rate from malaria throughout the world between 1955 and 1975.

2 Why are cholera and influenza usually thought of as epidemic diseases? What factors influence the spread of these two diseases?

3 Make a list of the diseases that occur most commonly in your country. How are they spread? What measures can be taken to reduce their spread? This information may usefully be recorded in the form of a table.

30

The Control and Prevention of Disease by Personal Hygiene

The best protection against disease is good health. This is not such an obvious statement as it may sound, since a person who is well-fed, clean and not overtired will usually resist infection better than one who already suffers from a number of minor complaints. Hygiene is the science and practice of maintaining good health.

The importance of an adequate, balanced diet has already been discussed in Chapter 6. The body's first lines of defence against invasion by bacteria and viruses are the skin and the mucous membranes lining the breathing system and alimentary canal. If these are to be effective barriers then the diet must contain adequate protein, fat and the appropriate minerals and vitamins for healthy cell growth.

Hygiene of hands and skin

Much of the food that we eat is handled at several stages between its production and the time when we eat it. Some aspects of food hygiene are dealt with in Chapter 34, but here we are concerned with the part played by our own hands in contaminating food.

Fig. 30.1 A sterile swab was rubbed over a lavatory seat and then over the left-hand side of the plate. A second swab was rubbed over the seat after it had been cleaned with disinfectant and applied to the right-hand side of the plate

(Domestos Hygiene Advisory Service)

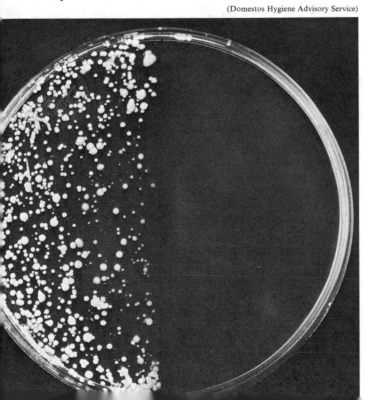

We are continually handling things such as furniture, implements and door handles that have been touched by other people, and many of us handle domestic animals and stroke our pets. These all carry micro-organisms that, in turn, stick to the skin of our hands, as is demonstrated in the practical work on p. 228. Our fingers touch our food, our mouths and other parts of our bodies and the micro-organisms are again transferred. We build up a resistance to many of the germs spread in this way (see p. 238) and for much of our lives we are unaware of any risk of infection being spread, especially if our hands do not *look* dirty. Nevertheless there are in Britain each year outbreaks of a mild form of dysentery, particularly among school-children, that probably spreads because they are not taught to use nor are they provided with facilities for washing their hands after using the toilet (Fig. 30.1).

The use of soap or a similar detergent when we wash is important. Detergents have the effect of breaking the bonds between fats and our skin and, since many kinds of micro-organisms are held by oils and fats, these too are removed by detergent action (see Chapter 26).

Antiseptics and disinfectants are not usually used on the hands unless we know we have been in contact with pathogenic organisms. Thus, during an epidemic of cholera or any other disease for which diarrhoea is a sign, it is wise to wash the hands thoroughly with an antiseptic after touching a WC seat (toilet seat) or indeed after touching the walls or any other part of a lavatory.

The fingers can transmit other kinds of micro-organisms such as the bacteria causing septic spots, and if these are touched on breaks in the skin like cuts and grazes—and we do touch them when they itch or irritate—then infection can be caused. Clean hands make this less likely.

We are unlikely to contaminate food with organisms carried on our feet (unless we touch them!) but most of us walk barefoot at some time during the day and our feet are exposed to infection. The larvae of *Schistosoma* penetrate the body through the skin of the feet when people walk barefoot through infected water and larval hookworms enter the body in the same way. The wearing of shoes or boots gives protection.

On the other hand, poorly ventilated boots and shoes encourage the skin of the feet to sweat and this makes the skin soft and open to attack by fungi. The tiny fungus causing athlete's foot is usually caught by people walking barefoot in communal baths and changing rooms when fragments of the fungus, shed from the foot of an infected person, grow in the clefts between the toes. If unchecked, the fungus can produce

225

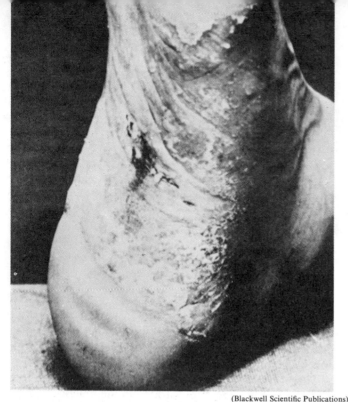

(Blackwell Scientific Publications)

Fig. 30.2 The fungal disease, athlete's foot, may spread to the whole foot

Clothing with a clean open texture is also absorbent and its ability to soak up sweat from the skin is an advantage. An accumulation of sweat may result in the skin condition known as *prickly heat*, which is accompanied by a fine rash and considerable irritation.

Hygiene of the respiratory system (Fig. 30.3)

We have read in Chapter 27 that many diseases are transmitted by droplet infection. We can breathe air into our lungs either through the nose or the mouth. Provided the nasal passages are not blocked with mucus or with catarrh or by swelling of the mucous membrane, we breathe through our noses except when we are talking or engaged in strenuous exercise such as running. Nose breathing ensures that air passes between the hairs in the nostrils and over the folds of mucous membrane in the nasal cavity. The surfaces of the hairs and membranes are normally moist and many germs and dust particles are trapped on these surfaces, though some of course pass on to the lungs. Since a minimum number of organisms must be present before disease symptoms will develop, it can be seen that any means of reducing the numbers by 'filtering' air before it reaches the respiratory passages and lungs should be helpful. Blowing the nose, preferably into a disposable handkerchief, is a means of removing the mucus and trapped organisms.

considerable discomfort and, because it causes areas of epidermis to be shed, may open the way to secondary infection. Regular thorough washing with soap and water followed by careful drying is essential to prevent the spread of this organism (*see* Fig. 30.2).

Clean underclothing is necessary if good hygiene is to be maintained over the rest of the body. A fungus similar to that causing athlete's foot produces the condition called dhobie itch or tinea cruris. This develops in the skin of the groin and can be spread by the casual use of another person's towel or underclothing that carries the fungus.

Most skin infections are spread by direct or indirect contact, which is not easy to avoid, but once established the speed with which these infections can be controlled is influenced by personal hygiene. Regular bathing and changing of underclothing helps to control infestation with lice and fleas. These are dangerous as vectors of disease (p. 236) and if they breed on our bodies or in our clothing then the risk of eventual infection through their bites is multiplied.

Skin parasites such as the itch mite, causing scabies, are less likely to attack the body if it is regularly washed. If the itch mite does penetrate the skin it forms burrows up to 1 cm long in which the female lays eggs. Hot baths with vigorous scrubbing of affected areas with soap, water and a nail-brush is the essential first stage of treatment, followed by very thorough washing of all underclothing.

Clean clothing, because of the airfilled spaces between the fibres, is a good insulator. It helps the body to retain heat in cool weather and equally gives protection against direct radiant heat from strong sunlight. When clothing is dirty, the air spaces become blocked and the insulating properties are reduced. Some bacteria are able to breed in the dirt and they are always a potential source of infection.

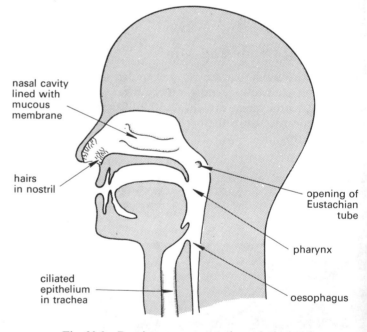

Fig. 30.3 Respiratory passages through the head

When we breathe through the mouth there is a more open passageway for air to reach the trachea and no effective filtration of the air. When we are running or making other efforts that result in heavy breathing we are not usually in crowded conditions and the risks of droplet infection are small. But we often talk when we are in crowds, and are standing very close to other people, and there is no doubt that the risk of inhaling germs is then greater than if we breathe through the nose.

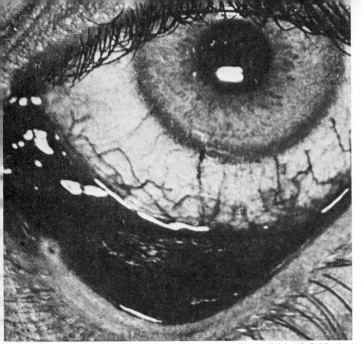

(Blackwell Scientific Publications)

Fig. 30.4 Conjunctivitis, inflammation of the membrane covering the eye

Even if we do breathe slowly and carefully through the nose the risk of catching droplet-transmitted viruses, such as those causing influenza, has been shown to be very much greater for people who have to travel close together in a crowded train or bus during an epidemic. Good ventilation of buildings and public transport reduces this risk (see p. 258).

Hygiene of the eyes and ears

The conjunctiva (see p. 133), the thin layer of cells covering the cornea of the eye, has an important protective function similar to that of the skin covering the soft tissues of the body. If the cornea is damaged, for example by the scratching action of sharp dust blown into the eye, then a break is made in the protection and pathogenic organisms may invade the surface tissues of the eye. Such pathogens include the rickettsia-like organism causing *trachoma*, a form of blindness common in some tropical countries, in which the conjunctiva becomes opaque and unable to transmit regular patterns of light rays. The pathogen is present in the discharge from an infected eye and is transferred on towels and by flies which alight on the eyelids to feed on the liquid film over the eye. The same methods of spread are responsible for transmission of a virus causing epidemic conjunctivitis (inflammation of the conjunctiva) and a bacterial conjunctivitis which is highly infectious (Fig. 30.4).

A continuous secretion of watery liquid from the tear glands bathes each eye. This lubricates the eyeball so that the eyelids can move freely over it and it washes away fine dust particles and bacteria. Sir Alexander Fleming first described an enzyme that he discovered in tears which is capable of *lysing* or breaking down the outer coat of bacteria, and which he called lysozyme. Clearly this enzyme does not destroy all pathogenic organisms but it is important in controlling many of them, just as a steady flow of fluid washes away many organisms.

The importance of vitamin A in the maintenance of good vision has already been described on p. 36 and the common defects in vision are dealt with on p. 138.

The middle and inner ear are encased in bone which provides protection against mechanical damage. The tube of the outer ear is less well protected. Wax is secreted from cells in the skin lining the tube, and its function, apart from being mildly antiseptic, is uncertain. If too much accumulates in the tube then hearing is less distinct, but care should be taken when trying to remove it since the careless use of any implement such as a matchstick could easily damage the ear drum, with the possibility of infection and deafness. Wax near the entrance to the ear passage should be removed in the course of washing; wax deep in the passage should be removed only by a qualified medical worker.

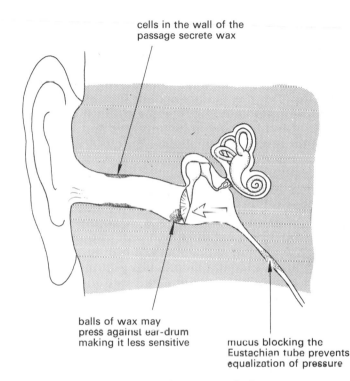

cells in the wall of the passage secrete wax

balls of wax may press against ear-drum making it less sensitive

mucus blocking the Eustachian tube prevents equalization of pressure

Fig. 30.5 Causes of temporary deafness

As far as possible the ear tube should be dried after swimming or bathing to prevent the germination of fungal spores, a condition more common in tropical than in temperate countries.

A short tube, the Eustachian tube, connects the middle ear to the pharynx (back of the mouth) and its function is to permit movement of air to equalize the pressure on each side of the ear drum (see Fig. 30.5). The drum then vibrates with maximum sensitivity. Secondary infections with bacteria following a cold sometimes spread into the Eustachian tube which may be blocked by the thick catarrh produced; if this happens, any change in air pressure between the two sides of the ear drum results in the drum bulging outwards or inwards and becoming tensed. It is less sensitive to sound vibrations and deafness is noticed. Treatment of the infection usually results in normal hearing being restored.

Earache arises when micro-organisms penetrate the Eustachian tube into the middle ear chamber and set up an infection there. The pain may be the result of the action of toxins on nerve endings or the result of the formation of pus which accumulates and builds up pressure. Such a condition can be dangerous if untreated by a doctor, since under pressure the pus and the germs it contains may burst through the ear drum.

This may cause permanent partial deafness as a result of the scar tissue that heals the wound. More seriously, the infectious matter may be forced into the bone tissue surrounding the brain.

People who work in conditions with very loud noise such as in heavy engineering works or men using pneumatic drills often become deaf. So do a considerable number of young people who listen to music played very loudly through powerful amplifiers. Such deafness is termed sensory deafness because it results from damage to the sense cells and nerves in the inner ear or cochlea. Whereas deafness through damage to the ear drum can often be repaired, there is no known treatment for deafness resulting from damage to the inner ear.

Hygiene of the genital organs

Because they are associated with the removal of body waste, usually carrying considerable numbers of micro-organisms, the genital organs need careful attention to cleanliness.

In males the opening of the urethra at the end of the penis is well separated from the anal opening and there is usually little chance of organisms normally present in faeces finding their way to the urinary tube. In females the two openings are only a few centimetres apart and carelessness in cleaning the body after either urination or defaecation may result in germs from the rectum being spread to the urethra. Quite how such germs make their way up the urethra is uncertain but they are able to enter the bladder where they may cause the inflammation known as cystitis. Careful, quite separate cleansing and drying of the region around each opening should become a habit.

In addition, in females, the cells lining the uterus and vagina produce a secretion of mucus that is mildly antiseptic when fresh and washes out micro-organisms. Those organisms causing venereal diseases seem able to survive in this fluid but most others do not. However, as the fluid accumulates in the vulva, the folds of flesh outside the vagina, chemical changes take place and many kinds of bacteria can now feed on the fluid, producing waste products with disagreeable smells. Thorough washing or bathing with soap and water at least once each day is the most effective way of maintaining the hygiene of this part of the body.

For males, apart from washing the anal region at least once every day, the penis, scrotum and groin should be thoroughly cleansed with soap and water. The sweat glands in the groin produce a sweat that differs in composition as well as being more abundant than that from most other parts of the body. When freshly secreted it is innocuous but if decomposed by bacteria on the skin and pubic hair can acquire a distasteful smell. It can also make the skin more hospitable for the growth of the fungus of dhobie itch and for certain bacteria that cause skin irritations.

Care should be taken to cleanse the end of the penis, particularly if this is covered by the foreskin, because germs can feed in the mucus produced by the glands under the foreskin. Recognition of the risk of infection from such bacteria is just one of the practical reasons for circumcision, in which the foreskin is drawn back and cut away from the penis, usually when a boy is very young (Fig. 30.6).

The term *venereal disease* (*see* p. 208) refers to two diseases transmitted during sexual intercourse or close sexual contact. The name is derived from the Latin, *Venus*, the goddess of love, and is associated with 'love-making'. Many kinds of organisms including bacteria, fungi and protozoa are transmitted in this way. In order to maintain sexual hygiene, a wise person would not expose himself or herself to the risk of infection through

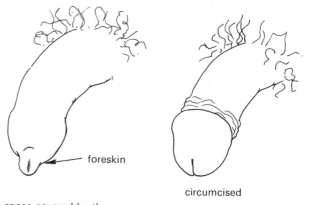
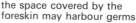
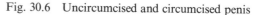

the space covered by the foreskin may harbour germs

Fig. 30.6 Uncircumcised and circumcised penis

intercourse with another person whose state of sexual health was not known. Even 'heavy petting', touching and stimulating the genital organs of the other person, carries a risk of the transfer of disease-causing organisms on the fingers.

Practical Work

Hands and bacteria

Prepare four agar plates (p. 202). Rub your fingers on the floor and then press them firmly on the agar jelly of the first plate and mark it 'Dirty fingers'. Now wash your hands with soap and water. Dry them by waving them in the air and *not* with a towel (why not?) and make a set of finger marks on the second plate, labelling it 'Washed fingers'. Scrub your fingers thoroughly for not less than half a minute and make a third set of marks. Label this 'Scrubbed fingers', and the fourth plate 'Control'. Incubate the four plates at 37 °C for not less than two days and then compare and discuss the growth of bacterial colonies on them. Destroy the cultures by sterilizing when you have observed the bacterial colonies.

Question

What do you think would be the most effective way of encouraging and developing personal hygiene in someone younger than yourself?

31
Control of the Vectors of Disease

A *vector* is an organism that acts as an agent in the transfer of a disease-causing parasite from one host to another. Sometimes this is purely mechanical, as when a housefly, having fed on the faeces of a dysentery sufferer, carries the causative organisms on its mouthparts and deposits these when it feeds on foodstuff prepared for human consumption.

Many vectors are involved in a more complete role in which the disease-causing parasite acquired from one host grows and sometimes reproduces within the body of the vector before being transmitted to a new host. This is illustrated by the anopheline mosquito, in whose body the malarial parasite must undergo reproduction and development before it can be successfully transferred to another human host.

The housefly illustrates *mechanical transmission* of cholera vibrios and dysentery bacteria, while the anopheline mosquito shows *cyclical transmission* of malarial parasites.

A further role is shown by the snail in which the parasite causing schistosomiasis undergoes its larval development. While not a vector in the sense of transmitting the schistosome directly to the next host, the snail plays an essential part in the transmission of the disease.

Insecticides

Not all the vectors of disease are insects, but since the majority are either insects or other arthropods, the chemicals used for destroying them are usually termed *insecticides* (insect killers). We are not concerned with the detailed chemistry of insecticides but an outline of their classification will be useful.

The insecticides in common use are separated into non-

residual and residual, depending on how stable they are in contact with air and, therefore, whether their effect is long-lasting or not.

Non-residual insecticides. Pyrethrum, and an extract from it called pyrethrin, is made from the dried powdered petals of *Pyrethrum* flowers. It can be used as a dusting powder or it can be dissolved in kerosine (paraffin) and used as a spray. It is the insecticide used in most domestic aerosols (Fig. 31.1).

When used as a fine spray in a closed room it kills most flying insects very quickly. However, when the room is re-opened, other insects entering will not be affected and their destruction can only be achieved by re-spraying. Pyrethrum, then, is a *non-residual* insecticide and a natural material.

Residual insecticides are stable chemicals that are usually sprayed or dusted on to surfaces on which insects alight or crawl. The active substance dissolves in the waxy outer layer of cuticle on the insect's feet and penetrates, slowly, to the nervous system, causing paralysis and death. The effectiveness of such chemicals may last for weeks or even months.

Most residual contact insecticides are synthetic compounds called chlorinated hydrocarbons and are more familiar as DDT, gamma BHC (also Gammexane and Lindane) and dieldrin. Gamma BHC is very toxic to insects but vapourizes easily so

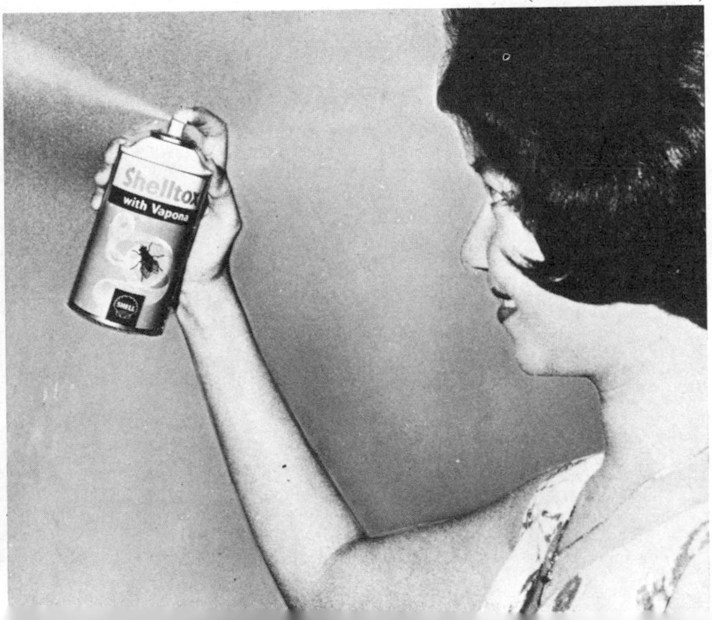

Fig. 31.2 Large-scale spraying of mosquito breeding grounds in a town

(Shell Petroleum Co. Ltd)

Fig. 31.1 Using an aerosol spray indoors

(Shell Petroleum Co. Ltd)

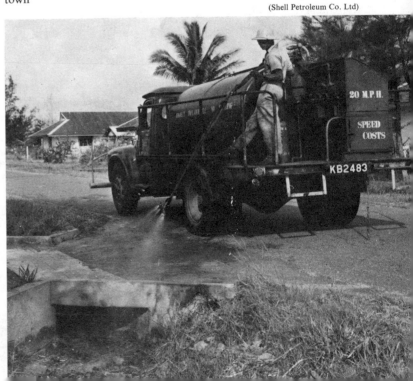

that it is not so long-lasting as DDT and dieldrin. All three substances are poisonous to humans if they enter the body in sufficient quantity. Most is known about DDT in this respect. It is not only stable in the atmosphere but resists breakdown by the normal process of detoxication in the liver (*see* p. 69). It is fat-soluble and accumulates in body fat. There is little evidence to show that it has caused death to humans except when consumed, perhaps deliberately, in large quantity, but its presence in the body fat of people who feed on vegetables treated with DDT insecticide or on animals fed on insecticide-treated crops is sufficient to keep health authorities alert (*see* Food chains, p. 58).

A further group of insecticides, the organic (or organo-) phosphorus compounds which include diazimon, malathion and DDVP, is in wide use. Some of the early organo-phosphorus insecticides were highly toxic to man and a few were considered for use as war gases. The three named are relatively safe, though people concerned with their use take rigorous precautions to avoid inhaling spray or dust or getting them on to their skin. Research to produce safer, longer-acting and more powerful insecticides continues.

Control of mosquitoes

Mosquitoes are found in most parts of the world. As adults they all feed on plant juices though the females of most species will also suck the blood of mammals and birds before producing eggs. It is these blood-sucking adults that are potential vectors for disease organisms. Whether they actually do transmit pathogenic micro-organisms depends on the capacity of the micro-organisms to survive inside the body of the mosquito as well as in the blood of the host animal from which they were sucked. A particular pathogen will usually be transmitted by one of a small group of related mosquito species, but not by all species.

Although there are some hundreds of species of mosquito the main features of their life cycles are surprisingly uniform and provide a basis on which the general principles of control can be established (Figs. 31.3–5).

The females lay their eggs on water either singly or in groups termed 'egg rafts' (Fig. 31.5*b*). Hatching occurs after two to three days in the tropics, though it may take longer in cooler climates. The larvae feed by filtering minute algae from the water and, with this protein-rich diet, they grow rapidly and wriggle actively. They breathe atmospheric air through a tube or siphon near the tail end. After a period of ten days to several

weeks the larva changes into an active pupa which still breathes air through a breathing tube, but at the head end. Metamorphosis, a dramatic change in body shape, takes place inside the pupa case which is eventually split to let the young adult emerge. While its wings expand and harden the newly emerged adult stands on the floating pupal case and then flies off in search of vegetation from which it proceeds to suck its first meal. For this purpose the mouthparts are arranged to form two channels with sharp, piercing ends. Saliva can be pumped through the smaller channel while liquefied food is sucked up through the larger. The table shows four important diseases and the more important kinds of mosquitoes that transmit them.

Disease	Causative organism	Mosquito vectors	Geographical distribution of disease
Malaria	protozoon	*Anopheles*	potentially world-wide
Dengue	virus	*Aëdes*	S.E. Europe, Middle East, North & West Africa, S.E. Asia, North Australia, Central & S. America
Filariasis	filarial worm	*Aëdes Culex Mansonia Anopheles*	Africa, Caribbean, India & Sri Lanka, S.E. Asia, North Australia, Polynesia
Yellow fever	virus	*Aëdes Haemogogus Taenorhyncus*	Africa, S. America, Caribbean

Although the life cycles of all these mosquitoes are similar, precise breeding sites vary greatly as do their feeding habits. For example *Anopheles gambiae*, the most widely distributed malaria carrier in Africa, will lay eggs in almost any sunlit water such as roadside puddles, wells, pools in river beds and even slightly salted water. *Anopheles claviger*, an urban mosquito found in Syria and Israel, lays eggs in wells and cisterns, while *A. plumbeus*, found in Britain and Northern Europe, lays eggs in tree holes. *A. punctimaculata*, which spreads malaria in Central America, will only lay in pools or sluggish water in shade.

Information about where eggs are laid, when the adult females feed on blood, and where they rest when not feeding,

(a) Eggs and larvae

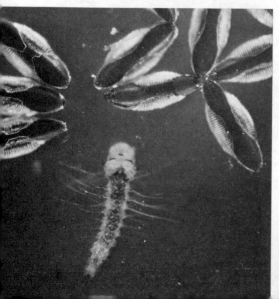

Fig. 31.3   Life cycle of *Anopheles*

(b) Pupae

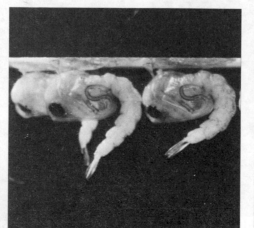

(c) Adult female

(Shell Petroleum Co. Ltd)

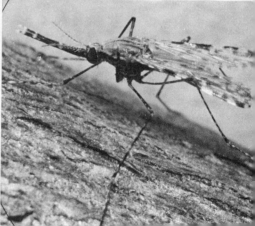

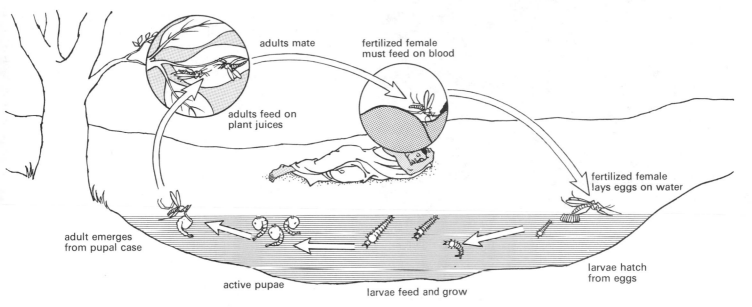

Fig. 31.4   Life cycle of a culecine mosquito

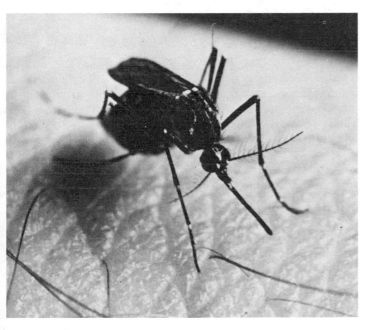

(a) Adult preparing to feed on human arm

(c) Larvae

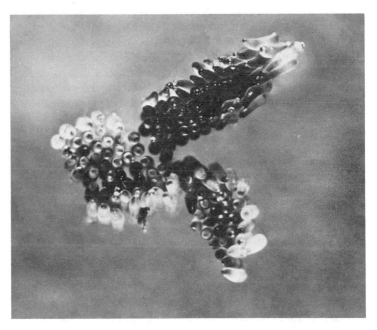

(b) Egg raft

Fig. 31.5   Stages in the life cycle of *Culex*

(d) Pupae

(Shell Petroleum Co. Ltd)

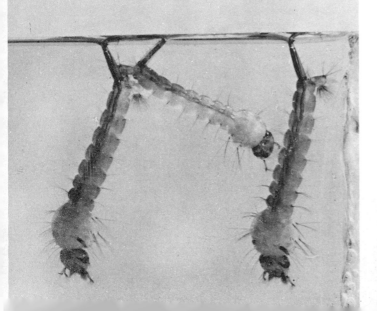

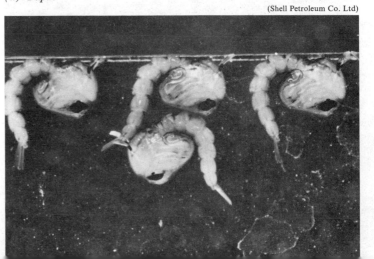

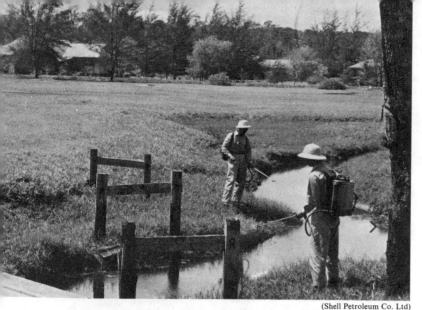

(Shell Petroleum Co. Ltd)

Fig. 31.6 Spraying breeding grounds of anopheline mosquitoes

is of importance in planning control measures. So is knowledge of the length of time that the adults spend between taking their first blood meal and when they stop feeding, and the frequency with which they feed.

With a carefully planned campaign based largely on the use of insecticides, as described on p. 215, malaria and yellow fever have been brought under control in many areas of the world where they were once endemic. Success in controlling filariasis has not been so spectacular, partly because species of *Culex* transmitting this disease are less susceptible to insecticides. However, in Sri Lanka (Ceylon), where filariasis is transmitted by *Mansonia*, control has been achieved by the use of a herbicide to destroy the water plant *Pistia stratiodes* to which the larvae attach themselves and on which they are dependent.

Once a vector has been destroyed in an area it is important to prevent its re-introduction. For example, since the eradication of *Anopheles* from the Mediterranean island of Cyprus, health authorities check and spray with insecticide all aircraft arriving from malarious countries.

In Guyana, S. America, *Anopheles darlingi* was systematically destroyed along the coastal belt by spraying houses with residual DDT to kill the adults. It is no longer necessary to maintain this spraying programme, provided that a narrow barrier zone is continuously treated between the cultivated and populated coastal zone and the high bush of the interior where the mosquito still breeds. People visiting the country

Fig. 31.7 Taking a blood sample to test for the presence of malarial parasites

(Shell Petroleum Co. Ltd)

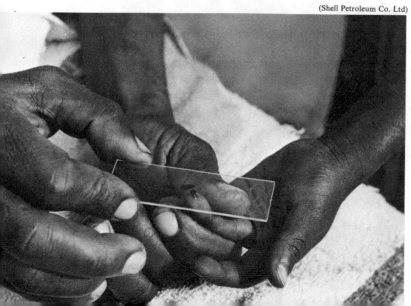

from known malarious areas have to provide a drop of blood to be examined for parasites (Fig. 31.7).

Where extermination is not possible, use is made of the knowledge that most mosquitoes bite at night. By reducing the area of exposed skin by wearing slacks and long sleeves, the risk for those people who must be out after dark is reduced. Indoors, spraying with an insecticide destroys mosquitoes that have entered the building during the day. Keeping windows covered with fly wire, while allowing ventilation, excludes the

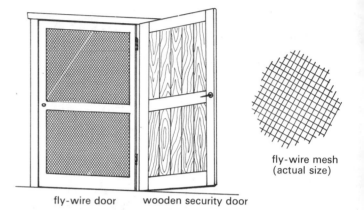

fly-wire mesh (actual size)

fly-wire door   wooden security door

Fig. 31.8 Fly wire is placed over windows and doors to exclude mosquitoes

vectors. Sleeping under a mosquito net is important in such circumstances, not only to keep mosquitoes from healthy persons but particularly from malarial or other patients. If such patients are bitten by the appropriate mosquito then the life cycle of the parasite is continued and other people are at risk.

A combination of methods is necessary for successful control and these may be summarized as follows:

(i) destruction of breeding grounds (p. 215);
(ii) killing adult mosquitoes and larvae with insecticides;
(iii) preventing mosquitoes reaching human hosts;
(iv) use of chemical prophylaxis (p. 215) appropriate for malaria and yellow fever.

Fig. 31.9 Spraying a doorway with residual insecticide to control mosquitoes in Taiwan

(Shell Petroleum Co. Ltd)

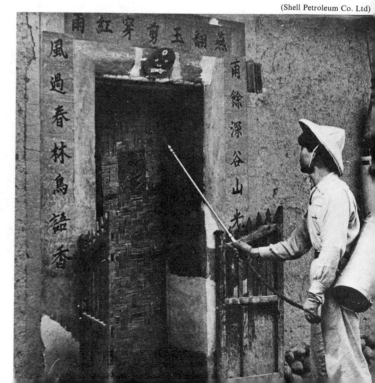

Control of houseflies

Houseflies of the genus *Musca* are world-wide in their distribution. A connection between flies and the spread of disease has been assumed since very ancient times. Moses' instruction to the children of Israel to bury their excrement suggests an awareness of this, and the Romans supposed that dysentery was spread by flies falling into or walking over food. Adult flies are attracted to and walk over and feed on foetid, decomposing material and, particularly, human faeces. More than a hundred different pathogens have been identified from the bodies of houseflies at one time or another, including those causing cholera, bacterial and amoebic dysentery and typhoid fever.

Adult flies are capable of feeding only on liquid food, that is, on food already in liquid form or else food which can be dissolved in the plentiful saliva that the fly secretes. In order to suck liquid the fly uses its proboscis which has a flap or labellum at the end. Bacteria can be shown to be present in the liquid on this flap and also in the saliva that the fly produces while feeding. When it is feeding on food destined for human consumption then contamination occurs. Sometimes partially digested food is regurgitated with the saliva, carrying still more micro-organisms (Fig. 31.10).

Flies drop their faeces as and when necessary and this frequently occurs as they walk over food. Many kinds of pathogens are unaffected by passage through the alimentary canal of the fly and are still capable of causing disease if ingested by humans.

Careful examination of an adult fly shows the body and legs to be covered with hairs. These are able to hold small particles of dust and bacteria in the same way that the bristles of a brush do, and they may be scattered from these hairs on to food as they walk over it.

In order to control this vector of disease it is necessary to know its life cycle (Fig. 31.11). During mating the female fly receives large numbers of sperms into her body and these will fertilize the eggs. Before laying she seeks out decomposing organic matter such as faeces, a manure heap or a dustbin. Flies are attracted to this material by its smell. Bacterial decomposition converts it into a liquefied state on which the larva will be able to feed easily after hatching. Hatching occurs ten to seventy-two hours after laying, depending on temperature. Bacterial decomposition results in release of heat energy and this accelerates development of the embryo within the egg.

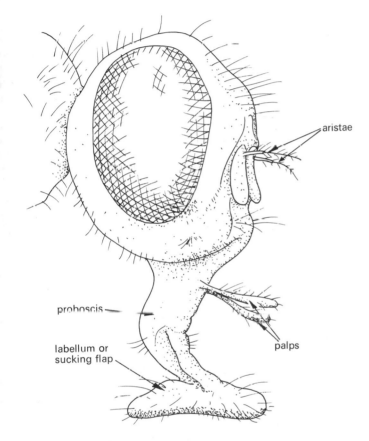

Fig. 31.10   Head and proboscis of housefly

Effect of temperature on the development of the housefly

| | Length of each stage | |
Stage	Warm climate 30 °C	Cool climate 10 °C
egg	10 hours	3 days
larva	3 days	8 weeks
pupa	3 days	4 weeks
adult	4 weeks	12 weeks

The larva has a white body, almost transparent when newly hatched, tapering from a blunt posterior to a small head (Fig.

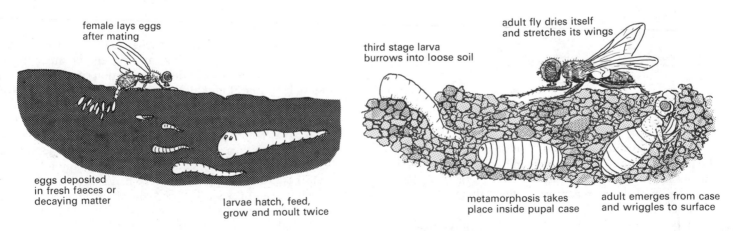

Fig. 31.11   Life cycle of the housefly

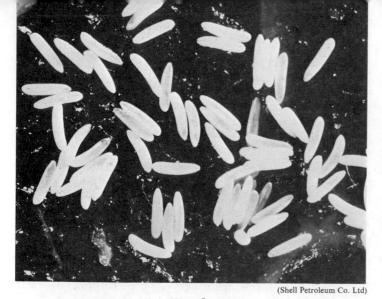

(Shell Petroleum Co. Ltd)

(a) Housefly eggs

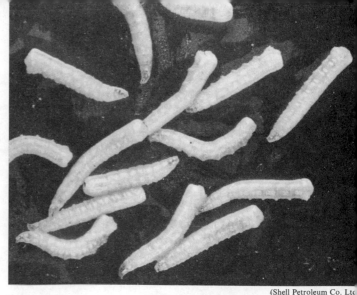

(Shell Petroleum Co. Ltd

(b) Housefly larvae

Fig. 31.12

31.12). Although it has no eyes the larva is sensitive to light and burrows into the decomposing mass away from light, thereby avoiding the risk of death through drying out. It grows through two moults to a length of about 1 cm and then changes its habits, seeking a dry situation in which it can pupate. The larval cuticle forms the pupal case inside which metamorphosis, or change to the adult shape, takes place. After three or four days the adult fly emerges, its wings expand and harden, and the adult then flies off to feed and mate.

Control can be gained by (i) preventing flies from breeding and raising more flies, (ii) killing flies, and (iii) preventing them from having access to food for human consumption.

1 Preventing flies from breeding. We have seen that flies are attracted to foetid, decomposing matter in which to lay their eggs. If faeces are buried or disposed of through a sewage system or in deep latrines then flies will not lay eggs in them.

Kitchen waste, which usually is wet and contains organic matter that can quickly decompose, should be kept covered, for example in a bin with a tight-fitting lid, to prevent flies reaching it. Bins should be emptied regularly and frequently (Fig. 31.13).

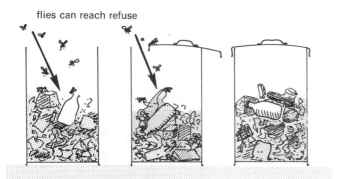

flies can reach refuse

Fig. 31.13 A dustbin (garbage bin) for kitchen waste must have a tight-fitting lid

When rubbish or garbage is collected for disposal it should be taken to a point well away from human habitation. Experiments in which flies marked with drops of paint have been released and later recaptured show that they can travel distances of over 2 km, so that while accepting that it is difficult to make a rubbish tip free from flies, the chances of their reaching an urban area should be kept to a minimum.

Where there is no local authority to collect and remove refuse, such waste can be either buried or else burned in a fire or an incinerator (a small furnace for reducing combustible material to ashes).

2 Killing flies can be effectively done by destroying them with a fly swat but insecticides, sensibly used, will destroy more flies in less time. At the present time, flies throughout the world are developing resistance to DDT, which had the advantage of being a residual insecticide (*see* p. 229). Similarly resistance to BHC and dieldrin is growing. For spraying rooms and other enclosed spaces a combination of pyrethrums and piperonyl butoxide is most effective, and there is no sign yet of resistance to these chemicals developing in houseflies. However since it is not a residual spray applied to surfaces this treatment has to be repeated frequently. Trials have been made of other substances that destroy flies, but in spray form there is the risk that the chemical may reach and affect other kinds of animals including humans. Some of these more dangerous compounds have been impregnated into cards and strips of absorbent material to be hung from ceilings. The best remain toxic to flies for up to six months and are useful in buildings such as dairies and lavatories where flies are attracted. But care must be taken while handling the strips when putting them in place

3 Protection of food. A shopkeeper wishing to sell goods will usually display them to his customers. Meat, wet fish and most perishable foods attract flies which may have come from feeding on faeces or putrefying matter. It is important to keep food on display covered, for example with butter muslin or gauze or better, behind glass or transparent plastic, to prevent flies from settling on it (*see* Fig. 34.3).

Similarly when such food reaches the home it is necessary to keep flies away. Wrapping in polythene or other flyproof material is not necessarily the best solution since impenetrable material of that kind also excludes air and thus provides conditions for any anaerobic bacteria already present to multiply to dangerous numbers. Where a refrigerator is not available perishable food should be stored in a ventilated cupboard or a meat safe, ventilation being provided through fine mesh gauze which excludes flies. (*See* Chapter 34.)

Of these various approaches, the first is the most important since if we can prevent or reduce the chances of flies breeding, there will be fewer adults to act as vectors. No country has eliminated houseflies but many have greatly reduced even the hot-season fly population, when breeding is most rapid.

234

Control of tsetse flies

Tsetse flies, which transmit the trypanosome causing sleeping sickness (*see* p. 197), are confined to tropical Africa. There are many species, though they all belong to one genus, *Glossina*. All have mouthparts for piercing and sucking, though the males feed on plant juices while the females suck blood. Only a few species transmit trypanosomes to humans (Fig. 31.14).

The fertilized eggs hatch within the female. Each larva develops rapidly, being nourished by a secretion from special glands in the abdomen of the mother. They are quite large when they are deposited by the mother in a place where they can burrow into dry sandy soil or under dry leaves to pupate. This stage takes three to four weeks. As adults, the flies live from three to six months during which time the female will produce between six and twelve larvae. Compared with mosquitoes and houseflies, they are slow breeders.

Certain species of tsetse breed only among vegetation in shady, humid conditions along river banks, while others breed in thickets of vegetation in open savannah country.

Control can be achieved by destroying the kinds of vegetation on which the male flies feed and among which the females deposit the larvae. This involves identifying the species of tsetse present and identifying the appropriate food plants.

For controlling those species breeding on river banks the technique most used is total clearance of trees, though elimination of only the type of tree on which the males feed would be as effective and would be less damaging to the environment. In savannah land it is possible to eliminate small patches of thorn scrub but where the thorn scrub is extensive another approach can be made. By removing scrub along a band two kilometres wide the tsetse can be contained in an infested area while development of grazing land takes place on the 'safe' side of the band. The band of cleared ground can be extended further into the thorn scrub as resources become available.

In East Africa barriers of evergreen thickets of shrubs unacceptable as food plants to the tsetses provide a method of containing the insects. Such barriers have to be 100 m wide.

Barriers and bands of cleared ground give protection around villages and water-holes but, with increased use of road transport, care has to be taken to avoid bringing tsetses into a community in or on cars or, indeed, simply following foot travellers, as flies do.

Burning of grassland is discouraged because, although it may drive out the flies temporarily, it is usually followed by the growth of a variety of plants which may include some that encourage the adult flies to re-enter the area.

No tsetse feeds exclusively on human blood and the destruction of game animals has been advocated as a means of eliminating alternative hosts in which trypanosomes may be present. Conservationists are reluctant to accept this approach and a solution in which game is confined to game reserves may be possible.

A modern method of control involves breeding tsetse flies in captivity and exposing the adult males to heavy doses of radiation. This renders the males sterile but they can still mate with females. The irradiated males are released among wild tsetses at a time in the year when the proportion of males in the natural population is low. Mating takes place and sterile seminal fluid is passed. The females rarely mate more than once and so, their eggs being infertile, produce no young. The method is as yet in use on an experimental rather than a widespread scale.

Control with insecticides introduced problems. Tsetse flies are very susceptible to the effects of chlorinated hydrocarbons such as DDT, but spraying from the air, essential if large areas are to be treated, must be done during daylight, and at this time most adult flies are resting on the *undersides* of leaves. In tall, dense forest, penetration of spray is inadequate anyway but small-scale experiments in riverside villages show that spraying dieldrin emulsion from the ground on to vegetation around the village reduces the fly population.

Control of traffic and the spraying of the insides of cars and aircraft with insecticide should be re-emphasized as a means of

Fig. 31.15 Domestic cattle infected with trypanosomes being treated by injection

(Shell Petroleum Co. Ltd)

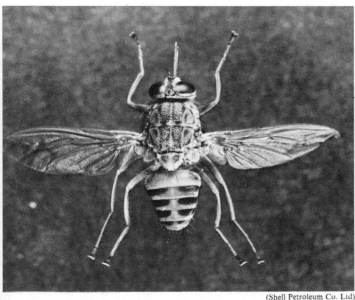

(Shell Petroleum Co. Ltd)

Fig. 31.14 Tsetse fly

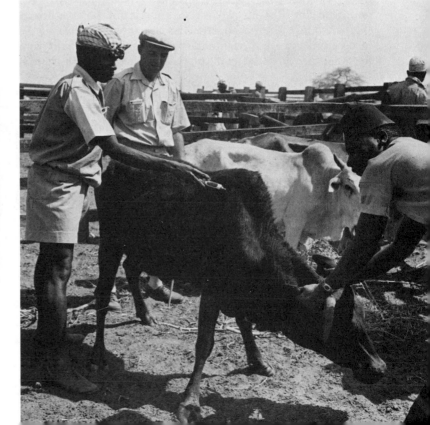

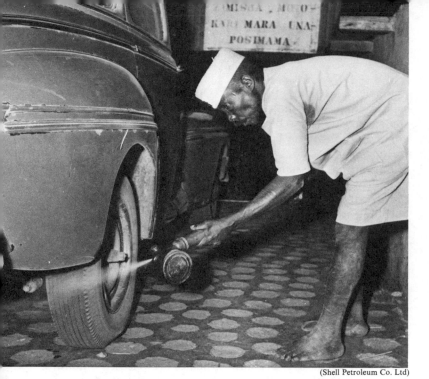

(Shell Petroleum Co. Ltd)

Fig. 31.16   Spraying a car to destroy tsetse flies

preventing the re-introduction of the vector, possibly carrying trypanosomes, into a cleared area (Fig. 31.16).

Body parasites

Bugs, fleas, chiggers (or jiggers), lice and ticks are all blood-sucking arthropods that live in close contact with the human body for at least part of their lives. Because they bite through human skin to suck blood they represent a means by which pathogenic organisms can gain access to the blood stream. In some cases pathogenic organisms complete a part of their life cycle in the body of the vector, while in other cases the blood sucker transmits pathogens mechanically on the outside of its mouthparts.

Bedbugs (Fig. 31.17) cause irritation through their bites but they are not known to be vectors of disease. Scratching the inflamed region around their bites often breaks the skin and allows pathogenic organisms to enter. The 'assassin bugs' of S. America (Fig. 31.18) transmit *Trypanosoma cruzi*, the pathogen causing Chagas' disease, but it is not the mouthparts that introduce the pathogens; the trypanosomes live in the insect's gut and are shed into the wound in a drop of fluid from the hindgut, expelled after the bug has finished feeding on blood.

There are many kinds of fleas, wingless insects whose laterally compressed bodies permit them to crawl between hairs and through fur. *Xenopsylla* the rat flea is a tropical flea that can survive in heated buildings in temperate countries and plays a part in the transmission of bubonic plague (*see* p. 222), as does the common human flea, *Pulex irritans*. Many mammals and birds harbour fleas which may occasionally feed on the blood of man and act as mechanical vectors.

Chiggers (Fig. 31.19) are a small group of fleas originating in S. America but now found also in West, South and East Africa and parts of India. The chigger is of importance not as a vector but because the female, after mating, burrows into human skin using her powerful, toothed mandibles. Her body swells as the eggs inside her develop and her presence irritates the skin which becomes inflamed. When the eggs have been laid the skin breaks and ulcerates and secondary infections are common. Before mating, the female chigger is similar to any other kind of flea and spends time in the dust and debris on floors. She is not a good jumper and is most likely to reach a naked foot. Wearing shoes reduces the chances of acquiring chiggers.

Unlike the animals so far described in this section, the louse (*Pediculus*) is obliged to spend most of its life in contact with its human host, and each species possesses curved claws for ensuring a firm hold on the skin (Fig. 31.20). The two varieties, the head louse and the body louse, can interbreed and the females in each case attach eggs to the shafts of hairs on the head or the body. The eggs are commonly termed 'nits'. The adults are vectors of the rickettsiae that cause epidemic typhus and relapsing fever, which are spread when the lice move from the body of one host to another. Transfer takes place when people sleep huddled together; during sexual intercourse; and sometimes as a result of changing clothes. A third louse, the crab louse, which lives mostly among pubic hair, is also transferred during sexual intercourse (Fig. 31.20b).

Ticks form a large group of arthropods, related to the spiders. The soft-bodied ticks transmit the spirochaete that causes relapsing fever. The spirochaete penetrates the gut wall of the tick, after being sucked in during a meal of blood, and multiplies in the body cavity. They are transmitted in saliva and other secretions from the tick and may also pass, in the eggs, to the next generation of vectors.

The soft-bodied ticks are quite large (females 12–14 mm long, males 8 mm long), but most of the hard-bodied ticks that parasitize man are less than 6 mm long. They are the vectors of

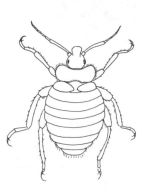

Fig. 31.17   Bedbug, *Cimex* (×6)

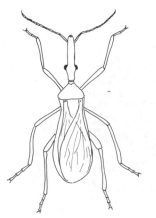

Fig. 31.18   'Assassin bug', *Rhodnius* (×2)

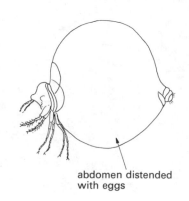

abdomen distended with eggs

Fig. 31.19   Female chigger, *Tunga* (×15)

236

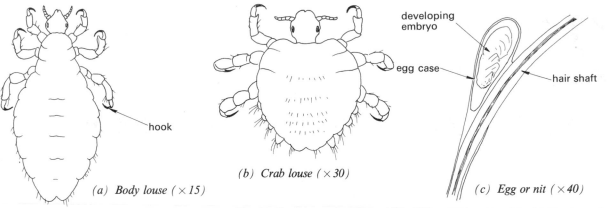

(a) Body louse (×15)   (b) Crab louse (×30)   (c) Egg or nit (×40)

Fig. 31.20   Lice and egg

tick-borne typhus and other diseases caused by rickettsiae. Certain of the hard ticks release a toxin into the blood stream while feeding. This toxin affects the endings of motor nerves, resulting in paralysis. Ticks producing this effect are found in western Canada and eastern Australia.

This brief survey indicates the desirability of controlling these body parasites which cause distress and disease both through their presence and activity and as vectors for pathogenic organisms.

Methods of control. Bedbugs hide in bedding and in cracks in floors and walls during the day. Thorough spraying of floors and walls with DDT or dieldrin–BHC in oil kills them. Bedding may be sprayed, but in this case pyrethrum is a safer insecticide to use on material that is likely to be in close contact with the skin.

The assassin or triatomid bugs are controlled by house spraying with gamma BHC. They are resistant to DDT.

In controlling fleas it is necessary to discover the haunts of the insect and treat these rather than to spray an entire house. Insecticide dust is most frequently used and applied to clothing, bedding, floors and rat-runs. Where there is no danger of humans or domestic animals coming in contact with the insecticide, high concentrations may be used since these seem to kill rats as well as their fleas. Domestic pets can have their bodies dusted with insecticides that are sufficiently weak not to harm the pets.

Chiggers in their mobile state are controlled by the same methods, but once under the skin they should be removed with a sharp, sterilized needle, the small wound that results being dressed with an antiseptic and covered to prevent the entry of dirt and germs.

Lice on the body are controlled by puffing DDT dust beneath the clothes with a plunger-type 'puffer' or by sprinkling it on the inside of clothing. This method arrested the spread of louse-borne typhus in areas of dense population such as Naples during the Second World War when an epidemic seemed imminent.

Head lice are more appropriately controlled by the use of a liquid preparation which should contain a substance to destroy the eggs (nits). Crab lice are treated in a similar way. Lice in many parts of the world are showing resistance to DDT. This resistance to DDT was first noticed during the war in Korea in the 1950s; as a result, pyrethrums are now being used, though their action is not so long-lasting as that of DDT.

Ticks are mostly sensitive to DDT with the exception of the soft ticks spreading relapsing fever in East Africa. Here BHC powder is dusted on to the floors of dwellings.

DDT or dieldrin sprays are used against hard ticks hiding in cracks in floors and walls and on vegetation.

The use of these various chemicals does not remove the responsibility of the individual for his own personal cleanliness and hygiene. Frequent and thorough washing of the body and wearing of clean clothing remain the most effective measures in ensuring freedom from blood-feeding body parasites.

Questions

1 Most of the vectors of disease are large enough to be seen clearly with the naked eye, yet the part they play in the transmission of disease organisms has only been understood within the last 50 to 100 years. Why do you think this was so?

2 Many insect vectors can be controlled by methods other than the use of chemical insecticides. Draw up a table to show what these other methods are and which vectors can be controlled by their use.

3 Why is a knowledge of the life cycle of a vector of particular importance in planning a programme to control an insect vector?

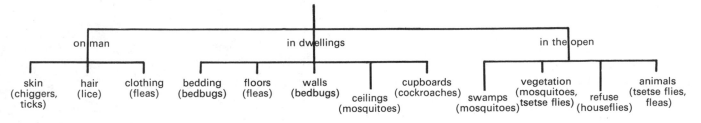

WHERE ARE DISEASE VECTORS FOUND?

Fig. 31.21   The distribution of disease vectors

32
Immunity and Immunization

Immunity to disease among certain people in a population was noted in mediaeval times. In the eighteenth century Edward Jenner, a country doctor in Gloucestershire, England, concluded that the immunity of some of his patients to smallpox, a disease that is usually fatal, might be due to a recent attack of cowpox, a much milder disease, which is transmitted from cattle to the people who handle and milk them. Jenner tested his hypothesis by infecting a young boy with cowpox and then, some weeks later, infecting him with scrapings from the pustules on a smallpox victim. The boy survived and showed no symptoms of smallpox (Fig. 32.1).

Jenner thought that cowpox was simply a mild form of smallpox. It is not, but the two diseases are caused by viruses that are essentially similar and when the body 'learns' to counteract cowpox virus it becomes able to counteract smallpox virus also. Since the material for producing this immunity to smallpox came from a cow, for which the Latin name is *vacca*, the procedure became known as *vaccination*. The disease-inducing substance with which a person is inoculated is called a *vaccine*. It is very unusual, however, to find an overlap of immunity to two diseases.

In studying immunity to pathogenic organisms we must consider again the ways in which the host can resist invasion by pathogens. These are listed in the table below.

Physical barriers to entry	Active agents within the body
Skin Mucous membranes Hairs (e.g. in the nose)	Secretions containing active agents (e.g. sweat, tears, gastric juice) Cilia in the trachea Lysozyme, interferon in cells Phagocytes in blood

These factors affect our *innate immunity*, that is, the natural immunity with which we are born. The effectiveness of these barriers varies from one person to another.

Invading microbes that get past the barriers listed above carry on their surfaces, or else secrete, large protein molecules which are termed antigens. These foreign protein molecules induce a reaction or response when they come into contact with lymphocytes (*see* p. 72) which form the second line of defence in the blood of the host. Immunity produced in this way is *acquired immunity* (Fig. 32.2). It is associated with the formation of complex chemicals called *antibodies* or *immunoglobulins* in the blood plasma. A particular antibody will react with a particular antigen forming a chemical link. These lead to a sequence of reactions which may destroy the pathogenic

organism or else neutralize the poisonous substances or toxins that it has produced. Each antibody is said to be specific to one antigen.

One of the reactions is termed *precipitation* because, as a result of interaction between an antibody and a soluble toxin a precipitate is formed.

Agglutination occurs when the antibody reacts with the pathogenic organisms, causing them to stick together.

Opsonization is the name given to the process of coating invading bacteria with antibody which makes them more attractive to phagocytes which then ingest them.

Acquired immunity may be gained when live organisms invade the body and disease symptoms follow. On recovery the ability to make antibodies remains and these become effective if the person is infected for a second time and thus the infection is overcome. Jenner's discovery was the possibility of anticipating or preparing for a disease attack by introducing

Fig. 32.1 Dr. Jenner inoculating James Phipps. Note the dairymaid, who has given the cowpox serum, binding up her wrist

(Wellcome Museum of Medical Science)

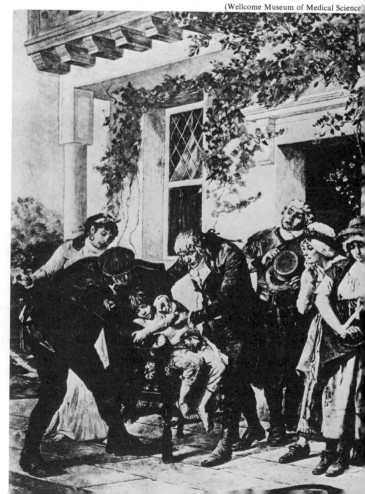

he pathogen into the body artificially and inducing the body o produce antibodies. Immunization has developed a great leal since Jenner's experiments and nowadays three kinds of antigen preparations or vaccines are used.

1 **Toxoids.** These are extracts of the toxins secreted by bacteria such as that causing diphtheria. The poisons are made harmless by the addition of formalin, and when a cell-free extract is injected into the body, stimulate the blood to produce antibodies. The immunity that results is active and persists for many years.

2 **Killed vaccines** are prepared from cultures of bacteria or from viruses grown in suitable host cells. Again, chemicals such as formalin are used to kill them and they are usually administered by injection. Protection against poliomyelitis is given this way and short-term protection against cholera is also provided by such a vaccine.

3 **Attenuated living vaccines.** These are prepared from cultures of organisms that have become less virulent (*see* p. 211) by growth in an unusual host, for example a horse. Strains of organisms arise that survive in the new host without causing disease symptoms. When injected into man they are no longer able to produce disease symptoms in him either but they do induce the body to manufacture antibodies, and so immunity is given against the active organisms, should infection take place. Protection against tuberculosis is given by this method using BCG (Bacille Calmette–Guérin) vaccine. Two French bacteriologists, Calmette and Guérin, discovered that while killed mycobacteria would not stimulate the formation of antibodies, the attenuated bacillus would. Immunity to yellow fever is produced by injection of the attenuated virus, grown in tissue culture.

Active acquired immunity is produced when the body reacts to the antigens of disease-causing organisms by producing antibodies. The immunity may last for a lifetime in the case of diseases such as measles or smallpox. In the case of cholera and influenza the immunity lasts only for a short time. Immunity to the common cold has never been developed successfully and this is probably because a large number of different strains of the causative virus are in circulation in a population.

Development of immunity

Immunity depends on there being a sufficient concentration of antibody in the blood stream to counteract invading antigens. With some vaccinations the level of antibody produced after the first injection is too low to give protection. In such a case a second injection is given, usually when the first response has reached its maximum. This second or booster injection causes a very high level of antibody to be formed and active immunity results (Fig. 32.3). Furthermore, the lymphocytes seem to 'learn' to produce antibodies and this 'memory' may last for many years. Further booster injections at intervals of three years in the case of smallpox and six years in the case of yellow fever step up the formation of antibodies and maintain immunity at a high level.

Passive immunity. If ready-made antibodies are transferred to a non-immune individual then he automatically acquires immunity. However, since no antigens are introduced the

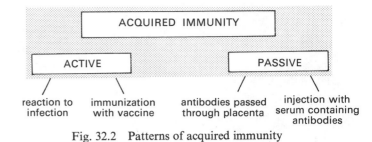

Fig. 32.2   Patterns of acquired immunity

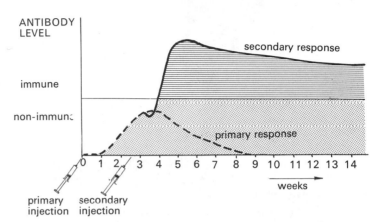

Fig. 32.3   Development of active acquired immunity

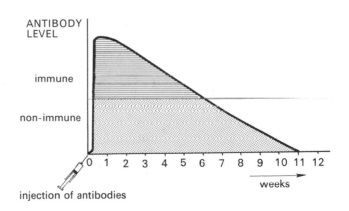

Fig. 32.4   Development and loss of passive immunity

recipient does not 'learn' to produce his own antibodies and the immunity is described as *passive*. There are two chief ways in which passive immunity may be acquired.

The antibodies present in the blood plasma of a pregnant woman diffuse through the placenta into the foetus which therefore, at birth, has immunity to the same diseases as its mother. The antibodies are slowly excreted and the immunity is short-lived but it accounts for the fact that newborn babies do not catch many of the diseases in the first few weeks of life that they are likely to contract during childhood.

The other way of acquiring passive immunity is by the injection into the body of a serum containing ready-made antibodies (Fig. 32.4). This is known as immune serum and is valuable as a precautionary measure when, for example, a person is likely to be exposed to the risk of the virus disease, infective hepatitis, through nursing sick people. It is the means

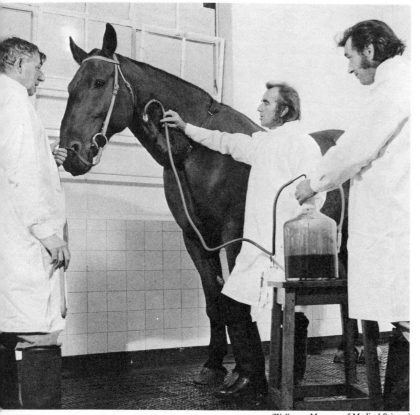

(Wellcome Museum of Medical Science)

Fig. 32.5   Bleeding a horse to obtain antitoxins

of protecting a person against tetanus after he has sustained a deep wound that has been contaminated by soil. To vaccinate with toxoids then would impose more strain on the antigen–antibody reaction mechanism, whereas to inject ready-made antibodies provides a direct means of counteracting the bacilli

of tetanus if, by chance, they have entered the wound. As with the antibodies received during pregnancy, these, too, are eliminated from the body.

While it is possible to acquire immunity to many viruses by the methods already described, it is interesting to note that cells that are invaded by a virus produce a protein called *interferon*. When a virus invades a susceptible cell it induces the cell to synthesize more virus. It is at this time that the cell also produces the interferon, which then interferes with virus synthesis. The production of interferon probably accounts for the suppression of virus in the case of natural recovery from a virus infection. It would be very helpful if we could inject interferon into tissues either before a virus infection or when it seemed that the body was not able to counteract the invading virus quickly enough, but at the present time it is not possible to produce and collect interferon in the quantities that would be needed.

Effectiveness of immunization

Although laboratory tests and carefully controlled studies of the effects on man accompany the introduction of any new vaccine, only the passage of time produces the evidence by which effectiveness can really be measured. In 1939 about 75 000 cases of diphtheria were notified in Britain. In 1940 mass immunization against the disease was introduced, and in 1970 fewer than 10 cases of diphtheria were recorded.

In a similar way the introduction of mass immunization against tuberculosis by the use of BCG vaccine has dramatically reduced the incidence of TB in many parts of India and Pakistan.

Questions

1   Write a paragraph to explain the difference between passive and active immunity.
2   Why do you think infectious diseases are most common in a class of schoolchildren one or two weeks after a new term has begun?

33
Drugs and Antibiotics

Many diseases can be treated and cured by the use of chemicals. Such treatment is termed *chemotherapy*. The chemicals used must be capable of destroying pathogenic micro-organisms without destroying or damaging human tissues. Before the present century most of the materials used in treating infections were obtained from plants, some of which contain very powerful drugs. The modern antibiotics are also extracted from plants, chiefly fungi.

By 1900 many of the organisms causing diseases had been seen under the microscope and classified. At the same time advances had been made in the understanding of the chemistry of carbon compounds (organic chemistry). A German scientist, Paul Ehrlich, who had knowledge of both chemistry and medicine, was at this time investigating the possible use of dyes in the treatment and control of the trypanosomes causing sleeping sickness. He shifted his researches to the study of certain compounds of arsenic and, in 1910, published his discovery of a chemical compound called *Salvarsan* that would kill trypanosomes not only in laboratory mice but in man. Furthermore, it would kill the treponeme bacterium causing syphilis. It had to be used with care, since too large a dose proved poisonous to the patient. Thus the need to calculate the size of dose of a drug that would prove effective against germs without harming the patient was recognized, and measurement of the safe dose was put on a scientific basis.

Intensive research led in the 1930s to the discovery of a group of chemicals which became known as *sulphonamides*.

These proved effective against many kinds of bacteria including the diplococci causing pneumonia, a disease that until then had commonly proved fatal.

In 1929 Fleming, working in a hospital in London, noticed that growths of a mould called *Penicillium* stopped the spread of staphylococci on a Petri dish (Fig. 33.1). He found that an antibacterial substance could be extracted from the mould and this substance he called *penicillin*. Tests carried out on laboratory animals and later on human patients showed that penicillin would kill many kinds of bacteria without damaging the tissues of the patient.

The term *antibiotic* is now used to classify penicillin and an increasing range of other substances which are extracted from living organisms and which kill bacteria or inhibit their growth. Antibiotics include *tetracycline* and *streptomycin*. Many of the naturally produced antibiotics are now made more effective or sometimes more stable by chemical treatment to alter the structure of the molecules. Advances in this field are sometimes the outcome of careful planning and prediction, but most frequently they follow chance intelligent observations, as in the case of Fleming noticing the destructive action of the mould on bacteria. Most antibiotics are effective against a variety of bacteria and are termed broad-spectrum drugs. Penicillin and chloramphenicol are good examples. The synthetic drug isoniazid is used exclusively to destroy the mycobacterium of tuberculosis and is a narrow-spectrum drug.

Broad-spectrum drugs that are taken by mouth usually have

Fig. 33.1 Growing *Penicillium*
(Beecham Research Laboratories)

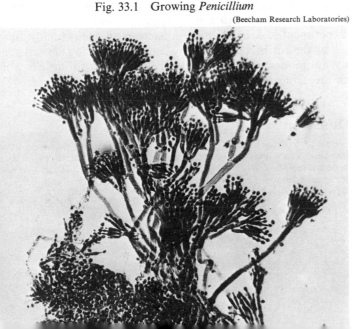

Fig. 33.2 Control panel for penicillin production on an industrial scale
(Beecham Research Laboratories)

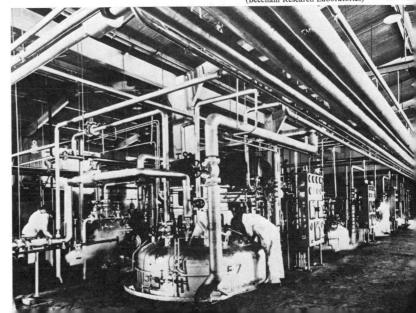

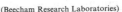

an effect on the bacteria that are natural inhabitants of the gut. Most of these are commensals, organisms that live harmlessly inside us, while a few perform useful tasks such as synthesizing riboflavin and vitamins B_{12} and K. If our diet contains these vitamins then the destruction of the bacteria by antibiotics is not important, but for a person on a limited diet the killing of the gut bacteria may mean an inadequate supply of vitamins B_{12} and K. We should note at the same time that many kinds of gut bacteria use up vitamins from our diet, and probably the effect of taking antibiotics orally, since it involves the destruction of these competitive bacteria as well as the vitamin synthesizers, is of less importance than was once thought. It is important to note that penicillin taken orally kills off susceptible strains of bacteria but leaves resistant strains to multiply and increase. These resistant strains of bacteria are capable of transmitting their resistance to other kinds of bacteria and if these others are pathogens then they, too, become resistant to penicillin. Diluted antibiotics or doses that are too small are most likely to have this effect.

It should be stressed at this point that all medicinal drugs whether naturally produced or synthetic *can* be harmful to man if too large a dose is taken. As commonplace a substance as aspirin (acetyl salicylic acid), used in many communities to relieve pain and to reduce fever at the rate of 20 milligrams of aspirin per kilogram of body weight (two tablets for an average adult person), will cause haemorrhage of the stomach and intestine at three or four times that concentration, and in appreciably larger quantity will be fatal.

Drugs such as penicillin are usually available only through a qualified doctor or with his approval. Even so, care has to be taken to use the drug only at the recommended dose-rate. Some people are more sensitive to drugs than others and the threshold concentration at which a particular drug harms them may be too low to destroy bacteria successfully. In such cases alternative antibiotics or synthetic drugs have to be used. In all cases, drugs should be used only under medical supervision.

Practical Work

Experiment 1   The action of antibiotics

Prepare a suspension of soil bacteria by just covering a quantity of fresh soil in a sterile beaker with distilled water. Pour off the first 5 cm³ of water into a sterile test-tube and use a sterile pipette to transfer 1 cm³ of this soil water to each of four agar plates or slopes. Tilt the jelly so that the soil water wets the entire surface and then pour off the surplus water. Incubate the cultures for one day.

Meanwhile collect moulds from four different sources such as the skins of ripe fruit and the rind of cheese. 'Blue' cheese is coloured by the growth of *Penicillium* and is a particularly interesting source of mould. If the cultures show bacterial growth, use a sterilized wire loop to transfer a small quantity of one mould to one plate, another to the second and so on. Incubate at room temperature for two days and observe whether there is any interaction between the mould and the bacteria. Remember that you are likely to have the same kinds of bacteria in each culture. Examine the results without opening the cultures, which should be re-sterilized after the experiment.

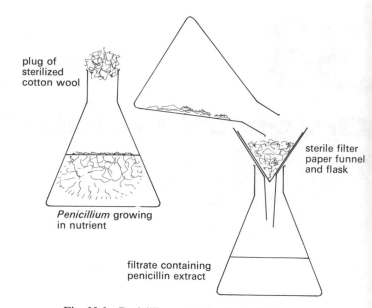

Fig. 33.3   Penicillin production in the laboratory

Experiment 2   Extraction of an antibiotic

Penicillium mould can be grown well in a liquid medium, made by dissolving 1 g of meat extract and 4 g of dextrose in 200 cm³ of distilled water and sterilizing it in a pressure cooker for 15 minutes. When cool the medium is inoculated with *Penicillium* spores and incubated at room temperature until a strong growth of mould is seen through the liquid, usually after one week. The medium is now filtered into a sterile vessel using sterile filter paper and funnel. Any antibiotic formed will be in the filtrate (*see* Fig. 33.3).

Experiment 3   Tests with an antibiotic extract

Prepare a fresh plate, as in Experiment 1. When bacterial colonies are apparent, cut out and remove a strip of agar. Use a sterile pipette to transfer about 0.5 cm³ of the antibiotic extract from Experiment 2 to the groove left by removing the agar strip. Incubate at room temperature for one day and observe whether there is any interaction between the bacteria and the extract.

Experiment 4   Response of different bacteria to an antibiotic

If during your experiments you have plates with different kinds of bacteria, use a wire loop to draw streaks of, say, four different bacteria on a fresh, sterile plate. Incubate the plate at 37 °C until strong streaks of bacteria can be seen. Remove a strip of agar so that the end of each streak reaches the groove. Place antibiotic extract in the groove and incubate, as in Experiment 3. Are the different bacteria affected equally, or at all, by the antibiotic? Since any bacteria surviving are resistant to antibiotics it is particularly important to destroy the cultures, unopened, by sterilizing.

Question

Several of the drugs used in the treatment of disease at the present time contain the same or very similar chemical substances to those found in the plants used in herbal remedies. What do you consider to be the most important advances in the use of modern drug treatment over the use of old herbal medicines?

34
Safe Food

We have seen in Chapters 26 and 27 that disease-causing organisms can enter the body through the mouth with food. We consume large numbers of micro-organisms of various kinds with our food every day. Most of these organisms are harmless but those that are active pathogens can in certain circumstances give rise to disease. They may be present in numbers too small to cause an infection, though some, such as *Clostridium welchii* which causes food poisoning, can multiply so rapidly in the alimentary canal that the minimum infective dose is only a few hundred bacteria.

Micro-organisms such as bacteria and fungi not only make food dangerous to eat but may cause it to decompose to the extent that it is unpleasant or unfit to eat.

Foods that contain a great deal of water, such as meat, fish, fruit and vegetables, are described as perishable. They may be spoiled very quickly, particularly in warm conditions, by the action of bacteria and moulds and also by the enzymes that are present naturally within the cells of the food material. Food preservation is any method of treating food that keeps it palatable and nutritious and prevents micro-organisms from using it as their own source of energy and growth material.

Foods from plants are often harvested in very large quantities and stored, in order to spread the use of such food over a long period of time, or it may be necessary to move the food over a large distance from the production area to where it will eventually be eaten; the food therefore requires preservation.

Foods with a high protein content are particularly attractive to bacteria, many of which do no more than make food unpleasant to eat by decomposing it and producing unpleasant tastes and smell or altering the texture. Other bacteria, including species of *Salmonella* and *Clostridium*, if they start multiplying in food which is then eaten, can cause serious illness and death. They may be dangerous even when their numbers are too small to produce noticeable unpleasant decomposition products affecting taste and smell.

Methods of preservation

Methods of food preservation are of two general kinds. The first is *bactericidal*, in which all micro-organisms are killed. This includes canning and any other process involving sterilization. The second group of methods is termed *bacteriostatic* since the bacterial activities are stopped, but without actually killing the organisms. Freezing, dehydration and pickling come in this group.

1 **Canning** was first introduced in America during the Civil War and was widely used in Europe by the time the First World War broke out in 1914. The principle was developed over a hundred years earlier by Appert in Paris. He discovered that if food is adequately cooked and then sealed, while hot, in jars or cans then it will remain safe to eat for a long time. In fact, roast veal canned in London in 1823 for a naval expedition was opened in 1958 and the meat found to be in good, wholesome condition.

Appert's principles are now applied on a commercial scale to a wide range of foods, including meat, vegetables, fruit and fish. Heat treatment at 90 °C or blanching is essential to destroy natural enzymes as well as to kill micro-organisms and is a form of sterilization. The food is then placed while it is still hot in cans made of tin plate (sheet steel coated with tin) that has been coated with lacquer to prevent the metal causing discolouration of the food. After sealing and cooling, the contents contract and a vacuum develops, causing the ends of

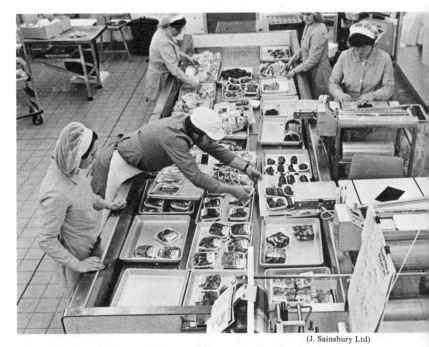

(J. Sainsbury Ltd)

Fig. 34.1 Prepacking food for sale in sterile containers reduces the chance of contamination through handling by customers

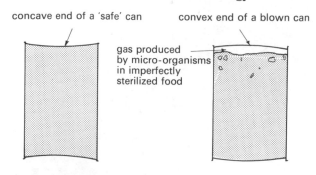

concave end of a 'safe' can   convex end of a blown can

gas produced
by micro-organisms
in imperfectly
sterilized food

Fig. 34.2   Sections through perfectly sterilized and 'blown' cans

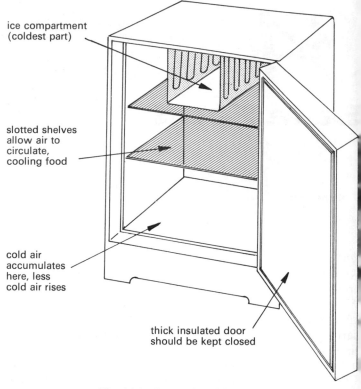

ice compartment
(coldest part)

slotted shelves
allow air to
circulate,
cooling food

cold air
accumulates
here, less
cold air rises

thick insulated door
should be kept closed

Fig. 34.4   Domestic refrigerator

the can to curve in slightly (Fig. 34.2). This vacuum is maintained as long as the food is free from micro-organisms and the seal is intact. On opening a can, one should hear a slight rush of air into the can when it is pierced. If the ends of a can bulge then there is a positive pressure inside and this usually means that anaerobic micro-organisms (p. 195) have been respiring, reproducing and feeding. The food is suspect and should be destroyed. Cans in this condition are said to be 'blown'.

Although the record for successful storage of veal in a can is 125 years, most meat products tend to deteriorate after 7 years and some acid fruits such as pineapple are likely to corrode the tin plate from the inside in less than 2 years, thereby destroying the seal and making contamination possible. It is wise therefore not to rely on keeping canned foods for indefinite periods of time.

2   Freezing. An increasing amount of food around the world is preserved by freezing. At sub-zero temperatures, bacteria and most moulds are unable to digest and decompose food or to reproduce. Natural enzymes in food are inactive also. Fishermen have preserved fish by packing it in ice or in brine (salt water) at sub-zero temperatures for over a hundred years, and refrigerated ships have carried meat safely through the tropics to be eaten thousands of miles away from where it was produced.

In recent years the technique of quick freezing has been applied to a wide range of foods from meat, fruit and vegetables to ready-prepared complete meals. The material to be preserved must be cooled very rapidly to a temperature of -18 °C

Fig. 34.3   Joints of meat to be sold are prepared under hygienic conditions and then placed in a refrigerated glass-fronted cabinet

(J. Sainsbury Ltd)

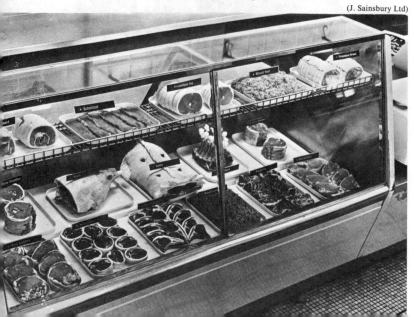

(0 °F). The food must be spread thinly on shelves or a conveyor belt in close contact with brine pipes at a temperature a little below -18 °C. Strong brine does not freeze at 0 °C like pure water. Thus brine at -20 °C can be circulated between the refrigerator unit and the chamber containing the food, so extracting heat from the food. An alternative method of freezing involves blowing very cold air from a refrigerator unit through the food on a conveyor belt in a tunnel. Once frozen, such food must then be stored at temperatures below 0 °C. Domestic refrigerators do not run at temperatures as low as those we have discussed. The icebox or freezer compartment will be at a temperature lower than 0 °C, but much of the space in the refrigerator will have a temperature between 0 °C and 5 °C. At such temperatures bacterial activity is slowed down but not completely stopped, and certain moulds seem to grow quite actively at such temperatures. This does not mean that refrigerators are useless, but it does mean that we should use our knowledge and sense in deciding what sorts of food can be kept safely in a 'fridge' and for how long they can be kept.

3   Dehydration. One of the reasons that perishable foods are so readily used for nutrition by micro-organisms is that they contain plenty of water. If this water were removed then the food would be preserved against the digestive action of enzymes, whether bacterial or those natural to the food.

The simplest method of dehydration is air drying. Fish, for example, can be split, the visceral organs removed, and then hung in the sun and wind to dry. Wind speeds up the rate of evaporation. The sun's rays provide the heat necessary and may kill bacteria through the effect of ultraviolet radiation. Vegetable foods such as peas, beans and split coconut can be dried in this way as can many fruits such as dates and plums. Dried foods are lighter and less bulky than fresh foods and, provided they are protected from humid conditions, may be

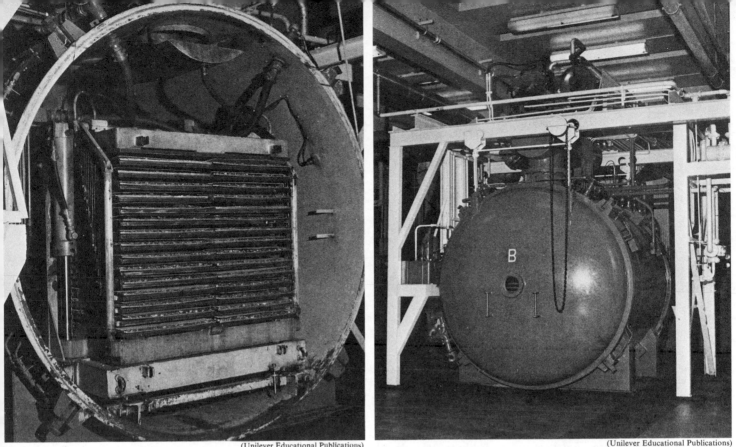

(a) *Peas have been arranged on shallow trays in the freeze-drying cabinet*

(b) *The cabinet is sealed before pressure is reduced*

Fig. 34.5 Accelerated freeze drying

kept for long periods. When placed in water they absorb liquid, swell up again, and may then be eaten.

Vacuum drying is a more modern method of preservation by dehydration. Use is made of the fact that water evaporates quickly at temperatures well below boiling point if the air pressure around it is reduced. Perishable foods such as eggs (taken from their shells), milk and several proprietary foods are treated in this way to reduce them to dry solids which can be powdered and packaged. If the water had been removed by boiling then the foods would have been cooked and changed in flavour. It is a curious fact that many kinds of bacteria can survive vacuum drying, even though the degree of vacuum would cause the death of all other kinds of organisms. Bacteria will not multiply in the food while it is kept dry, although they will resume activity when water is added.

Freeze drying is an even more up-to-date process in which food is first quick frozen, as described on p. 244, and then subjected to reduced pressure. The ice crystals evaporate directly, a process called sublimation, instead of first melting. As with any other dried food, material dried by this method can be stored at the normal temperature of the environment.

4 **Curing and salting** are very old methods of preserving meat and vegetables. Common salt, sodium chloride, dissociates in water (*see* ionization, p. 21) and the sodium and chloride ions attract water around themselves. If sufficient salt is added then all the available water in a piece of meat may be drawn out in this way. The resulting solution is osmotically active (p. 22), and if bacteria are present then water may be drawn out through the bacterial membrane by the salt solution, thus killing the organisms. Many kinds of fish are preserved in this way and so are beef and pig meat (bacon and ham).

5 **Pasteurization** is the name given to a process devised by Louis Pasteur to prevent the souring of wine by bacterial action. The French scientist observed that when wine was exposed to the atmosphere, microbes (micro-organisms) appeared in it, which he believed were the cause of chemical changes that spoiled the wine. He discovered that boiling the wine killed these microbes, but boiling also destroyed the fragrance (or bouquet) and removed the alcohol. Further experiments showed that the microbes could be killed by heating the wine to a temperature of 50–60 °C for thirty minutes. At this temperature the quality of the wine was not very much altered. This treatment does not kill all possible kinds of micro-organisms, and is a partial sterilization.

The term *pasteurization* was first used in connection with the partial sterilization of beer, but nowadays we think of it in connection with the treatment of milk produced for human use.

Fig. 34.6 Pasteurization plant. Milk is passed through stainless steel pipes to the heater units, one of which is seen in the lower right-hand corner. From these the milk passes to the cooler units

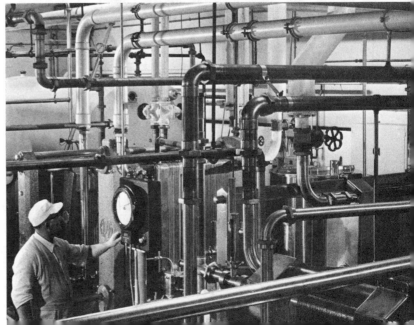

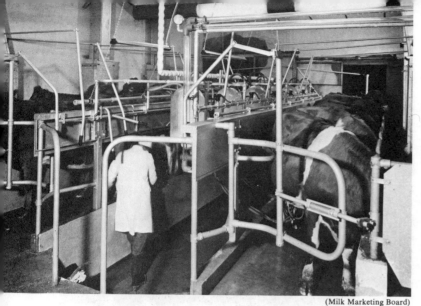

(Milk Marketing Board)

Fig. 34.7   Cows being milked in hygienic conditions

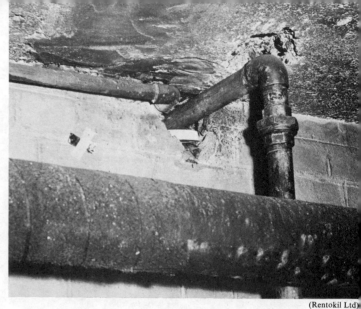

(Rentokil Ltd)

Fig. 34.9   Cockroaches are tropical insects. In temperate countries they seek warm protected environments such as this passage for hot-water pipes through a wall in a hospital basement

Raw milk from a cow is an excellent medium for bacterial growth. Most of the kinds of bacteria commonly found in milk do not cause disease but several of them alter the flavour of the milk and others cause it to curdle. However clean the cows and the dairy are kept it is not possible to exclude all bacteria from the milk. Some come from within the mammary glands or udder of the cow. If the milk is either heated to 63 °C for thirty minutes and then cooled, or else passed between metal plates heated to 80 °C for about half a minute and then cooled rapidly, then most of the contaminating bacteria are killed. We now know that this treatment destroys *Mycobacterium tuberculosis*, the pathogen causing TB which is often transmitted in milk.

Pasteurized milk is safe to drink and should 'keep' for several days if kept cool; but with pasteurized milk, as with any other preserved food, once fresh micro-organisms have been allowed into it, deterioration may take place and further sterilization may become necessary.

Storing food in the home

When storing food at home we have to take into account the nature of the food. Deterioration by enzyme action, whether the enzymes are those occurring naturally in the food or are produced by micro-organisms, is slowed down at low temperatures. Food should be stored in as cool a place as possible. Shade is often the first consideration in siting a food store, since direct sunlight has a marked heating effect.

A closed food store will be unlikely to allow any movement of air, which consequently becomes saturated with water vapour, derived from the food. In such saturated conditions moulds, in particular, germinate readily and become active, decomposing food. A store in which air can circulate may not prevent mould from growing, but makes it less likely. The presence of fresh air with the normal 20 per cent oxygen content inhibits certain kinds of harmful bacteria (*see* Chapter 37).

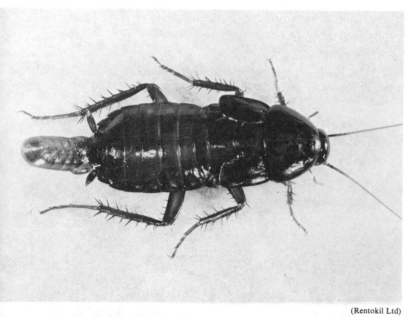

(Rentokil Ltd)

Fig. 34.8   Common cockroach. This female is carrying an egg case which will be deposited in a crevice

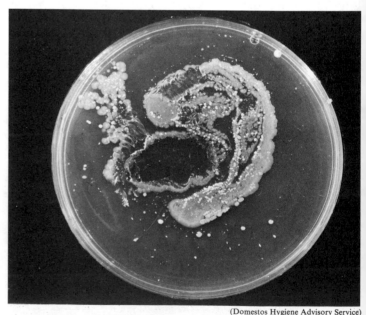

(Domestos Hygiene Advisory Service)

Fig. 34.10   Growth of bacteria on nutrient agar twenty-four hours after a cockroach had walked over the plate

246

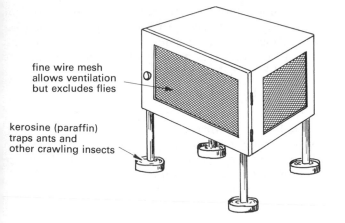

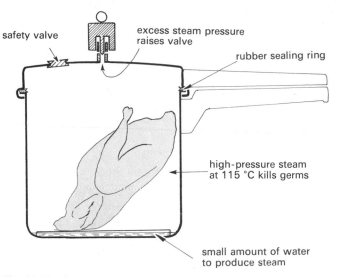

Sausages are made by chopping up or mincing meat and putting it into skins. If the meat contains tapeworm larvae then these may survive the chopping. Frying the sausages or lightly cooking them will not destroy the larvae and this is one of the ways in which tapeworm infections begin (p. 200).

Fig. 34.12 A pressure cooker can be used to cook food rapidly and to sterilize food and utensils

Fig. 34.11 Ant-proof meat safe

The size of the store depends on the space available as well as on the amount of food to be stored, and may range from a 'meat safe' (Fig. 34.11) with fine wire gauze in the sides, to a cupboard or even a room with air intakes and outlets. Whatever the type of store, it is desirable to exclude flies, cockroaches, ants, rats and other rodents. Flies contaminate food with bacteria carried on their bodies and in their saliva and faeces (p. 208). Cockroaches contaminate food similarly, and also damage packaging and leave their droppings in dry food, such as flour, giving it an objectionable taste (Fig. 34.8). Ants are generally destructive, though of less importance as vectors, while rats transmit germs on their bodies and in both their urine and faeces, which may be shed on food.

Flies can be excluded by covering ventilation openings with fine wire gauze and by keeping the doors of the store closed.

Cockroaches and ants can crawl through small cracks, and it is difficult to exclude them by purely physical means (Fig. 34.9). Sealing up cracks and then spraying a contact insecticide around the gap between the door and its frame probably gives the best protection when crawling insects are a serious nuisance. Small storage boxes and meat safes can be stood with the legs in dishes of kerosine with DDT or of water containing disinfectant. The liquid acts as a barrier to crawling insects.

Rats are able to gnaw their way through wood, and while it is wise to keep them out of the house altogether, it is particularly necessary to prevent them gaining access to food. If dry foods such as flour, grain and beans are stored in jars with lids, or in tins or metal bins with lids, then rodents are excluded.

So far we have discussed some of the more important methods of preserving and storing wholesome food. The ultimate aim of storing food is to eat it, and while primitive man no doubt ate all his food raw there are good reasons for cooking much of the food that we eat. This applies particularly to food that is rich in protein since, as mentioned earlier in this chapter, such food provides a breeding ground for many kinds of pathogenic organisms.

Although cooking is often a means of adding flavour to food and making it easier to eat, adequate cooking is also a means of sterilizing food (Fig. 34.12). Boiling meat and vegetables for a minimum of ten minutes kills most active bacteria, but not all bacterial spores. Roasting is less reliable since while it usually sterilizes the outside of a chicken or a piece of meat, the temperature in the middle of the meat may never reach a level that ensures sterilization.

All the utensils used for preparing, holding and serving food should be washed in hot water, preferably with a detergent to remove grease. Careful washing can be made pointless by drying dishes and utensils with a dirty cloth. Once washed they are better left to drain and dry in a place where flies will not land on them (Fig. 34.13).

The main points about safe food may be summarized as follows.

(i) Food may contain bacteria or micro-organisms that cause it to decay or which introduce serious intestinal infections.

Fig. 34.13 Ordinary washing up does not always destroy bacteria. This newly washed glass was placed on sterile nutrient agar and incubated for twenty-four hours. The colonies of bacteria are quite obvious

(Domestos Hygiene Advisory Service)

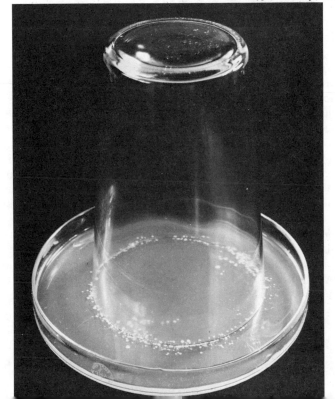

(ii) Fresh food may be treated by methods such as drying, which prevent micro-organisms from reproducing and altering the food chemically.

(iii) Some of these preservation processes, for example canning, also destroy any micro-organisms already present.

(iv) Methods of storing and preserving food are aimed at excluding both the micro-organisms that cause decay and disease and organisms such as flies, which may introduce such microbes.

(v) Cooking may be used as a means of sterilizing food before it is eaten, provided that the method exposes all parts of the food to a high enough temperature for long enough to destroy all the micro-organisms.

Practical Work

Experiment 1 **The effect of cooking on food**

Prepare three agar plates or slopes (p. 203). Take a small piece of fresh meat and divide it into two. Use sterile forceps to rub one of the pieces of meat on the surface of one of the plates or slopes. Label the culture. Boil the other piece of meat in a small quantity of water in a test-tube for twenty minutes. If the test-tube is plugged with cotton wool, steam can escape but

bacteria will not enter while the meat cools. When it is cool, remove the meat with sterile forceps and rub it over the surface of the second plate. Label the container and keep the third as a control. Incubate at 37 °C for two days. Does cooking influence the number of bacterial colonies developing?

Experiment 2 **The effect of refrigeration**

Take two agar plates or slopes and moisten the surface of the jelly with milk, noting whether the milk is pasteurized or not. Incubate one plate at room temperature for two days and place the other in a refrigerator for the same time. Compare the two cultures, noting the appearance of each.

Now allow both cultures to incubate at room temperature for a further two days. What does this suggest about the effect of refrigeration on bacteria in milk?

Question

In what ways are personal hygiene (Chapter 30) and a knowledge of the habits of insect vectors (Chapter 31) important in ensuring that food is prepared and then stored in ways that will keep it safe for people to eat?

35

Pure Water

Clouds form as a result of the condensation of water vapour evaporated from the sea and any other wet surfaces (Fig. 35.1). The rain that falls from clouds is, therefore, biologically pure. Once having reached the ground, the water collects in rivers and lakes and these form the chief natural sources of water for drinking, cooking and washing. Unfortunately, rivers and lakes are often convenient places in which to dump waste water, including sewage and industrial outfall. Since sewage often contains the pathogens of such intestinal diseases as typhoid and cholera, its presence in water that is to be used for drinking and washing is a hazard to health. Lake Nakuru in Kenya has been affected by herbicide. This is killing off the plankton—tiny plants on which flamingoes feed.

When small communities spread their waste into large volumes of water, the harmful material is diluted so much that there is not very much risk to health. However, when the sewage from a town is run into a river or lake the number of disease organisms present in the water reaches dangerous

proportions. So, either raw sewage must *not* be discharged into water that is likely to be used for drinking (*see* p. 253), or the water must be artificially purified (Fig. 35.2).

On a small scale, contaminated water can be made safe to drink by boiling it, but this is not practicable when treating large volumes of water for use by a village or town community. Of course, when possible, town water supplies are taken from unpolluted sources among hills where rainfall is plentiful. But with the increasing demand for water, authorities are being forced to take water from polluted rivers and lakes and such water has to be made safe for domestic use. Depending on how dirty it is, water may first be pumped into settling tanks to allow large particles of debris to drop out. It is next pumped through a filter which should remove particles of any size greater than 0.002 mm in diameter. The design of filters varies with the volume of water with which they are expected to deal. *Slow sand filters* are usually very large and rely on a gelatinous film formed on the sand layer. This film is produced as a jelly-

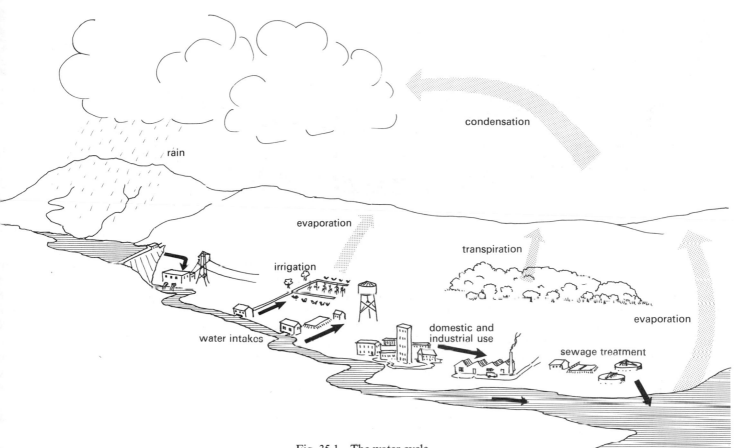

Fig. 35.1   The water cycle

like secretion from millions of protozoa and other micro-organisms. It traps bacteria which are then consumed as food by the protozoa. The film is supported on a layer of sand which is, in turn, carried by pebbles or grit resting on larger stones.

Rapid sand filters are similar in principle, except that filtration is brought about by an artificial jelly made from finely divided alumina (aluminium oxide). The construction of the filter bed is more elaborate to make possible a much faster rate of filtration.

Chlorination

Filtration should make water crystal clear, but it will still contain bacteria that are small enough to pass through the filter. These are destroyed by the addition of chlorine gas to the water as it passes from the filter to storage tanks. Chlorine is a very poisonous gas, but its action on bacteria depends on the fact that it combines with water to form hypochlorous acid. This is very unstable, and decomposes in contact with

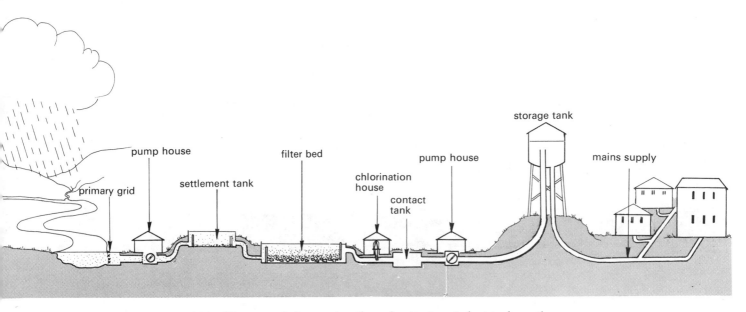

Fig. 35.2   Water supply from a river through a treatment plant to domestic users

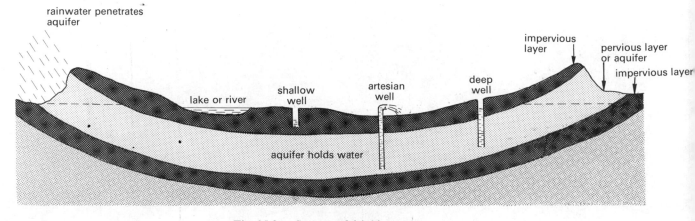

Fig. 35.3   Sources of drinking-water

bacteria to release a very active form of oxygen that destroys them. Other organic matter in the water would cause the hypochlorous acid to decompose wastefully, and this is a good reason for filtering the water carefully before chlorinating it.

The amount of chlorine needed to ensure total destruction of all bacteria in a given volume of water can be calculated, and a small surplus is added to form residual chlorine, a safeguard against any small contamination that may follow treatment.

Ideally the treated water should be stored where there is no risk of contamination, and the careful design of pipe-lines and storage tanks ensures this. The water is pumped to high-level storage tanks or to reservoirs on hills, from which it can flow under gravity to the houses, hospitals and factories that require a supply.

Within the home, water is often stored under the roof in a tank of 200 to 500 litres capacity, and this tank may be a source of re-contamination if birds, rodents or germ-bearing insects have access to it. Drinking water is usually taken from the main supply pipe coming into the house.

When no piped supply is available water may have to be taken from a well. This may mean a shaft or hole sunk deep into the ground, or it may simply be a shallow depression. Provided care is taken to prevent run-off water from the surrounding ground surface running into it, the water from a deep well should be safe to drink, since it is extensively filtered as it passes through the earth before entering the well and ideally should have percolated through permeable rock from sources some distance away from human habitation (Fig. 35.3).

Artesian wells are even more germ-free as a water source than deep wells, since the water they provide must have travelled a considerable distance from high ground through permeable rock. Water comes to the surface of the well under pressure which may be sufficient to force it through pipes to the houses where it will be used.

Surface wells are fed with water which has drained through a shallow layer of soil to an impervious layer of rock or clay where it forms a *water table*. The filtering effect of the shallow soil is rarely sufficient to remove bacteria. If human or animal waste is deposited on the ground or even in latrine pits near such wells, the water is very likely to be polluted (Fig. 35.4).

The supply of piped, treated water in the City of London in the nineteenth century brought an enormous improvement to health and the elimination of cholera as people abandoned the use of contaminated surface wells. A similar improvement in health is taking place in most countries of the world as the provision of piped, treated water becomes a community responsibility.

Questions

1   Why do you think the cholera epidemics in London in the 1840s and 1850 were associated with drinking-water? Why do you think they occurred in the summer months?

2   Water taken from a lake or a river is not always unsafe to drink. In what circumstances is such water likely to be safe for drinking?

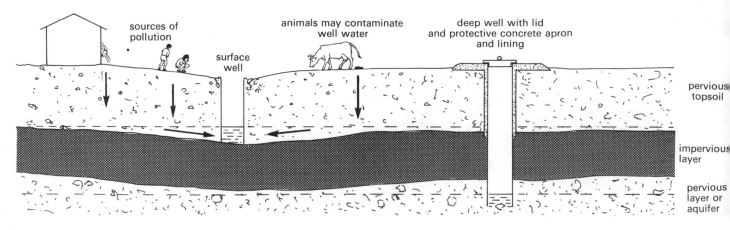

Fig. 35.4   Comparison between a shallow surface well and a protected deep well

36

The Disposal of Sewage and Refuse

Sewage is the name given to human urine and faeces when collected together. Very often it is diluted with the water used to flush WCs and with water carrying organic waste from kitchens and washrooms. It may also contain industrial waste or effluent.

Refuse and garbage are names given to solid waste that accumulates as a result of domestic and industrial activity. It includes paper, cartons and cans, and may also include unused food material that can harbour micro-organisms and feed creatures such as flies and rats which act as disease vectors. The methods of disposing of sewage and refuse differ.

Sewage

As explained on p. 205, urine and faeces carry bacteria and these organisms may be pathogens. By urinating and defaecating carelessly about the place, people can make it easy for such vectors as houseflies, cockroaches and rats to become infected with pathogens which can then be spread to other, healthy people.

In country districts where the population is widely dispersed the risk of the spread of intestinal diseases by vectors is less than in a densely populated town. When people live close together in large numbers, flies and other vectors have only a short journey from a source of disease-causing organisms to the food which may be eaten by a large number of people. Thus one person suffering from dysentery, thoughtlessly defaecating near a food market, could spread dysentery amoebae by flies to the food and infect a considerable population.

The number of people travelling from one town to another as traders or casual visitors increases the risk of the introduction of a disease to a healthy community. This can be seen clearly in the spread of cholera. However, the arrival of an infected visitor will only result in the spread of cholera if he is careless over the disposal of his faeces or if the sewage system is at fault.

In isolated houses and small villages both urine and faeces may be disposed of safely in a pit latrine, provided that the soil is permeable to water and that there are no wells within 100 metres that are likely to be contaminated by seepage. Such a latrine or privy should be dug as deep as the soil will allow and provided with a floor of concrete, brick or stone that can be cleaned easily and will not hold puddles of stagnant water. If the upper part of the pit is lined with concrete or brick then the chances of rats entering to feed on the faeces will be less. A cover over the pit keeps out flies, which are attracted by faeces and feed on them, gathering micro-organisms as they do so (Fig. 36.1).

When a good water supply is available then a flush privy or WC can be installed and connected to a water carriage system. This means that a flow of water is used to carry the excrement to the sewage disposal point. It is usual to instal one or more WCs in a house. The lavatory pan is made of earthenware or china with a shiny, glazed surface that makes it easy to clean. Urine and faeces are flushed away into the drainpipe and sewer by the rapid release of 10 to 15 litres of water from a cistern. Some of this water remains in the pan, forming a seal that prevents unpleasant-smelling gases from the sewer passing back into the house. A simple pattern of WC pan is shown in

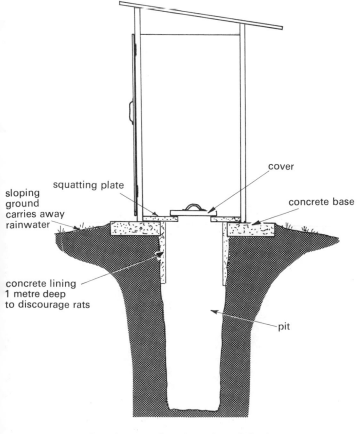

cover

squatting plate

sloping ground carries away rainwater

concrete base

concrete lining 1 metre deep to discourage rats

pit

Fig. 36.1   Section through a pit latrine

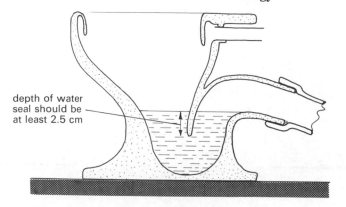

depth of water seal should be at least 2.5 cm

Fig. 36.2   WC or lavatory pan

Fig. 36.2 and an alternative to this, the squatting plate, is shown in Fig. 36.3.

The operation of both pieces of equipment depends on the rapid flow or flushing action of the water from the cistern. This flushing generates a fine spray which is not easily seen and most people are unaware of it. Like any fine spray or aerosol, these droplets float in the air and settle on the seat, on any fitting in the lavatory and on the person who has just used it. Normally the danger from this is not great, but when the WC is used by a person suffering from diarrhoea, germs from the liquid stools are spread all too easily by the spray. It is because one cannot avoid touching things such as handles that are contaminated by the spray-borne bacteria that so much importance is attached to washing the hands carefully after using the lavatory.

In a small village or an isolated house, the sewage may be carried by water flow to a septic tank (Fig. 36.4). This consists

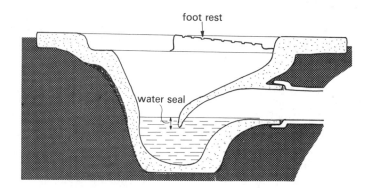

foot rest

water seal

Fig. 36.3   Squatting plate, an alternative to the WC pan and flushed in the same way

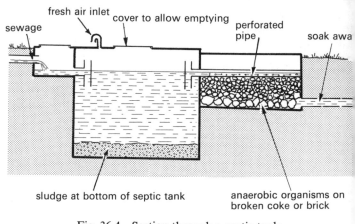

fresh air inlet
cover to allow emptying
sewage
perforated pipe
soak away
sludge at bottom of septic tank
anaerobic organisms on broken coke or brick

Fig. 36.4   Section through a septic tank

of two large chambers lined with waterproof concrete and built below the level of the house. Solid matter settles out in the first chamber after which the liquid flows into the second chamber which is filled with broken stone or brick on which live large numbers of bacteria and ciliate protozoa which, between them, break down the organic waste to harmless materials.

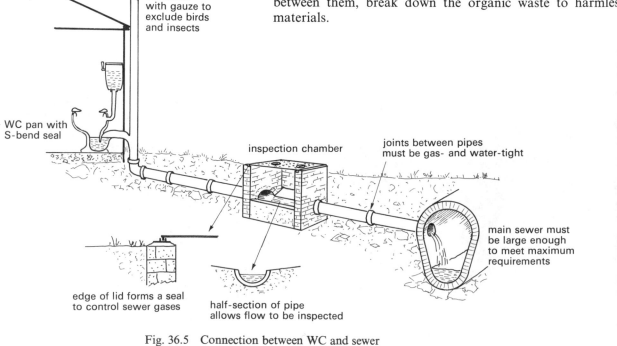

ventilator with gauze to exclude birds and insects

WC pan with S-bend seal

inspection chamber

joints between pipes must be gas- and water-tight

main sewer must be large enough to meet maximum requirements

edge of lid forms a seal to control sewer gases

half-section of pipe allows flow to be inspected

Fig. 36.5   Connection between WC and sewer

The term septic tank implies that the tank contains bacteria and, since these are necessary for its proper working, it is a mistake to put disinfectant into the water running into the tank. It is necessary to remember this when cleaning the WC or privy. Soap and water are recommended when there is risk of the cleansing fluid getting into the system.

From time to time the sediment or sludge in the first and second chambers has to be cleaned out. It may be removed into a mobile tank provided by a local health authority or, in a remote locality, it may have to be taken out and buried in trenches dug for the purpose. Always, care must be taken to prevent contamination of crops and water supply with germs in the sludge. The fluid is allowed to soak away underground.

A cesspool is a simpler construction, built of brick or concrete. It should be impermeable to water to prevent seepage and contamination of the surrounding ground. It must be emptied from time to time as it becomes full.

In towns and cities nowadays it is usual to find a community sewage system (Fig. 36.5). Waste is flushed from individual houses and other premises into sewers. These may be large glazed earthenware pipes in a small town, or large tunnels of brick and concrete in a city. Very often there is a separate system to remove rainwater run-off from roofs and streets, since this could seriously overload the sewage system.

When raw sewage is discharged into a lake or river, not only does it constitute a health hazard but it provides so much food for bacteria that they increase to vast numbers. These are aerobic bacteria which make such a demand on the oxygen dissolved in the water that fish and other aquatic creatures are deprived of oxygen and die (p. 52). One of the aims in sewage treatment, therefore, is to reduce the material available for feeding these deoxygenating bacteria before the sewage is discharged. The other principal aim is to render harmless any pathogenic bacteria in the sewage and this, in times of epidemic cholera, dysentery, typhoid or other intestinal diseases, can be of enormous importance. In fact if sewage treatment is

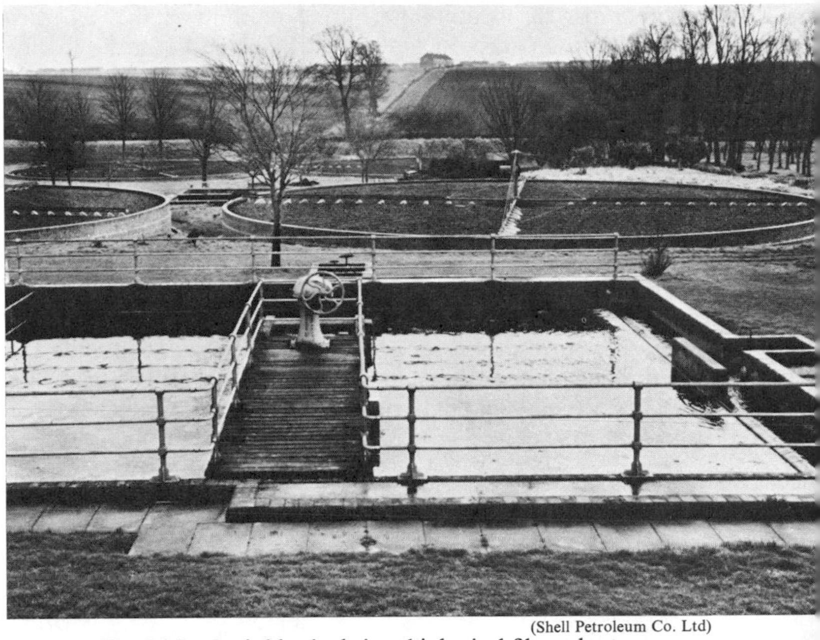

(Shell Petroleum Co. Ltd)

Fig. 36.7 Sprinkler beds in a biological filter plant

liquid is pumped through a perforated pipe that either rotates or moves backwards and forwards, sprinkling the sewage over a bed of coarse stone or coke. As in the septic tank, the stone or coke provides surfaces on which protozoa and bacteria can live. The large gaps between the surfaces ensure good aeration, so that bacteria thrive. When the liquid reaches the bottom of the bed any suspended solids will have been removed, together with dissolved organic matter. The liquid is now safe for discharge into a river (Figs. 36.6 and 36.7).

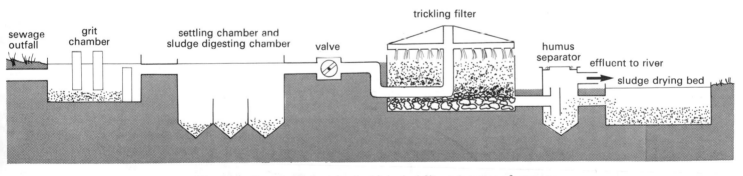

Fig. 36.6 Layout of plant for the biological filter treatment of sewage

effective and sanitary methods of disposing of faeces are being used properly, then epidemics of these diseases can usually be controlled or even prevented.

Treatment of sewage begins with screening, which traps large objects such as bottles and cartons, which sometimes are carried along with sewage. The next stage is sedimentation, in which solid matter settles out while the sewage stands in large tanks. Ferric chloride is often added at this stage to speed up the settling of the finer particles by a process called flocculation. The chemical forms a jelly which traps the particles.

Further treatment follows one of two courses. The older process is called the *biological filter method* in which the

The sediment or sludge from the sedimentation tank is transferred to a large tank for *digestion*. The term has the same meaning as when applied to our digestive systems, that is, solid materials such as proteins, fats and carbohydrates (including cellulose) are hydrolysed into simpler materials that are then used by the digesting micro-organisms. This stage may take up to thirty days, after which the digested sludge is spread on beds of sand and gravel to be dried. Once dry, the sludge can be carted away and used as fertilizer, though preferably on crops that will not be eaten raw since the sludge, unlike the liquid effluent, still contains large numbers of micro-organisms.

The most important alternative method is the *activated sludge process* (Figs. 36.8–10), in which the liquid, following sedimentation, is pumped into long channels together with a small quantity of sludge, which contains a variety of protozoa. The main feature of this process is the bubbling of air under pressure through a diffuser or perforated pipe along the bottom of each channel. This air both agitates and mixes the sewage and sludge and also maintains a high oxygen level in the water. This accelerates digestion by micro-organisms of the dissolved solids and consequently the plant can treat sewage at a faster rate than the biological filter method. The quantity of sludge builds up during the process. Some is recirculated while the remainder is digested with the sediment that settled out earlier in the treatment. The material left after digestion is dried and used as fertilizer.

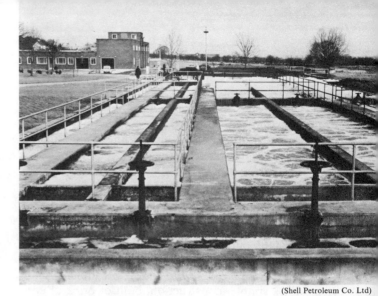

(Shell Petroleum Co. Ltd)

Fig. 36.8 Aeration tanks in an activated sludge treatment plant

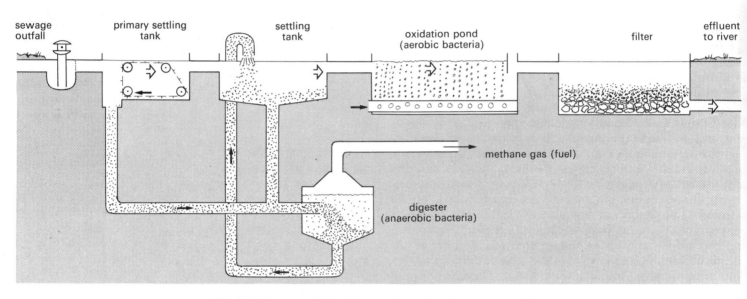

Fig. 36.9 Layout of plant for the activated sludge treatment of sewage

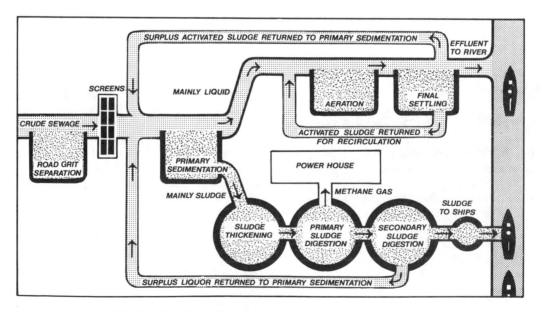

Fig. 36.10 Alternative arrangement for activated sludge treatment

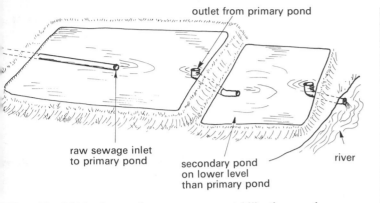

Fig. 36.11   Sewage lagoons or waste stabilization ponds

In many countries with flat land available and no more than moderate rainfall, sewage may be treated in sewage ponds or oxidation ponds. These are between 1 m and 1.5 m deep. The area depends on the quantity of sewage to be treated each day. Sewage provides nutrients for microscopic green algae as well as bacteria. In light the algae carry out photosynthesis and release oxygen which is promptly used by the bacteria. Wind movement produces small waves on the pond which mix the surface water with that lying near the bottom and this hastens the decomposing activity of the bacteria. This liquid is run off from time to time into one or more secondary ponds where further oxidation completes the process of rendering the material harmless and ready for discharge into a river or stream. Such sewage ponds are cheap to maintain and work with very little unpleasant smell provided they are not overloaded.

Disposal of domestic refuse

Dustbins or garbage cans are used for the collection of waste from the kitchen and other parts of a house. They are made of galvanized steel or of strong plastic and should have a lid that fits closely to exclude flies which breed quickly in decomposing

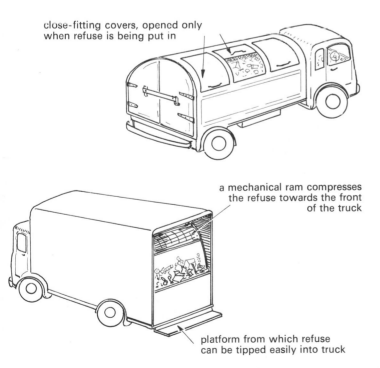

Fig. 36.12   Two types of refuse collection trucks

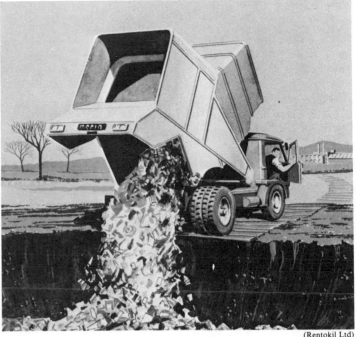

(Rentokil Ltd)

Fig. 36.13   Tipping rubbish from a modern refuse collection truck

rubbish (p. 233). The lid should also be heavy enough (or else held on by clips) to prevent scavenging dogs and cats from tipping it off. If the dustbin is washed out from time to time and dried out in the sun before being used again then the number of bacteria present is kept low.

In isolated villages and households the contents of the dustbin should be either burned or buried in pits or trenches in which the organic content will be decomposed. Such pits should be 1 m deep and the refuse should not be less than 0.5 m below the surface of the ground when the pit is filled in, so that rats are discouraged from burrowing into it and using it for food.

Communal incinerators or refuse pits may be set up by health authorities in villages and towns. Health authorities in larger towns usually organize the collection of refuse from dustbins into special lorries in which the rubbish can be carried, covered from rain, wind and flies (Fig. 36.12). The details of large-scale disposal of refuse are beyond the scope of this book but the principles are similar to those used on a domestic scale—burn or bury. When it is not practicable to burn or bury the rubbish, it is packed together very tightly by a bulldozer and left to decompose slowly. Tight packing makes it difficult (though, unfortunately, not impossible) for rats and fly larvae to burrow into it. A vigilant health authority keeps a check on the rat population near sewage and refuse disposal plant and takes steps to see that the numbers of rats are kept low (see p. 265).

Questions

1   The frequency with which certain intestinal disorders, such as summer diarrhoea, occur is often greater when people go camping in the countryside in large groups than when the same people are living in town. Why is this so? What precautions should be taken to guard against this?

2   Why is it desirable to have domestic refuse removed from a house at shorter intervals in hot weather than in cold weather?

37

Good Housing

Houses are not merely buildings but homes, in other words places where people live, and as such they should be hygienic and comfortable. Many of us have little choice in the matter of where we live or the kind of house or flat in which we live, but an awareness of the criteria of good housing may be helpful when a choice does have to be made and in any case may help us to improve and get the best out of existing housing.

Site

Ground that is well drained is preferred to damp or marshy land. Dryness can often be achieved by building on a raised site, which can be an artificial mound, provided this is well compacted to make the ground firm. Permeable soil means good drainage as a rule. When it is necessary to build on water-logged ground or on land subject to flooding it is desirable to raise the house on piers or stilts. This is often seen on river-bank sites (Fig. 37.1).

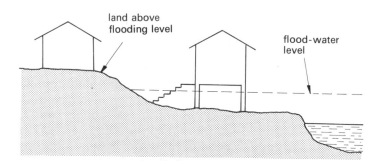

Fig. 37.1   Houses near a river may be built on stilts to avoid flooding

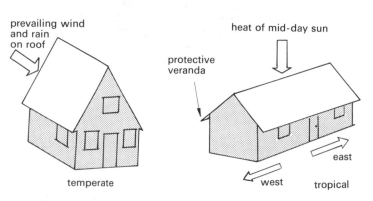

Fig. 37.2   Siting houses in temperate and tropical regions

Account should be taken of the prevailing wind, since this may carry smells from factories and flies from places where rubbish accumulates and decomposes. Where rainfall is heavy, a driving wind may blow water into openings that would be unaffected by rain falling vertically downwards. In this case the house should be sited so that the windward side either has no openings such as doors, windows and ventilators, or else these should be protected by a generous, overhanging veranda.

In temperate climates sunshine may be an asset, and a house with windows facing the sun may be very comfortable. In the tropics, too, such a siting is ideal, since for much of the day the sun will be overhead and not likely to shine into doors and windows, to overheat the rooms (Fig. 37.2).

Larders and store-rooms are best placed on the north side of a house in northern temperate countries so that they are cooler. In the tropics such rooms should also be away from direct sunlight but accessible to ventilating air currents.

The number of rooms will be decided by the size of the family and the money available for building. Since all human beings require privacy on occasions, one room per person is ideal but not often possible.

Construction of the house

Construction is determined by the materials available. Wood, bricks, fired-clay bricks and concrete are used in different parts of the world. The qualities looked for are permanence and durability, and insulating properties.

Foundations. Unless foundations are firm a house is unlikely to be very permanent. The depth to which foundations are sunk below ground level depends on the nature of the ground, whether it is rock, clay or sandy soil. They have also to be suited to the weight which they are expected to carry. Most building materials allow water to travel through them by capillary action like oil travelling up a wick, so a *damp course* is placed in the walls above the foundations and above ground level. This must be an impermeable material such as slate, glazed tile, bituminized felt or heavy-gauge polythene strip (Fig. 37.3).

Walls. Brick walls and concrete block walls usually are built with an air cavity between two layers of material. The air is a good insulator both against heat loss and against excessive heating by the sun. If the outside wall is made damp by wind-driven rain then the air cavity prevents the damp affecting the inner wall.

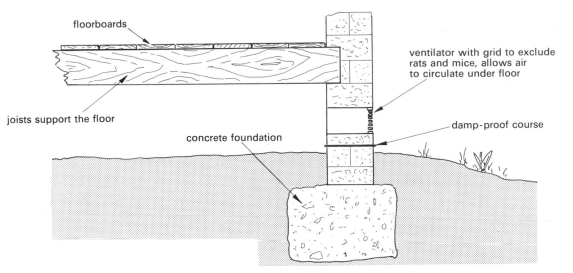

Fig. 37.3 Foundations and damp course

The avoidance of damp is important since moisture favours the growth of fungi which destroy wood and many other materials that we put inside a house.

Floors. Floors may be made of wood resting on joists which are secured in the walls above the level of the damp course (*see* Fig. 37.3). An alternative method is to level the earth between the wall foundations and put down broken stone or brick (termed *hard core*) covered with sufficient sand to fill the spaces. A continuous sheet of waterproof polythene is placed over the sand and a concrete floor is poured over this, levelled and smoothed. This makes a very strong, dry and durable floor. Wood can be laid over the concrete to give heat insulation (*see* Fig. 37.4).

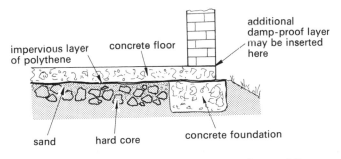

Fig. 37.4 Alternative construction for damp-proof ground floor

Roof. A strong, durable and watertight roof is essential. The pitch or slope of the roof is determined often by tradition but really should take account of climate. A steep pitch is desirable in countries experiencing heavy snowfall since a thick layer of snow may add a great weight to the roof supports. On the other hand, snow is quite a good heat insulator and in regions of moderate snowfall a strong roof with a snow 'blanket' on top may lose less heat to the atmosphere than a steep roof with no snow. Rainfall also has to be taken into account. In countries with low or sporadic rainfall a flat roof may serve to collect rainwater which can be led off to storage tanks. A gutter around the edge of any roof is desirable to prevent rainwater running on to the walls and making them damp. In Europe, roofs have traditionally been made waterproof by laying overlapping slates or tiles on the roof timbers. Asbestos sheeting and corrugated galvanized steel may be used. Sheet aluminium is particularly useful in tropical countries because it reflects the heat of the sun. Although less durable, a thatch of palm or other leaves, skilfully laid, gives a waterproof roof with good insulating properties. The roof frame and the fixing of the covering should be sufficiently strong to resist wind action.

The space under the roof is important. In the temperate zone, heat is lost through the ceiling into the loft in cold weather, and a layer of insulating material such as glassfibre wadding or granulated asbestos or polystyrene will reduce heat wastage (Fig. 37.5). In the tropics the space under the roof is often kept open to give extra height and a greater volume of air. This helps to produce a circulation of air, with a cooling

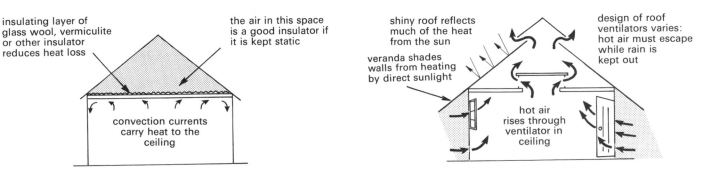

Fig. 37.5 Roof design in temperate and tropical regions

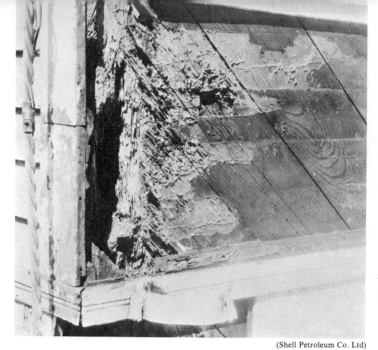

(Shell Petroleum Co. Ltd)

Fig. 37.6   Termite damage to the timber frame of a house

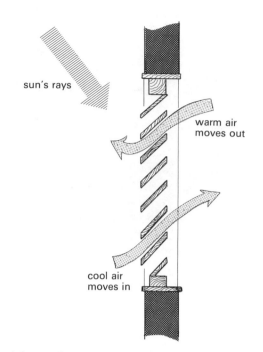

Fig. 37.7   A louvre shutter prevents direct sunlight from overheating a room while permitting ventilation

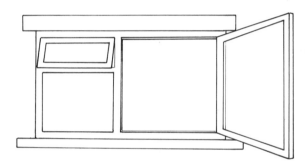

Fig. 37.8   Windows should have sections that can be opened and adjusted to control ventilation

effect. Where the under-roof space is closed it can be a dead space in which pests may breed, such as wasps or mice. There should be a trap-door giving access for inspection of this space.

Timber construction and termites

In many tropical countries termites cause extensive damage to buildings constructed of timber (Fig. 37.6). These insects use their powerful jaws to bite into wood, chewing it to a pulp. This pulp is digested, not by the termites themselves but by protozoa living in their gut. One kind of termite, *Macrotermes*, differs in that the wood pulp is laid down as food for a fungus, cultivated in the underground nests of the termite.

Because of the large numbers of termites in a colony and their enormous capacity to chew wood, these creatures can do immense damage to wooden buildings, eating timbers such as pillars, door and window frames and floor joists, resulting in the collapse of the structure.

Complete protection against damage is difficult to achieve. Concrete piles or pillars help by raising a timber building clear of the ground, but many species of termite can build covered, tunnel-like runs over the concrete to the timber above. Impregnation of timber with proprietary insect-killing chemicals such as Rentokil fluid gives long-lasting protection. Alternatively the ground around the house may be treated with BHC or a similar persistent insecticide to prevent the insects from reaching the house.

Ventilation and draughts

Fresh, oxygen-rich air is desirable for the comfort and well-being of the people living in a house. In hot weather in any country a free movement of air also aids the evaporation of perspiration or sweat. The cooling effect thus produced adds to one's feeling of comfort.

In hot countries louvre shutters permit movement of air in and out of a room while preventing the direct rays of the sun from overheating the room. They also provide privacy (Fig. 37.7). In cooler climates ventilation must be achieved without simply admitting rushes of cold air and losing warm air.

Adjustable ventilation is preferred and this may be obtained by having different-sized sections in a window that can be opened to varying extents (Fig. 37.8). Ventilator or air bricks in an outside wall allow air in but should carry an adjustable shutter or grille inside the room. In rooms with an open fire or a gas fire connected to a chimney the flue ensures a natural movement of air, as shown in Fig. 37.9.

Where central heating radiators are used, however, more positive action has to be taken to ensure ventilation. Extractor fans may be used to draw out excessively humid (steamy) air from a kitchen while a meal is being cooked, and they can also be used to ventilate other rooms such as bathrooms and lavatories where there is no natural air movement.

Good ventilation should ensure a slow, gentle movement of air through a room without any direct, concentrated air stream. Anybody sitting in a draught or stream of air is likely to be chilled either because the air is cold or, more usually, because moving air accelerates the evaporation of perspiration from the skin. Excessive cooling could result in hypothermia—lowering of body temperature below the normal range (p. 99). People do not *catch* cold through sitting in a draught, but chilling reduces the body's resistance to disease organisms.

Heating

In cold climates a great deal of money can be spent on heating a house, so wastage of heat should be avoided. The influence of the choice of building materials on insulation has already been mentioned (p. 257) and so has the effect of excessive ventilation on heat conservation.

What constitutes an ideal living temperature is a matter of opinion, related to feelings of comfort. This is related to the rate at which the body loses heat (*see* Chapter 14). People are usually less active physically inside a house than out-of-doors and therefore generate less heat. Loss of heat from the body to the surroundings is reduced by wearing clothes that act as insulators. A living-room temperature between 15 °C and 20 °C (60 °F and 69 °F) is considered comfortable in temperate regions and light clothing provides adequate insulation.

The sources of heat include open fires, burning coal or a smokeless fuel; central heating, in which heat from the burning of fuel in a boiler is carried by water (which has a high specific heat capacity) through pipes to radiators; electric heaters, in which electric current either heats a coil to such a high temperature that it glows and throws out radiant heat, or else heats a different type of coil enclosed in special bricks—a storage heater, so called because, once heated, the bricks emit heat over a long period; gas fires, in which burning coal gas or natural gas (methane) heats clay elements to a high temperature so that they glow and radiate heat; and finally oil heaters, in which the hot products of the burning of kerosine (paraffin) circulate in the room.

All of these methods involve some heating by convection, as well as by radiation. The proportion of heat transferred by the two methods varies with the design of the heating equipment used. In a fan heater, for example, most of the heat from an electric coil is dispersed by air currents, increased by the

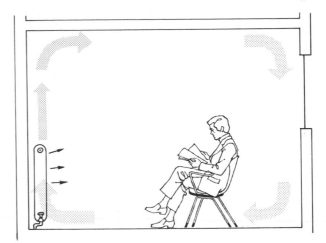

Fig. 37.10 Most of the heat from a central heating 'radiator' is dispersed by convection

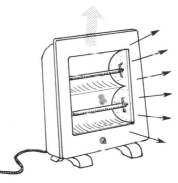

Fig. 37.11 Most of the heat from an electric fire is radiated while some is spread by convection

action of a fan. Most of the heat from a central heating radiator is dispersed by convection, while a high proportion of heat from an electric fire is radiated (Figs. 37.10–11).

Whatever kind of heating is used, there is a tendency for the humidity of the atmosphere to be reduced, acutely in the case of electric and central heating because the air temperature is increased without moisture being added, less so in the case of gas fires and oil burners where one of the products of combustion is water.

While reduced humidity may be an advantage when drying clothes or when the air temperature is very high, it is not always an advantage where health is concerned—lung disorders such as bronchitis are accentuated by very dry air—and some means of increasing atmospheric humidity may be desirable. This can be achieved by placing an open container of water on a radiator or near an electric fire.

In tropical countries and in high summer in temperate regions it may be desirable to cool the air in rooms rather than to heat it. Increased ventilation often produces this effect but sometimes air-conditioning equipment is installed. This usually involves passing air over the cooling coils of a refrigeration unit and then blowing it into the room. While cool air can be a pleasant contrast to the heat out-of-doors, it can produce rapid cooling of the body with risks of chilling already mentioned on p. 258. Acceptable cooling can be obtained in all but the most humid climates by good ventilation, the circulation of air cooling the body by speeding up the evaporation of sweat.

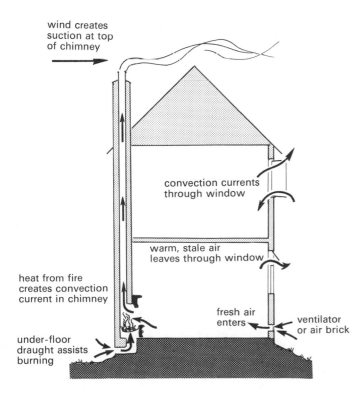

Fig. 37.9 An open fire assists ventilation

Lighting

Natural lighting is desirable whenever possible because it is more intense than all but the most sophisticated and expensive forms of artificial lighting. The human eye is able to adapt to seeing under a wide range of light intensities (*see* p. 135), but many of the activities that depend on acute vision—reading, writing and fine manipulative skills—are often carried on indoors and under artificial lighting. In designing housing, windows should occupy not less than one-tenth of the wall surface. In practice window areas may be much greater than this, but in the tropics large unshaded windows can certainly lead to overheating of a room and even in temperate areas such as Britain a large window area can be a source of heat intake during sunny weather. Of course, a window may be a considerable source of heat loss in cold weather.

Electric lighting is the accepted source of artificial lighting in many parts of the world and, in homes, is provided either by filament lamps or by fluorescent tubes. Filament lamps depend on the emission of light energy from a coil or filament, heated by the electric current. Such lamps are cheap but in terms of light output for the energy consumed are not very efficient. Fluorescent tubes are more expensive but have a longer working life and are certainly more efficient. They also provide a more even or diffused light. The siting of lamps depends very much on the use to be made of a particular room. For reading, it is helpful to have lamps so sited that light falls directly on the pages of the book. For general lighting, a lamp suspended from the ceiling is often adequate though a softer illumination is obtained when light is reflected from the walls and ceiling. Such light is termed indirect light.

Whatever the source of light, natural or artificial, it should produce no sense of strain or discomfort in the person using it. It should not produce intense shadows in the room. Although shadows look interesting in photographs, they produce an undue strain on the eyes when the gaze is shifted from a brightly lit object to one in shade. Fluorescent lamps sometimes flicker as they age and they should be replaced, since this flicker is harmful to the retinal cells and irritating to the nervous system.

Lavatories and washing facilities

When lavatories can be connected to a water carriage system (Chapter 36) it is usual to install WCs or lavatory pans inside the house. Ideally the WC should be located in a small room used for no other purpose, though quite often a WC is located in a bathroom. Since, however careful the users are, a lavatory is always a source of germs, it is wise to locate it well away from the kitchen and food store. Building regulations in Britain require that a lavatory shall not lead directly off a kitchen or living room. There must be a passageway between the two. The WC should be sited where there is a natural fall from the lavatory pan through the pipes to the main drainage system. The same applies to the siting of the bathroom or washroom. By modern standards a house should have a bath or a shower so that a person can wash his whole body easily.

Kitchen facilities

The kitchen should be a light, airy, well-ventilated room, and the surfaces on which food is prepared, whether a table or the tops of cupboards, should be made of a material that can be cleaned easily and thoroughly. Modern plastic laminates covering wood have a hard, smooth surface that can be kept free from germs provided there are no cracks. Wooden surfaces eventually become porous and may carry large populations of germs (Fig. 37.12). If there is no alternative, then wooden work surfaces should be washed daily with a powerful (but nontainting) disinfectant. Bleach solution, suitably diluted, is one of the best.

The type of cooking facilities and whether a refrigerator is provided or not will depend on circumstances, but a cool, airy food store is necessary (*see* p. 246).

Care in the design and equipping of a kitchen and food store may be of no avail if vermin such as rats, mice, cockroaches, ants or houseflies invade the place. If any of these creatures is found in the neighbourhood then excluding them from houses can be surprisingly difficult. Rats and mice can enter through open doors or windows even if a house is otherwise rat-proofed. Rat-proofing involves making ground floors of

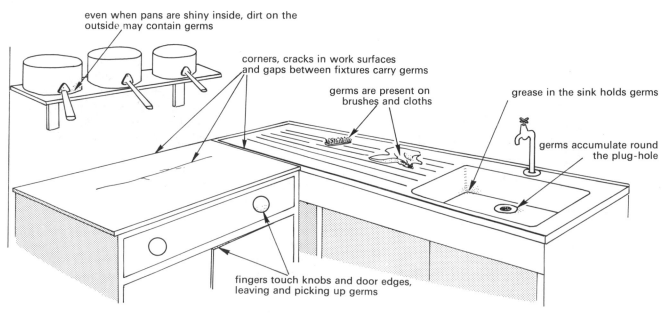

Fig. 37.12 Some of the sources of germs in a kitchen

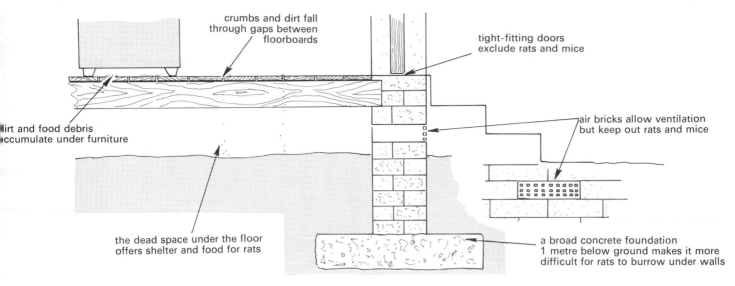

crumbs and dirt fall through gaps between floorboards

tight-fitting doors exclude rats and mice

dirt and food debris accumulate under furniture

air bricks allow ventilation but keep out rats and mice

the dead space under the floor offers shelter and food for rats

a broad concrete foundation 1 metre below ground makes it more difficult for rats to burrow under walls

Fig. 37.13   Where rats are numerous, special precautions must be taken to make houses rat-proof

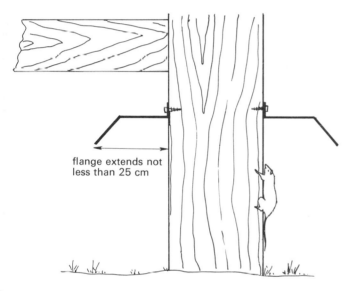

flange extends not less than 25 cm

Fig. 37.14   A metal flange prevents rats from climbing walls and wooden piers

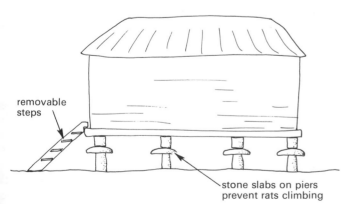

removable steps

stone slabs on piers prevent rats climbing

Fig. 37.15   Grain stores require special protection against rats and mice

concrete, continuous with the walls, or else sinking the foundations sufficiently deep into the ground so that rats cannot burrow underneath (*see* Fig. 37.13).

Tight-fitting, well-maintained doors are essential and, in regions where rats are numerous, additional precautions may be necessary. A metal flange will form a barrier to prevent rats and mice from climbing walls and gaining access to open windows (Fig. 37.14). Such a flange is particularly important where houses are made of wood. When houses are built on piles or stilts a flange should be fitted around each pile. In many parts of the world, grain stores have been built on piers with slabs of stone to prevent rats climbing up. The steps used for entering the granary are removed when not in use (Fig. 37.15).

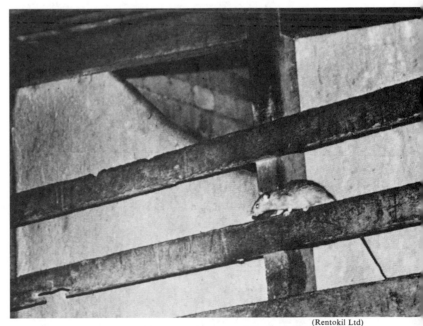

(Rentokil Ltd)

Fig. 37.16   Rats are good climbers and use roof timbers as routes from one part of a building to another; routes are stained with oil from the rats' fur

Cockroaches and ants are primarily crawling insects, but whereas ants form their nests usually in the earth under or near a house and crawl in to find food, cockroaches live and breed inside houses. In Britain they are often mistakenly called black beetles. They spend the hours of daylight under floorboards, behind cupboards and in the gaps where hot-water pipes pass through walls. They often gain access to houses in boxes and baskets and apart from killing them with DDT or pyrethrum powder, the principal preventative measure is to reduce the number of cracks in floors and other small gaps in which they can hide. The dead space under a wooden floor provides an ideal breeding ground, with crumbs and other food accumulating through the cracks between floorboards (*see* Fig. 37.13), and this space is usually difficult to disinfest.

Ants are rarely a serious problem in temperate regions but in the tropics they can be a considerable nuisance. The design of a house rarely prevents their entry and when the path of entry is noticeable it should be sprayed with a residual DDT spray.

Flies and mosquitoes can be excluded by covering window openings with fine wire mesh, and doors that are left open for ventilation in hot weather can also be protected by a second, light frame door covered with wire mesh. Kitchens and food stores in particular should be protected in this way since free air movement is desirable, especially in hot weather. It is also helpful to make bedrooms or sleeping rooms free from insects in the same way, partly because they can be irritating and particularly because most biting insects, many of which are night fliers, are also vectors of disease organisms.

Rainwater gutters and drains

Many insects breed in surprisingly small amounts of water. A badly laid rainwater gutter around a roof may hold water for a sufficient number of days after rainfall for hatching and larval development of an insect to be completed.

Where possible, drains around the house should be of the type shown in Fig. 37.17. The grid allows water to pass through but excludes leaves and other large pieces of material that might block the drainpipes. The grid also deters flies and mosquitoes from entering the drain, though it is not always 100 per cent effective in this respect. The space below the grid traps grit and also provides a seal to prevent gases from the drainpipe seeping back. The grit trap needs to be cleaned out at intervals, depending on the amount of water passing through the drain and the amount of grit and sediment deposited.

Practical Work

Experiment 1 Heat transfer

Take two jam jars or two tin cans of equal size. Paint one black or cover it with black paper and paint the other white or cover it with white material. Place an equal amount of cold water at the same temperature in each. Read the temperature on a thermometer and record it.

Now place the two containers either in strong sunlight or in the rays from an electric fire. Measure the temperature of the water after ten minutes and after twenty minutes. Which container warms up more rapidly? What does this result suggest about the choice of colour for the outside of a house in a hot, sunny climate?

Now place equal quantities of hot water in each of the two containers and put them in a cool place. Which *loses* heat more rapidly? What does the result suggest about the choice of colour for the outside walls of a house in a cold climate?

Experiment 2 Capillary action

Collect a variety of the materials used in building. Some suggestions are shown in Fig. 37.18 but you could add many more. Place them in shallow water in a tray or tank—the depth of water is important and should not exceed 2 cm; the container could be a sink or a bath.

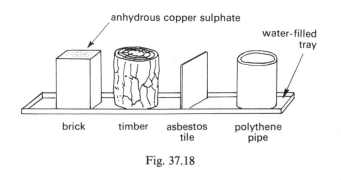

Fig. 37.18

Place a small amount of white anhydrous copper sulphate on the upper surfaces, as shown. Anhydrous copper sulphate turns from white to blue when it absorbs water. On which materials does the copper sulphate change colour? Which materials conduct water by capillary action? Which materials could be used to form a damp course?

(*Note*. In humid climates, anhydrous copper sulphate will absorb moisture from the atmosphere, if left, and it will be necessary to put fresh powder on the materials after, say, 2 hours, 1 day, 2 days.)

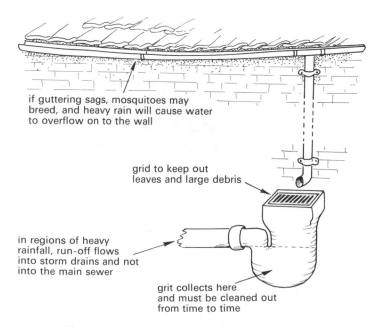

Fig. 37.17   Design of rainwater guttering and drain

Experiment 3 Convection currents

Convection currents in air, important in heating and ventilation, can be studied by using smoke. Provided care is taken to avoid accidentally setting fire to things, smoke can be produced from a short piece of smouldering rope or a smouldering loose roll of paper or cardboard. Notice that the smoke from smouldering rope itself rises by convection, due to the heating of the air around the burning end. Changes in the *speed* as well as the *direction of movement* of the smoke indicate air movements (Fig. 37.19).

Test the movement of air near open and closed windows, around the edges of doors, over cracks in floor boards, near ventilators and radiators. It is not easy to measure the point at which air movement constitutes a draught, but make a list of the positions in which you carry out your tests and grade them in order. You may find that an open window or door, for example, gives the strongest air movement.

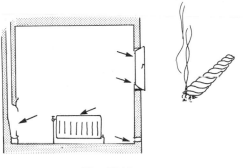

Fig. 37.19

Experiment 4 Sources of bacteria

Consult the suggestions for practical work in Chapter 25, p. 202, for information about setting up culture plates. Use a sterile wire or, preferably, a sterile swab to collect micro-organisms from work surfaces, corners between walls and shelves, handles, taps and other locations in a kitchen (*see* Fig. 37.12). Incubate the culture plates and observe which sources produce the greatest number and the greatest variety of colonies of micro-organisms.

Be careful to wash your hands thoroughly after doing this experiment. Do not open the cultures, but sterilize them carefully before disposing of them.

Question

Explain how an elementary knowledge of the physics of conduction, convection and radiation is helpful in designing a house.

38
Local Health Services

The health of a community cannot be left to chance. In Britain the Government, through the Department of Health and Social Security, has organized a number of Regional Health Authorities as part of the National Health Service. Under them a total of 90 Area Health Authorities control the hospitals, public health services and the provision of doctors to serve the community. At a more local level Family Practitioner Committees are responsible for family doctors, dentists, pharmaceutical services to provide drugs and medicines, and ophthalmic services to see to the care of eyes. These Practitioner Committees have to coordinate the services under their control and one of the key people is the District Community Physician (commonly referred to as the DCP). He has largely taken over the duties once carried out by the Medical Officer of Health or MOH, and he organizes the services in his district. His department analyses health statistics (pp. 186 and 190) to see whether patterns of health are changing and to ensure that the medical services are being put to best use. He takes charge of the coordination of resources in the event of an epidemic and this may include the vaccination of the local population, the tracing of contacts and the arrangement of emergency hospital services. He is expected to notify the National Health Organization of the nature and extent of the outbreak.

The provision of safe drinking water (Chapter 35) and the efficient removal of sewage and domestic refuse (Chapter 36) are also matters of public health and in Britain they are the concern of the Environmental Health Officers who also arrange for the inspection of food processing plant, slaughterhouses and catering establishments as well as for the control of rats, mice and other pests.

Ante-natal care

Provision of maternity and child welfare services forms an important part of the DCP's responsibilities. One of the objects of these services is to teach mothers and mothers-to-be about pregnancy and the care of babies. A pregnant woman is encouraged to attend an ante-natal ('before birth') clinic where routine tests are carried out month by month to check her health and that of the foetus. These include tests on her urine, to discover whether she is diabetic. Diabetes could affect the unborn child but, if detected early, can be controlled. Blood pressure, too, is checked regularly. High blood pressure can be harmful to both mother and baby. A blood test is taken early in pregnancy and if disease organisms are found to be present then remedies can be applied. The blood sample enables the mother's blood group to be identified and also whether she is rhesus positive (Rh +) or rhesus negative (*see* Chapter 11).

Advice is given about diet, for although the mother does not, literally, have to eat for two people, her choice of diet can have a considerable effect on the health and development of the foetus. She is also given advice on feeding and caring for the baby after its birth. Guidance on family planning is provided. This is sometimes assumed to involve only the prevention of pregnancy by contraception but it really amounts to positive planning of the size of a family and the time spacing between babies, as well as knowing the stages in life when it is safer for a mother to have babies. Fig. 38.1 shows that the risk to health is lowest at twenty-five. The shaded areas indicate the ages when health risks are greatest.

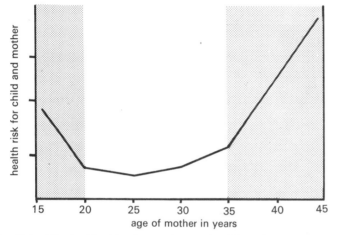

Fig. 38.1   The health risks for mothers and children from pregnancy are lowest when the mother is between 20 and 30

A midwife normally supervises the birth, whether this takes place at home or in hospital, and she is able to judge whether the assistance of a doctor is necessary. A health visitor may take over duties a few weeks after the baby has been born, visiting the mother in her home and reminding the mother at the appropriate time about vaccinating the baby against small-pox and immunizing against diphtheria, whooping-cough and polio.

Child health

At school, children are seen by the school medical officer. The frequency of medical inspections varies but in most countries, at least, takes place when a child starts school and on changing from one school to another. It includes testing of eyesight and hearing and a dental inspection. In addition, a school nurse will usually see each child more frequently than the school doctor and check cleanliness of the hair and scalp, hygiene of eyes, ears and mouth, as well as noting the child's posture and whether the shoes worn allow the feet to grow without becoming deformed. When defects are observed, a report to the school medical officer and the community health service should ensure that remedial steps are taken. Ideally the school, the medical services, parents and children should all co-operate.

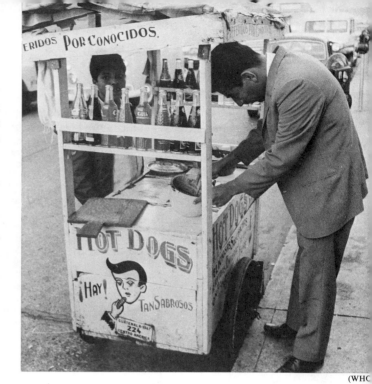

(WHO

Fig. 38.2   An environmental health inspector in Guatemala checks the food on a street vendor's stall

Community health

The DCP is usually concerned with analysing the vital statistics (p. 185) for the community since these provide him with valuable information concerning the state of health of the population.

Environmental health inspectors (sanitary inspectors) are appointed by the authority to supervise aspects of public hygiene (Fig. 38.2). These include the standards of cleanliness and hygiene of food markets and shops, and of restaurants, communal kitchens and catering establishments. In most countries laws are enacted either at national level (statutes) or at community level (bye-laws) which require food dealers and caterers to observe certain minimum standards of hygiene. Where such standards are not observed the chance of epidemics of food-borne disease increases and community health is at risk.

Fig. 38.3   A meat inspector wearing sterile overalls examines sheep carcases before their distribution to shops; each carcase is labelled with its origin

(J. Sainsbury Ltd

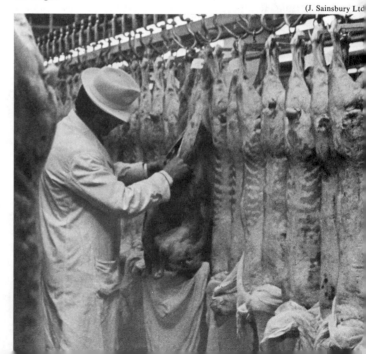

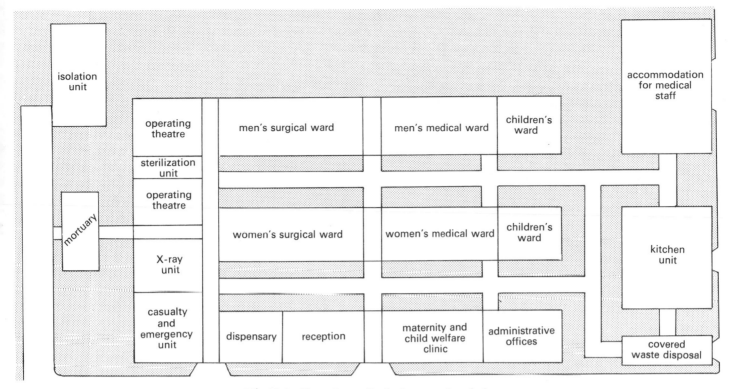

Fig. 38.4 Plan of a small, single-storey hospital

Fig. 38.5 A small operating theatre, designed for easy construction in remote areas

(Central Office of Information)

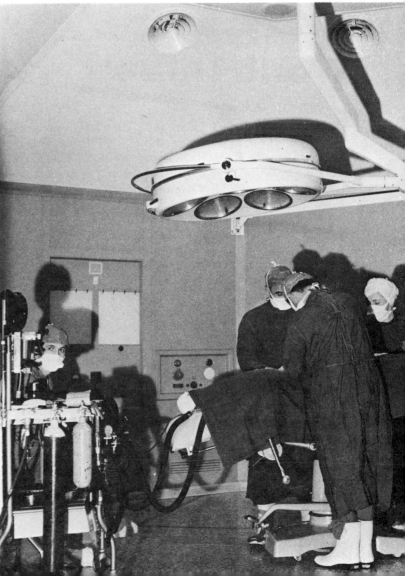

Public health inspectors are particularly concerned with the conditions under which animals are slaughtered for human consumption and with the way in which carcasses are handled and stored before being bought by members of the public. Animal flesh provides a nutritious breeding ground for a wide variety of pathogenic organisms. It is also necessary to check that the animal was healthy before it was slaughtered (*see* Tapeworm, p. 200, and Fig. 38.3).

The community health service has as another of its duties the extermination of rats. The breeding and feeding areas have to be discovered and then methods devised for the destruction of rats that do not put the human population at risk. Thus gassing of rats may be appropriate in a warehouse that can be sealed off and isolated, but it is a dangerous method in houses or flats.

Hospitals

The provision of hospitals is usually a national rather than local responsibility, but the pattern varies throughout the world. In some countries hospitals are run by private concerns such as religious orders. Certain hospitals cater for the training of doctors as well as nurses and are known as teaching hospitals. They form part of a medical school and may be very large with several hundred beds.

Whether a hospital is large or small, it is usual to treat the patients in wards—large, airy rooms with several beds. In order to organize the treatment efficiently the patients are separated into *surgical* and *medical* cases, according to whether a surgical operation is necessary or treatment with drugs and medicines alone is required. Patients suffering from infectious diseases are usually isolated in rooms with a single bed or, in large communities, in special *isolation hospitals*. Apart from these divisions it is usual to separate male patients from female, and children are usually treated in children's wards or in children's hospitals since the patterns of medical care they require are often quite different from those appropriate to adults.

In addition a hospital will usually have a *casualty unit* for the immediate treatment of injured persons and, close to this, an X-ray unit so that the state of a patient's bones can be studied. Using modern techniques it is also possible to study many of the soft tissues and organs of the body by X-ray. One or more operating theatres are located near to the surgical wards and close to the casualty department. Fig. 38.4 shows the layout of a small modern hospital in which the distances that patients have to be moved and nursing staff have to travel between one department and another have been kept to a minimum through thoughtful planning.

In many countries the provision of medicines prescribed by a doctor to out-patients is made from the hospital. The department concerned is called the *dispensary* and it also provides and checks the medicines used for treating the in-patients, those patients being treated in the wards.

The organization of health services is an expensive business and it is an unfortunate fact that the resources available both in terms of material facilities—hospitals and health centres— and trained medical personnel vary a great deal between one country and another. More is said about this in Chapter 39. The money to pay for medical services is usually provided through taxation and, in some countries, by levying a contribution from all employed people and also from their employers, as happens in Britain. The introduction of the National Health Service into Britain in 1948 resulted in a general improvement in the health of the population. It marked a further step forward in a pattern of progress that began more than a hundred years ago with the discoveries and energetic action of men like Jenner p. 238), Pasteur and Snow (p. 190). As a result, most of us can look forward to longer and healthier lives than our great-grandparents.

39

World Health

Mutual help between countries in tackling health problems is by no means new. In the nineteenth century the discoveries of Pasteur in France, Koch in Germany and Lister in Britain were being made known throughout Europe and through much of the rest of the world. Quarantine was already operating between many countries. This involved the isolation of travellers for a period of time, originally forty days, in which any disease organism would incubate so that the person concerned would show recognizable signs of the disease. There were, however, only sporadic attempts to standardize methods of promoting health.

In 1948 the first World Health Assembly met in Geneva, Switzerland and established the headquarters of what is now known as the World Health Organization or WHO. The activities of WHO are many and are organized under divisions, for example the Divisions of

> Education and Training
> Public Health Services
> Health Protection and Promotion
> Communicable Diseases
> Malaria Eradication
> Environmental Health
> Health Statistics

The Division of Public Health Services co-ordinates developments in such fields as maternal and child health, nursing, organization of medical care, and public health administration. It makes funds available for the setting up of health services in countries where resources are limited, and provides expert knowledge on the methods of organizing such services. The influence of WHO in the field of maternal and child health has led to a very noticeable reduction in the infant mortality rate (*see* p. 186) in all the countries in which the Organization has been active.

The Division of Communicable Diseases runs the Epidemiological Intelligence Service. This grand name implies that information is collected about the spread of disease around the world. In particular, reports are collected in Geneva about outbreaks of cholera, plague, relapsing fever, smallpox, typhus, and yellow fever—the internationally *notifiable diseases* (p. 189). Member states of WHO are bound by the International Sanitary Regulations to send in this information. The division publishes quarantine regulations which, if put into practice, help to check the spread of these diseases to other parts of the world. The same division also publishes vaccination requirements for travellers who have to carry a certificate of vaccination when journeying from countries where a given disease is endemic (Fig. 39.2). For example, visitors to the Caribbean islands from South American and people travelling from other parts of the world to the Caribbean via South America must carry a valid certificate of vaccination against yellow fever, signed by a qualified doctor. This is checked on entry to the country.

The present campaigns to control TB throughout the world and to eliminate smallpox from the African continent (p. 218) are sponsored by this division of WHO.

Malaria is a disease that as recently as 1955 killed millions of people every year as well as making many millions more seriously ill. The disease was considered to be of such world-wide significance that a special Division of Malaria Eradication was set up in that year. By providing an international scientific team to study the parasite and its mosquito vector and in particular the ways in which the vector can be controlled using insecticides, many former malarial regions are now free from the disease. By 1970 over 60 per cent of the population of areas formerly with malaria were no longer at risk.

Where mosquitoes have developed resistance to a particular insecticide, international knowledge enables an alternative chemical to be suggested and used swiftly. Control is still being extended and new antimalarial drugs are being tested to control the parasite inside the human body. However, as long as the disease exists anywhere in the world and people travel from one country to another in which a suitable vector exists, there is the chance of the disease being re-established. One of the tasks of this division therefore is to check all reports that indicate the possible spread of the disease and to maintain mosquito control measures, even when indigenous malaria has been eliminated from a country.

The Division of Environmental Health is concerned with such matters as community water supply, sanitation and environmental pollution. Much has been achieved in the matter of providing safe drinking water and co-operation is growing. When a new dam is being built for the purpose of providing water for irrigation WHO provides expert guidance on the measures to be taken to prevent the spread of, for example, bilharziasis (schistosomiasis) and cholera—two diseases whose continuance has marred the benefits of several imaginative, large-scale irrigation schemes.

Other fields in which WHO is active include the standardization of drugs so that the degree of purity as well as the size of dose has an international uniformity.

Fig. 39.1 A stewardess sprays the passenger compartment of an international aircraft in a WHO-sponsored campaign to reduce the transmission of insect-borne disease

(WHO)

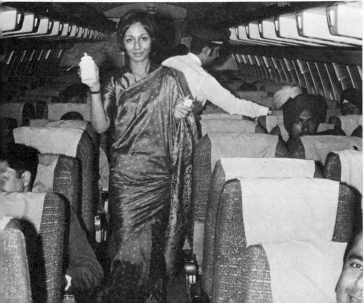

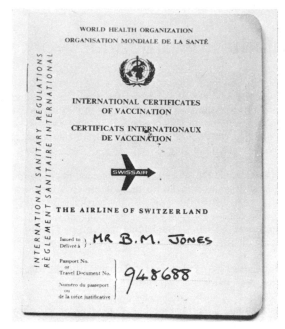

Fig. 39.2   International Certificate of Vaccination

WHO works in close collaboration with FAO, the Food and Agricultural Organization, in planning food production programmes in countries where undernourishment undermines community health. Merely to produce more food will not improve health if the resulting diet is deficient in protein or vitamins. WHO investigators determine whether illness is in any way due to such deficiencies and advises the Food and Agricultural Organization.

There are, of course, other organizations that help to promote international health. Christian Aid, for example, provides seeds, fertilizers and farm machinery such as tractors and ploughs to help increase food production in areas where famine threatens. Research organizations such as the School of Hygiene and Tropical Medicine in London and the Institut Pasteur in Paris undertake work for very many countries around the world and many of the international pharmaceutical companies, manufacturing medicines, also conduct intensive research programmes and make their results available for use in other countries. This emphasis on international co-operation to raise the standard of health throughout the world is one of the most encouraging features of the twentieth century.

Fig. 39.3   International co-operation is essential to prevent the spread of rabies by domestic pets; all pets must be placed in quarantine on arrival at the owner's destination

(WHO)

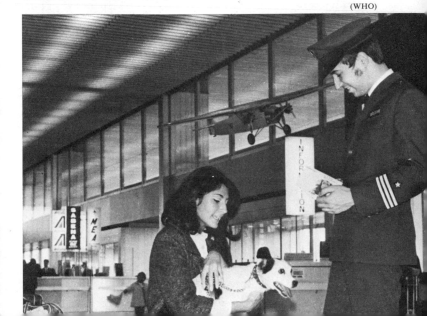

Reagents for practical work

Benedict's solution. To make 1 litre, dissolve 170 g sodium citrate crystals and 100 g sodium carbonate crystals in 800 cm³ warm distilled water. Dissolve separately 17 g copper(II) sulphate(VI) crystals in 200 cm³ cold distilled water. Add the copper sulphate solution to the first solution with constant stirring.

Ethanoic (acetic) acid (M/10). Place 6 cm³ glacial ethanoic (acetic) acid in a graduated flask and make up the volume to 1 litre with distilled water.

Hydrochloric acid (M/10). Dilute 10 cm³ concentrated hydrochloric acid with 990 cm³ distilled water.

Hydrochloric acid (2M). Dilute 100 cm³ concentrated hydrochloric acid with 400 cm³ tap water.

Hydrogencarbonate (bicarbonate) indicator. Dissolve 0.2 g thymol blue and 0.1 g cresol red powders in 20 cm³ ethanol. Dissolve 0.84 g 'Analar' sodium hydrogencarbonate (sodium bicarbonate) in 900 cm³ distilled water. Add the alcoholic solution to the hydrogencarbonate solution and make the volume up to 1 litre with distilled water. Shortly before use, dilute the appropriate amount of this solution 10 times, i.e. add 9 times its own volume of distilled water.

To bring the solution into equilibrium with atmospheric air, bubble air from outside the laboratory through the diluted indicator using a filter pump or aquarium pump. After about ten minutes, the dye should be red.

Iodine solution. To make 100 cm³ stock solution, grind 1 g iodine and 1 g potassium(I) iodide in a mortar while adding distilled water. Pour the solution into a measuring cylinder and dilute to 100 cm³. Do not store in polythene bottles because the solution will become decolourized. For experiments with enzymes, dilute 5 cm³ of the stock solution with 100 cm³ water.

Lime water. Shake tap water with an excess of calcium(II) hydroxide and allow to settle overnight. Decant the clear liquid.

Methylene blue. Dissolve 0.3 g methylene blue in 30 cm³ ethanol and add 100 cm³ distilled water.

Millon's reagent (1½ litres).

Solution A (1 litre). Add 100 cm³ concentrated sulphuric acid carefully to 900 cm³ distilled water and allow to cool. Dissolve 100 g mercury(II) sulphate(VI) (*poison*) in the diluted acid by grinding a little at a time in a mortar with successive portions of acid.

Solution B (500 cm³). Dissolve 5 g sodium(I) nitrate(III) (sodium nitrite) in 500 cm³ distilled water. Mix two volumes of solution A with one of B just before use. The mixed solutions will keep for two or three weeks.

Phenolphthalein solution. Dissolve 1 g phenolphthalein in 200 cm³ ethanol.

Sodium carbonate solution (M/20). Dissolve 5.3 g anhydrous sodium carbonate in 1 litre of distilled water.

Starch solution. Shake the appropriate quantities of starch powder and cold water together until the powder is dispersed completely. Heat the mixture while stirring constantly, until the liquid becomes translucent.

Water cultures (Experiment 4, p. 48). Either purchase the Sach's water culture tablets or prepare the solutions as follows, using chemicals of the highest purity available and freshly distilled or deionized water. Store the stock solutions in stoppered Pyrex flasks and mix and dilute them when required as described in table 2. The three solutions selected have been found to give the most consistent and reliable results with wheat.

Table 1: stock solutions†

Solution	Compound	Formula	Mass/ g	Volume of water/ cm³
A	calcium(II) nitrate(V)	$Ca(NO_3)_2.4H_2O$	9.5	100*
B	calcium(II) chloride	$CaCl_2.2H_2O$	4.5	100
C	magnesium(II) sulphate(VI)	$MgSO_4.7H_2O$	15.5	300
D	sodium(I) nitrate(V)	$NaNO_3$	6.9	100
E	potassium(I) dihydrogen-phosphate(V)	KH_2PO_4	8.5	300
F	iron(II) chloride	$FeCl_2.4H_2O$	1	200

*Add one drop of concentrated nitric(V) acid to prevent the carbonate forming.

To make up 500 cm³ of each culture solution (enough for about 16 experiments) add the solutions in the volumes indicated in table 2 to 485 cm³ distilled water. If the mixed culture solutions are to be kept for more than a week, add a further 0.5 cm³ iron(II) chloride solution to each 500 cm³ just before use. Set out the culture solutions in labelled containers and also a container of distilled water.

Allow 30 cm³ of each solution per experiment.

Table 2: culture solutions†

	Full culture	Lacking calcium	Lacking nitrogen
Solution A *calcium*(II) *nitrate*(V)	5 cm³	no calcium	no nitrate
Solution B *calcium*(II) *chloride*			5 cm³
Solution C *magnesium*(II) *sulphate*(VI)	5 cm³	5 cm³	5 cm³
Solution D *sodium*(I) *nitrate*(V)		5 cm³	
Solution E *potassium*(I) *phosphate*(V)	5 cm³	5 cm³	5 cm³
Solution F *iron*(II) *chloride*	0.5 cm³	0.5 cm³	0.5 cm³

†These tables have been selected from *Wellington Hydroponics Solutions* worked out by D. J. Angwin of Wellington College.

Books for further reading

The number of pages is given in brackets at the end of each entry, in order to indicate the scope of the book.

Genetics

Human Heredity, C. O. Carter (Penguin, 1970) [266]

Human Genetics and Medicine, C. A. Clarke (Edward Arnold, 1970) [74]

Mankind Evolving, T. Dobzhansky (Yale U.P.) [381]

Heredity and Evolution in Human Populations, L. C. Dunn (Oxford U.P.) [157]

Genetics and Man, C. D. Darlington (Penguin, 1966) [413]

Heredity and Human Affairs, J. J. Nagle (Mosby) [337]

Outline of Human Genetics, L. S. Penrose (Heinemann, 1973) [146]

Principles of Human Genetics, C. Stern (Freeman, 1973) [753]

Your Environment and Heredity, A. Scheinfeld (Chatto & Windus, 1965) [830]

Physiology

Textbook of Physiology and Biochemistry, G. H. Bell, J. N. Davidson, H. Scarborough (Livingstone, 1972) [1065]

A Companion to Medical Studies, volume 1. *Anatomy, Biochemistry and Physiology*, R. Passmore and J. S. Robson (Eds) (Blackwell, 1968) [1100]

The Life of Mammals, J. Z. Young (Oxford U.P., 1957) [820]

An Atlas of Histology, W. H. Freeman and Brian Bracegirdle (Heinemann, 1966) [140]

Human biology

Man in Nature, Marston Bates (Prentice Hall) [116]

The Study of Man, E. J. Clegg (E.U.P., 1968) [212]

Human Variation and Origins – Readings from *Scientific American* (Freeman, 1967) [297]

An Introduction to the Study of Man, J. Z. Young (Oxford U.P., 1971) [719]

An Introduction to Social Biology, Alan Dale, ed. Susan Dale (Heinemann, 1971) [496]

Growth, J. M. Tanner (Time-Life International, 1968) [188]

Food supply, population and the environment

Survival, Man and his Environment, Don R. Arthur (E.U.P., 1969) [218]

Environments of Man, J. Bresler (Addison-Wesley, 1968) [289]

Biology and the Social Crisis, J. K. Brierley (Heinemann, 1967) [260]

A Natural History of Man, J. K. Brierley (Heinemann, 1970) [184]

World Agriculture (Food and Agriculture Organization) [42]

A Strategy for Plenty (Food and Agriculture Organization) [63]

Human Populations, David Hay (Penguin, 1972) [96]

World Population and Food Supply, J. H. Lowry (Edward Arnold, 1970) [122]

Pesticides and Pollution, K. Mellanby (Collins/Fontana, 1969) [219]

The Biology of Pollution, K. Mellanby (Edward Arnold, 1972) [60]

The Biology of Affluence, G. Smith and J. C. Smyth (Eds) (Oliver & Boyd, 1974) [126]

Man and his World, John Burton (Blackie, 1974)
1 *Population* [56]
2 *The Conservation of Wildlife* [56]
3 *Pollution* [56]
4 *Resources* [64]
5 *How Would You Like to Live?* [70]

Human Nutrition, V. H. Mottram (Edward Arnold, 1972) [264]

Malnutrition and Disease (World Health Organization, 1973) [47]

Population and History, E. A. Wrigley (World University Library, 1969) [254]

An Essay on the Principle of Population, T. Malthus (Penguin, 1971) [291]

Sex and Fertility, Clive Wood (Thames & Hudson, 1970) [216]

Treatment and Disposal of Wastes (WHO Technical Report No. 367)

Community Water Supply (WHO Technical Report No. 420)

Health and disease

Man against Disease, A. G. Clegg and P. C. Clegg (Heinemann, 1973) [381]

Disease and World Health, Nance Lui Fyso (Batsford, 1974)

Natural History of Infectious Disease, J. A. Boycott (Edward Arnold, 1971) [44]

Drugs, Medicines and Man, H. Burn (Unwin, 1963) [235]

A Companion to Medical Studies, volume 2: *Pharmacology, Microbiology and General Pathology*, R. Passmore and J. S. Robson (Eds) (Blackwell, 1970) [860]

Manson's Tropical Diseases, P. H. Manson-Bahr (Ed) (Bailliere Tindall, 1972) [1176]

Malaria (WHO Technical Report No. 357)

Parasitic Protozoa, A. Wiseman, J. R. Baker and B. J. Gould (Hutchinson Educational, 1969) [176]

Food Poisoning and Food Hygiene, B. C. Hobbs (Edward Arnold, 1974) [262]

The Venereal Diseases, R. D. Catterall (Evans, 1967) [160]

Techniques with Bacteria, R. K. Pawsey (Hutchinson Educational, 1974) [160]

Doctors and State Medicine, G. Forsyth (Open University/Pitman, 1973) [224]

Practical work

Experimental Work in Biology, D. G. Mackean (John Murray)

This series of booklets contains collections of well-tried experiments known to produce effective results. The instructions given to the students are carefully programmed so that time is not wasted in incorrect procedure, but the expected results are not stated. Instead, the student is asked questions about the experiment and its outcome to make him think about the adequacy of the experimental design and the scientific interpretation of results. The books which are considered suitable for a course in Human and Social Biology are:

1 *Food tests*
2 *Enzymes*
3 *Soil*
4 *Photosynthesis*
6 *Diffusion and osmosis*
7 *Respiration and gaseous exchange*

Questions from past examination papers (1970–74)

The authors would like to thank the following examination boards for permission to reproduce questions from past papers:

University of Cambridge Local Examinations Syndicate
   Human Biology O level (AO), home centres [CA]*
   Human and Social Biology O level, overseas (some questions from pre-1972 Health Science papers have been included) [CO]
Joint Matriculation Board
   Human Biology O level [J]*
University of London Schools Examinations
   Human Biology, home and overseas centres [L]
Oxford Local Examinations
   Human Biology O level, home centres [O]

Chapters 1 to 9

1 (a) Use diagrams to help you to describe not more than *two* experiments that would show the difference between diffusion and osmosis. (b) Give *one* example of simple diffusion and *one* of osmosis occurring in the human body. [CO]

2 Distinguish between 'breathing' and 'tissue respiration'. Explain how a molecule of oxygen present in an alveolus of the lung later becomes part of a molecule of carbon dioxide in a similar position. [L]

3 Why is plant life necessary for man's survival? (Your answer should include reference to the carbon and nitrogen cycles.) [O]

4 (a) Why are fertilizers and manures used in farming? Illustrate your answer by reference to the removal and replacement of soil phosphorus. (b) How may this phosphorus be used eventually by you? [CO]

5 Name *six* constituents of a balanced diet. For each, indicate its importance to your body and name *two* foods which contain it. What is a suitable diet for a pregnant woman? Give reasons for your choice. [O]

6 Suggest a menu for a nutritious meal for yourself and justify the inclusion of the foods you have chosen. [L]

Chapters 10 to 19

7 Make a diagram to show the organs concerned with human digestion. Describe the changes that a piece of bread undergoes when it is eaten. What use is made by your body of the products of this digestion? [O]

8 Why is the liver so important to body functions? [O]

9 Proteins occur in all living things. Explain, then, why digestion of proteins in our food is necessary and how this is brought about. [CA]

10 What are the main components of human blood? Indicate briefly the function of each. Compare the composition of lymph and blood. Explain why we need these different body fluids. [O]

11 Make a *large, labelled* diagram to show the structure of the human heart and the associated great blood vessels. Indicate on the diagram the route taken by the blood through the heart. Describe briefly how glucose in the blood reaches your brain cells and how *two* waste products of brain cell activity are removed from your body. [O]

12 (a) Explain how air is drawn into and expelled from the lungs during normal breathing. (b) What type of muscle is responsible for the respiratory movements? (c) Describe an experiment to show that there is more carbon dioxide in expired air than in the atmospheric air. [J]

13 (a) The kidney filters a solution from the blood that contains glucose. Why does urine *not* normally contain glucose? (b) Explain how you would test a urine sample to discover whether it contained glucose or not. [CO]

14 (a) How is heat produced in the human body? (b) How is a man able to maintain a body temperature of 37 °C when his surroundings are at a temperature of 40 °C? [CC

15 Draw and label a diagram to show the structure of the human skin. Briefly explain the function of the structures you have drawn. Why is regular washing important for the health of the skin? [L

16 Make large labelled diagrams of (a) the human female reproductive organs, (b) the male reproductive organs indicating the route taken by the sperm. What changes occur in the male at puberty? What is fertilization, and how and where does this process occur in humans? [C

17 (a) Explain with the help of a large clear diagram how a foetus obtains food from its mother. (b) What part does the foetus's own blood system play in the feeding process? [CC

18 Describe the ovary and its functions. What effect does the pituitary gland have on the ovary? [L

19 Describe the menstrual cycle and its control by hormones. What hormonal changes occur following conception? [L

20 Make labelled illustrations to show (a) the structure of a named hinge joint, (b) the relationship between muscles and bones leading to movement of this joint.

What effect does exercise have on skeletal (voluntary) muscles, the heart and the lungs? [L

21 In man, the upright animal, good posture is a valuable quality. Show how the arrangement and properties of bones and muscles enable a good standing posture to be maintained. [CA

22 (a) Why is a cardiovascular (circulatory) system necessary to the body? (b) What are the principal requirements of muscles engaged in the performance of vigorous exercise? (c) Record two beneficial effects to other systems resulting from regular exercise. (d) Give a general account of the changes occurring during exercise within the circulatory and respiratory systems. Explain how they enable vigorous exercise to be carried out successfully. [L

23 Trace the steps leading to the occurrence of tooth decay. Indicate the measures you can take to prevent dental caries, stating the biological significance of each. [CA

24 Make a *large, labelled* diagram to show the structure of a tooth. What is the composition of (a) the milk dentition, (b) the permanent dentition? What are the functions of the different types of adult teeth? How can a mother help her child to have healthy teeth?

25 Make a large diagram to show the structure of your eye. Explain how you can see a tree in daylight. What differences would occur in your eye when looking at the tree after dusk? [C

26 What information is our skin able to receive concerning the environment? How is this accomplished, and how are appropriate responses to the information brought about? [CA

27 (a) How are sound waves transmitted from the ear drum to the sensory cells of the cochlea? (b) How does the blockage of the Eustachian tube result in deafness? Make a sketch to illustrate your answer. [CC

28 Describe briefly the situation and appearance of (a) the thyroid gland, (b) the pituitary gland. Choose one of these glands and indicate its importance to your health. What do we call this group of glands and what do their products have in common? [CC

29 When an insect stings you on your leg what movements may your body make? Describe the part the nervous system plays in any *two* of these responses. [L

30 Outline the pathway and mechanism by which information received through *one* (named) sense organ is both interpreted and acted upon. [CA

31 List the general functions of a nervous system. Indicate which parts of man's nervous system perform them. [L

32 What bodily changes can you observe in yourself during and at the end of a spell of unusually vigorous physical activity? Explain how these are brought about and how they serve your needs. [CA

*The questions are designed with first-year sixth-form students in mind.

Chapters 20 and 21

3 From your knowledge of heredity explain the following: (*a*) approximately equal numbers of male and female children are born. (*b*) Identical twins are always of the same sex, whereas fraternal twins may be of the same or different sexes. (*c*) A husband and wife with normal colour vision may have a colour-blind son. (*d*) Two brown-eyed parents may have a blue-eyed son or daughter.   [J]

4 Discuss the mechanism whereby blood group A is transmitted from one generation to another. Explain why an individual of blood group A is not necessarily homozygous for that characteristic.   [CA]

Chapters 22 and 23

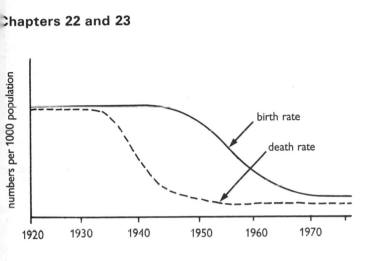

5 The graph above gives information about the changes in the population of a certain country over a period of fifty years. (*a*) Comment on the changes in population size between the years 1920 and 1930, and between 1940 and 1950. (*b*) How would the information be obtained for producing such a graph? (*c*) What use could be made of the information from the graph? (*d*) What is meant by the term 'crude death rate'?   [CO]

Chapters 24 to 31

6 At the present time the incidence of tuberculosis and rickets in Britain is much lower than at the beginning of the present century. The incidence of colour blindness remains unchanged. Explain (*a*) what causes each of these three conditions; (*b*) the reasons for decrease in the incidence of the first two, and (*c*) the absence of any change in the number of people suffering from colour blindness.   [J]

7 What is meant by the term 'droplet infection'? What precautions can be taken to reduce the risk of such infection?   [CO]

8 (*a*) If you had no microscope, how would you demonstrate experimentally that dust from the floor contains micro-organisms? (*b*) What sorts of micro-organisms would you expect to remain alive in dry dust?   [CO]

9 Describe the parasitic association between man and either (*a*) the tapeworm or (*b*) the malarial parasite. Explain two methods of preventing this association in the example you choose.   [L]

40 What changes take place in your skin if you cut your hand? What part is played by these changes in preventing infection?   [CO]

41 Summarize the methods of prevention of diseases spread by (*a*) food and (*b*) water.   [L]

42 Explain the dangers to health of (*a*) stagnant water, (*b*) spitting.   [CO]

43 How may humans contract (*a*) tuberculosis, (*b*) poliomyelitis, (*c*) smallpox, (*d*) typhoid? Why have these diseases become less common in Britain during the last hundred years? (Deal with each disease separately.)   [O]

44 Give the name of a disease which rats help to spread. Describe the disease cycle and explain methods of preventing the spread of the disease.   [CO]

45 (*a*) Explain how a person suffering from acute diarrhoea may lose more water from his body during the day than he takes in during that time. (*b*) How is cholera spread rapidly through a community? (*c*) What precautions can be taken to prevent its spread?   [CO]

46 Describe experiments you would carry out to show that washing your hands with soap and water (*a*) reduces the number of micro-organisms on your fingertips but (*b*) does not kill all the micro-organisms.   [CO]

47 Name a disease transmitted by houseflies. Explain how the behaviour of the insect enables it to transmit the disease organism. How can houseflies be controlled?   [CO]

Chapters 32 and 33

48 What do you understand by 'immunity'? Describe the ways in which immunity may be acquired and thus employed to safeguard the health of children.   [CO]

49 What is meant by immunity? Name four types of immunity and describe how each occurs. By which four routes may disease organisms enter the body? Name two commonly occurring diseases for each route. Choose one route and indicate how such infections can be prevented.   [O]

50 Malaria and yellow fever are both spread by infected mosquitoes. One of these diseases can be cured by chemical drugs, the other cannot. Why is this so? If it is not possible to take preventive action against mosquitoes, what other methods are available to counteract the onset of these two diseases?   [CO]

Chapters 34 and 35

51 What are the chief kinds of organisms that cause the decomposition of food? Choose examples to show that some of the organisms that decompose food are pathogens while others are saprophytes deliberately used by man.

Name one kind of food, rich in protein. Describe the methods that are used to preserve this food and explain the biological principles involved.   [CO]

52 Describe the various ways of preserving and storing foods and indicate the danger of faulty food storage in the home. For five named methods of preservation, state one food suitable for each.   [O]

53 Devise a code of hygiene that would be practical for the worker in a school kitchen. Explain briefly why you have included each point.   [L]

54 Imagine that you have been asked to inspect a restaurant. State and explain ten considerations that would guide you in deciding whether the restaurant provided for the health and safety of the customers and staff.   [J]

55 Give five properties of good domestic water. Describe how such water may be obtained from a mountain stream. Name five common contaminants of natural water and indicate their possible effects on health.   [O]

Chapters 36 and 37

56 Give (*a*) three uses of water to the body, and (*b*) three ways in which drinking water may be contaminated/polluted. Explain how tap water is made safe to drink for homes in our cities.   [L]

57 What are the dangers of faulty sewage disposal? Describe a water-carriage system of sewage disposal and include simple diagrams of house drainage and public processing. What use can be made of the final products?   [O]

58 Explain, with the aid of clear diagrams, the action of a water closet for the removal of domestic sewage (details of drains and sewers from the house are not required). How has its use made a major contribution to improved health?   [CO]

59 Describe the various methods in use for the disposal of kitchen waste. What are the dangers from improper disposal? What measures should a housewife take to maintain a hygienic kitchen?   [O]

60 Why is it necessary for local health authorities to make regulations about sewage disposal in towns while in country districts such regulations often do not exist? Explain briefly a system for the disposal and treatment of town sewage, once it has been collected.   [CO]

61   Name four diseases that can be contracted as a result of contamination with untreated sewage. Name four methods of sewage disposal and describe one of them in detail. What use can safely be made of treated sewage?

62   In designing and building a house, care should be taken to make it difficult for rats to gain entry. (*a*) Use drawings to help to explain how this can be done. (*b*) How can food stores in the house be protected from rats that do enter the house? (*c*) Why are rats considered a danger in the spread of disease?   [CO]

63   What is the importance of sunlight to housing? Discuss the principles involved in lighting, ventilation and heating of either an office building or a school or a hospital.   [O]

64   What factors which would influence your health would you consider when buying a house? Explain your choice.   [L]

65   State five major deficiencies common in poor housing and describe their probable effects on the residents.   [L]

66   Describe, with its interior fittings, a house which would provide a healthy environment for a small family in your area. Use the following headings: (*a*) structure; (*b*) temperature control; (*c*) light; (*d*) wate (*e*) sewage disposal; (*f*) ventilation.   [

Chapters 38 and 39

67   Describe briefly a visit you have made to a clinic, hospital or oth socially beneficial organization and explain how this organization (benefits the individual, (*b*) benefits the community and (*c*) could prol ably be improved without further excessive spending.   [

68   Describe how the work of a maternity and child welfare clin benefits both mothers and their babies.   [

69   Health in a small community may be the responsibility of tl individual but in a town it is necessary to have a health authority wil power to impose health measures. Discuss this statement with particul: reference to vaccination and the notification of infectious diseases. [CC

70   Write a paragraph on each of the following and justify their prvision as beneficial to the community as a whole as well as to those whuse them: (*a*) antenatal clinics; (*b*) immunization clinics for pre-schochildren; (*c*) hospitals for tubercular patients; (*d*) swimming baths (football pitches.   [

Glossary

The explanations of terms given in this glossary are meant to be reminders rather than formal definitions, and are restricted to the context in which these terms are used in the book. The numbers in parentheses are page references.

abdomen the part of the body below the diaphragm and above the legs.

absorption (63) uptake of a substance, usually in solution, by a tissue or organ.

accommodation (136) an automatic adjustment made by the eye enabling it to focus effectively on either close or distant objects. The curvature of the lens is altered in doing this.

active transport (29) a hypothetical method by which substances are taken up or expelled by living cells other than by simple diffusion. It is an energy-consuming process.

aerobic respiration (28) the production of energy in cells by removing hydrogen atoms from food substances and eventually combining them with oxygen to make water.

agglutination (75) clumping together of cells such as bacteria or red blood cells.

allele (175) one of a pair of genes controlling the same characteristic but not necessarily producing the same effect. Genes *B* and *b* are alleles both affecting coat colour in mice but *B* results in black fur and *b* in brown fur. The alleles occupy corresponding positions on homologous chromosomes.

amino acid (18) a chemical compound containing a –COOH (acid) and an –NH$_2$ (amino) group both attached to the same carbon atom. Proteins consist of many amino acids joined together in long chains.

anaerobic respiration (28) a process in which energy is made available by breaking down food inside a cell, but oxygen is not used in the reactions.

antibiotics (241) chemical substances produced by some bacteria and fungi, which destroy certain other bacteria, but do not harm man. The antibiotic chemicals are extracted from the organisms and used to treat disease in man and animals.

antibodies (74) chemicals made in the blood and tissues which counteract harmful organisms or substances.

antigen (238) a foreign chemical, tissue or micro-organism which, if it gains access to the body, causes it to produce antibodies. The antibodies act against the antigen.

calcification (111) the deposition of calcium salts in a living tissue, usuall cartilage, altering its physical properties and making it harder.

capillary action (**attraction**) (256) the force that causes water to be drawn be tween surfaces which are close together, e.g. making it spread into blottin paper or between soil particles.

carcinogen (194) a substance capable of causing cancer if eaten, inhaled o applied to the skin over a period of time.

catalyst (27) a chemical which alters the rate of a chemical reaction (usuall speeding it up) without being used up in the reaction.

centriole (159) a small body in an animal cell which participates in cell division It divides into two and the two parts separate early in cell division, contribu ting to the spindle. The term *centrosome* is sometimes used to describe th paired centrioles before they separate.

centromere (160) the part of the chromosome which becomes attached to th spindle and by which the chromatids appear to be pulled apart at ce division.

centrum (117) the solid cylindrical part of a vertebra.

cerebellum (155) the large outgrowth from the roof of the hindbrain which plays an important part in controlling co-ordinated movement.

cerebral hemisphere (153) a large outgrowth from the roof of the forebrai which is associated with intelligent behaviour, memory and consciousness

chiasma (170) a region of close contact between homologous chromosome in the early stages of meiosis. When first formed the chiasma indicate where the exchange of portions of chromatids is taking place.

chromatid (160) the product of replication of a chromosome. During ce division the chromatids are separated into the daughter cells.

chromosomes (162) structures which appear in the nucleus at cell division They carry the genetic information (genes) which controls the activity of th cells and the development of the entire organism.

collagen (125) a substance produced by the body in the form of tough fibres These fibres contribute to many tissues throughout the body, providin strength and flexibility.

combustion (57) the chemical term for burning, in which a substance combine with oxygen from the air and releases energy as heat and light.

commensal (204) one organism living in close association with another, sometimes actually inside it. The commensal organism is harmless and may even benefit its host.

concentration (20) the quantity of a substance that is present in a given volume, e.g. how much oxygen is dissolved in a fixed volume of water.

conservation (44) the preservation of a stable environment. It does not imply an unchanging environment, but one in which organisms and resources are not totally destroyed in the course of change.

contagion (208) transmission of disease organisms by contact with an infected person, his clothing or bedding, etc.

contamination (206) the introduction of harmful chemicals or organisms into food or water.

contraception (109) the prevention of conception. Sperms are prevented from fertilizing an ovum, or the fertilized ovum is prevented from implanting in the lining of the uterus.

convection (259) when a gas or liquid is heated it expands, becomes less dense and consequently rises. This movement is called 'convection'.

co-ordination (145) the way in which the organs and systems of the body work together to maintain life and efficient activity.

cortex (93) the outer layer of certain organs in the body.

crossing over (179) the exchange of portions of chromatids which takes place during the cell division giving rise to reproductive cells. It results in new combinations of characteristics in the offspring.

culture (195) the provision of ideal conditions for the growth of selected organisms.

deamination (69) the removal of the amino ($-NH_2$) group from an amino acid, leaving a compound which can be used to provide energy or changed to a carbohydrate.

deficiency disease (35) an illness which results from lack of a substance in the diet. It cannot be 'caught' or transmitted, and can usually be cured by adding the missing substance to the diet.

dehydration (66) excessive loss of water from tissues.

demography (185) a study of changes in population.

denaturation (18) an irreversible chemical change undergone by proteins when heated above 50 °C or treated with certain chemicals.

dialysis (25) a controlled process of diffusion by which dissolved substances can be extracted from a mixture through a membrane.

differential permeability (22) a property of a membrane that allows some substances but not others to pass through it.

diffusion (22) the natural movement of a gas or dissolved substance from a region of high concentration to a region of low concentration.

diploid (163) the number of chromosomes in non-reproductive body cells. The name reflects the fact that each chromosome is represented twice, one of each pair coming from the male and one from the female parent.

dissociation (21) the separation of the components of a compound into ions, usually when it is dissolved in water.

DNA (166) the abbreviation for deoxyribonucleic acid, a chemical present in the nucleus of all cells and which controls the cell's activities.

dominant (169) when two contrasting genes (alleles) are present in an organism, the one which produces observable effects is called 'dominant'.

droplet infection (207) the inhaling of disease organisms in droplets of water from the exhaled air of an infected person.

drug (241) a chemical taken into the body to alter the metabolism in such a way as to counteract an illness or relieve its symptoms.

effector (149) an organ which does something in response to a nervous or hormonal stimulus.

embryo (104) the developmental stage of an organism, from a single cell to the stage when all its organs and systems are functioning.

endemic (189) the continuous presence of a disease in a population.

endocrine system (156) a number of glands in the body which secrete chemicals (hormones) directly into the blood stream. These chemicals regulate the level of activity of the body's systems.

enzyme (16) a protein made in the protoplasm of cells that speeds up the rate of chemical reactions in them.

epidemic (189) a rise in the number of cases of a disease in a population far above the level normally expected.

epithelium (11) the layer of cells lining the surface of internal organs.

erosion (53) the removal of topsoil by the action of wind or rain.

eutrophication (52) an excessive growth of plant life in inland waters as a result of a high level of nutrients. The eventual decay of the plants removes nearly all the oxygen from the water.

excretion (2) removal of harmful or excess substances from cells and from the body.

F_1 generation (175) the offspring resulting from the mating between two individuals. The first filial generation.

F_2 generation (175) the offspring resulting from a mating between the individuals of the F_1 generation. The second filial generation.

feedback (141) information about the functioning of the body's systems which

is sent to the central nervous system or endocrine system, helping to maintain precise control over the bodily functions.

fertility (186) the numbers of offspring produced by an individual or a population.

fertilization (100) the joining together of reproductive cells, e.g. sperm and ovum, to produce a zygote which can develop into a new individual.

foetus (105) the developmental stage of a mammal from the time its organs are formed to the time it is born.

gamete (100) a reproductive cell. Gametes from opposite sexes must meet and join together in order to produce a new individual.

gastric (63) any structure or function related to the stomach.

gene (164) a sequence of DNA molecules on a chromosome, inside the nucleus of a cell. It controls the chemical processes in the cell and the development of the organism produced from a zygote. The genes are hereditary units passed on from parents to offspring, and determine the characteristics of the offspring.

genetics (159) the study of the way in which characteristics are inherited.

genotype (159) the genetic constitution of an organism, i.e. all the genes present in a cell of that individual, whether or not they have an observable effect.

gland (11) a group of cells, some or all of which produce a chemical which is released and used by other parts of the body.

haploid (170) the number of chromosomes in the gametes. This is half the number present in the other cells of the body.

hepatic (65) any structure or function related to the liver.

herbivore (58) an animal that feeds on vegetation.

heterozygous (175) carrying a pair of contrasting genes (alleles) for any one characteristic, e.g. *Bb*, where *B* determines black fur and *b* determines brown fur.

homeostasis (92) the maintenance of stable conditions inside the body. The temperature and composition of the body fluids are not allowed to fluctuate outside certain limits.

homoiothermic (98) the maintenance by an organism of a constant temperature independent of the temperature of its surroundings.

homologous chromosomes (163) the corresponding chromosomes of a pair, alike in shape and size. One is derived from the male and the other from the female parent.

homozygous (163) carrying a pair of identical genes (alleles) for a given characteristic. Breeding true for this character.

host (200) the animal in, or on, which a parasite is living or feeding.

hydrolysis (16) the breaking down of a compound by reacting with water.

immunity (74) the ability to resist disease organisms as a result of possessing chemicals (antibodies) made by the body, which counteract the organisms.

implantation (103) after an ovum has been fertilized it sinks into the lining of the uterus. This is implantation, and the zygote will undergo all further development in this position.

inoculation (74) introduction of antigens, usually by injection, into the body to stimulate it to produce antibodies. This gives the body immunity to a particular disease.

insecticide (229) a chemical that kills insects.

insulation (257) a method of reducing the transfer of heat or electricity.

involuntary action (118) an action that is not consciously controlled, such as blinking, sneezing or swallowing.

ion (21) an atom or small group of atoms carrying an electrical charge and having different properties from the uncharged atoms.

ionization (21) the splitting up of a compound into ions, usually when it dissolves in water to make a solution.

irrigation (42) the artificial supply of controlled amounts of water to agricultural land.

larva (198) an immature stage in the development of certain animals from the egg. It is independent of its parents but different from them in appearance and activities.

latent heat (99) the amount of energy (number of joules) needed to turn a liquid into a vapour.

leguminous plant (51) a plant whose fruits are pods, e.g. beans and peas. Leguminous plants have nodules on their roots containing nitrogen-fixing bacteria.

linkage (179) the presence of genes on the same chromosome. Genes which are close together on any one chromosome tend to be passed on together to the offspring.

lipids (27) fats and fat-like substances; often a fat combined with other chemicals, e.g. phospho-lipids.

lymph (83) a body fluid derived from the blood and tissue fluid and returned to the circulatory system in lymphatic vessels.

lymphatic (83) a thin-walled vessel in the body which returns lymph from the tissues to the circulatory system.

macrophage (74) type of white cell present in most kinds of connective tissue. It can ingest foreign particles.

malnutrition (32) general term for illnesses resulting from inadequate feeding. Usually due to lack of one or more essential components of the diet.

meiosis (170) type of cell division which results in the production of gametes. The chromosome number after meiosis is halved (haploid).

menstruation (108) the breakdown of the lining of the uterus at intervals of about twenty-eight days. This occurs about fourteen days after an ovum has been released but not fertilized, and is recognized by the loss of a small amount of blood through the vagina.

metabolism (30) all the chemical changes in the body that contribute to the living processes.

metamorphosis (230) the drastic changes that take place when the larval form of an animal changes into an adult, e.g. caterpillar to butterfly.

micro-organisms (193) very small animals and plants such as protozoa, bacteria and moulds.

mitosis (160) the events taking place at cell division which result in an equal distribution of chromosomes to the daughter cells and a maintenance of the diploid number of chromosomes.

motor (146) in biology, the term implies some positive action in response to a stimulus, e.g. a muscle contraction or secretion by a gland. *Motor* nerve fibres carry the impulses from the central nervous system to the organ that produces such action.

mucous membrane (60) the layer composed of epithelium, mucous glands and connective tissue, which lines the alimentary canal and breathing passages.

mucus (10) the viscous lubricating fluid produced by glands in the food canal and breathing passages.

mutation (168) a spontaneous change in a gene or chromosome which alters the metabolism of an organism.

nephron (93) one of the microscopic units in the kidney which filters the blood and reabsorbs some of the products.

neural (153) a term relating to structures associated with the nervous system.

neurone (146) a nerve cell. The cell has two or more processes which can conduct nervous impulses.

nitrogen-fixing (51) the ability, possessed by certain bacteria, to use atmospheric nitrogen to make organic compounds of nitrogen such as amino acids.

nitrogenous (73) containing compounds of nitrogen.

nutrient (20) a substance having food value, or able to be used by plants to make food.

nutrition (32) the intake, digestion, absorption and effective use of food.

obesity (33) being overweight. Caused by accumulating fat to the point where health is likely to be affected.

olfactory (132) a term describing structures and activities to do with the sense of smell.

oogenesis (171) the production of mature ova (eggs).

optic (133) biological term describing structures and functions related to the eye.

optimum (27) literally, the best. Usually refers to the best conditions for some biological activity.

osmo-regulation (94) adjustments made to the concentration of the body fluids, usually via the blood, to maintain their concentrations within narrow limits.

osmosis (22) the diffusion of water through a membrane from a weaker to a stronger solution.

osmotic pressure (23) the pressure built up as a result of the diffusion of water into a system by osmosis.

ossification (111) gradual replacement of cartilage by bone.

ovulation (102) the release of a mature ovum (egg) from the ovary.

ovum (102) the female reproductive cell; the egg.

pandemic (190) the spread of an epidemic disease from one country to a number of other countries.

parasite (196) an animal or plant living in or absorbing food from another living organism without necessarily killing it.

pathogen (193) a micro-organism that lives in or on another plant or animal, causing disease.

permeable (22) allowing a gas or liquid to pass through.

pesticides (58) chemicals that destroy plant or animal pests which threaten crop plants or the health of communities.

pH (21) a measure of how acid something is. When accompanied by a figure it indicates the concentration of hydrogen ions in a solution.

phagocyte (71) a type of white blood cell which can ingest foreign particles such as bacteria.

phenotype (175) the observable characteristics cf an organism. Usually contrasted with *genotype*. A genotype may contain genes for both black fur, *B*, and brown fur, *b*, but the phenotype is black fur.

placenta (105) a structure formed between an embryo and the uterine lining which enables the embryo to obtain food and oxygen from its mother's blood.

plankton (59) microscopic organisms living in the surface waters of ponds, lakes and oceans.

poikilothermic (98) having a body temperature the same as or a little above that of the surroundings. The temperature rises and falls with that of the environment.

pollution (248) accumulation of harmful substances in the environment.

polymerization (41) the formation of very large molecules by combining together numerous small molecules of the same type.

predator (56) an animal that kills and eats other animals (prey).

prophylaxis (214) taking measures to reduce the chances of catching a particular disease.

proprioceptor (131) an internal sensory organ, usually in a muscle. It is sensitive to stretching and sends impulses to the brain which enable one to judge the position of limbs and the tensions in muscles.

protein (17) complex chemicals used in building protoplasm, and hence cells, tissues and organs. Consequently it is essential that the diet contains some protein.

protoplasm (8) the living contents of a cell. The cytoplasm and the nucleus.

protozoa (195) single-celled animals.

recessive (167) the gene which, in the presence of its contrasting partner (allele) is not expressed in the observable characteristics of the organism.

reflex (148) a rapid, automatic response to a stimulus.

renal (77) a term relating to any structure or function to do with the kidney.

replication (168) the production of an exact copy of a structure.

respiration (27) the release of energy from food molecules and its transfer to molecules which play a part in the vital chemistry of the cell.

RNA (166) abbreviation for ribonucleic acid, a chemical which helps to convey the 'instructions' from the nucleus to the cytoplasm.

saprophytes (196) organisms, usually fungi or bacteria, which derive nourishment from dead or decaying organic matter.

selective permeability (22) allowing some substances but not others to diffuse through a membrane.

sensory (129) to do with detecting stimuli and sending impulses to the brain.

serum (74) blood plasma from which fibrinogen has been removed. Sometimes it contains antibodies which are used to combat a disease when the serum is injected into the patient.

soluble (20) able to be dissolved in a liquid.

solubility (20) a measure of how much of a substance can be dissolved in a given quantity of liquid.

solution (20) a mixture of a substance in a liquid in which the substance is dissolved and uniformly dispersed throughout the liquid.

specialization (10) the development of a cell or a structure so that it carries out one particular function more efficiently than any others.

spermatogenesis (171) the production of mature sperms from sperm-mother cells.

spore (195) a reproductive or resistant body formed by a micro-organism.

sterilization (202) destruction of bacteria and viruses in food or on medical or experimental equipment.

stimulus (129) a physical or chemical event in an organism or its environment which makes it alter its pattern of activity.

subcutaneous (96) beneath the skin.

thorax (88) the upper part of the trunk, from the neck to the diaphragm.

thoracic (117) a structure or function having something to do with the thorax.

toxin (74) a poisonous chemical produced usually by a bacterium.

urea (92) a chemical compound containing nitrogen. It is a product of metabolism and is excreted by the kidneys, forming one component of urine.

ureter (92) the tube conducting urine from the kidney to the bladder.

urethra (93) the tube conducting urine from the bladder to outside the body.

urine (94) the solution of nitrogenous waste products and salts which is produced in the kidney, stored in the bladder and expelled at intervals through the urethra.

uterus (100) the female organ in which the embryo develops.

utriculus (139) an organ of balance in the inner ear.

vaccination (238) the introduction of a disease-causing antigen into the body, which makes an antibody against the antigen and so develops immunity to an attack of the disease.

vaccine (238) a preparation of an antigen from a disease-causing organism, which is rendered harmless or incapable of reproduction but if introduced to the body will stimulate it to produce antibodies.

vector (192) an animal that carries a disease-causing organism from one host to another.

virus (222) a submicroscopic particle that can reproduce inside living cells and cause disease.

vitamin (35) a chemical taken in with the food that plays an essential part in chemical reactions in cells, but has no energy or body-building value.

zygote (100) the single cell resulting from the joining together of male and female gametes. It can develop into a new individual.